Vascular Occlusion: Epidemiological, Pathophysiological and Therapeutic Aspects

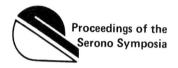

Proceedings of the Serono Symposia

---

*At the time of going to press these titles were in preparation.

Vascular Occlusion:
Epidemiological,
Pathophysiological
and Therapeutic Aspects

Proceedings of the
Serono Symposia, Volume 37

Edited by

M. Tesi

Department of Angiology
Main Hospital of S. Maria Nuova
Florence, Italy

J. A. Dormandy

St. James Hospital
London, England

1981

ACADEMIC PRESS

A Subsidiary of Harcourt Brace Jovanovich, Publishers

London New York Toronto Sydney San Francisco

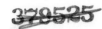

ACADEMIC PRESS INC. (LONDON) LTD.
24–28 OVAL ROAD
LONDON NW1

U.S. Edition published by
ACADEMIC PRESS INC.
111 FIFTH AVENUE
NEW YORK, NEW YORK 10003

British Library Cataloguing in Publication Data

Vascular occlusion. – (Proceedings of the Serono
  Symposia, ISSN 0308 – 5503; no 37)
  1. Cardiovascular system – Diseases – Congresses
  I. Tesi, M.   II. Dormandy, J. A.
  III. Series

  ISBN 0-12-685380-0

  LCCCN 80-42408

Typeset by Reproduction Drawings Ltd., Sutton, Surrey
Printed by T. J. Press (Padstow) Ltd., Padstow, Cornwall

PREFACE

This volume is a collection of the works presented at the First International "Colloquy" of Angiology in Florence from 23 to 26 October, 1979. The "Colloquy" was organized by the Department of Angiology of the Main Regional Hospital of Santa Maria Nuova of Florence and made possible by the generous help of Serono Symposia.

The function of the vascular system is to conduct blood. This is why this volume is entitled *Vascular Occlusion* as most pathological processes, on both the arterial and venous side of the circulation, are manifested by narrowing of the vessels and subsequent decrease in blood flow. The management of these patients must necessarily be based on a proper understanding of the aetiology and pathophysiology, as well as the medical and operative treatment of vascular occlusions. In many cases, arterial or venous occlusion means thrombosis. From this stems our interest in genetic and acquired predisposing conditions, whether they be biochemical, haematological or rheological. Atherosclerosis, the other principal cause of occlusion, is considered in the same way.

The many original contributions to the symposium have been selected to illustrate and explore these many areas of interest. They have been classified into five sections: epidemiology and primary prevention, pathophysiology, diagnostic techniques, medical treatment and surgical treatment. We hope this book will combine the latest concepts based on fundamental research as well as the most current ideas about the investigation and treatment of these patients. We hope that the contents of this volume will be both interesting and useful to all interested in vascular disease. If this hope is indeed fulfilled, it will be more than sufficient reward and satisfaction for all our work.

March 1981   M. TESI
                                                          J. A. DORMANDY

CONTENTS

Section II

Pathophysiology

Section V

Surgical Therapy

SECTION I
EPIDEMIOLOGY AND PRIMARY PREVENTION

EPIDEMIOLOGY AND PREVENTION OF ARTERIOPATHIES IN A MALE INDUSTRIAL POPULATION

Z. Reiniš, J. Pokorný and V. Bazika

Laboratory of Angiology, Charles University, Prague, Czechoslovakia

The major risk factors related to aetiology and pathogenesis of ischaemic heart disease (IHD) and peripheral atherosclerotic disease (PAD) have stimulated cardio-vascular prevention programmes in various coutries (Stamler, 1978; Turpeinen, 1979). It is generally accepted that the main risks of atherogenesis are represented by lipid metabolic errors. On the other hand, haemodynamic stress and low capacity for oxygen transport to the myocardium and the brain play the most important roles in infarctogenesis. For this reason attention on the primary pre-vention of IHD and PAD was focused on lowering atherogenic serum lipoproteins, on the elimination of cigarette smoking, on increased physical activity and on medical prophylaxis in hypertension.

These basic principles were embedded in the long-term educational prevention programme for the male industrial population of North Bohemia.

METHODS

Using the method of epidemiological trials of seven countries (Keys, 1970), the prevalence and incidence of IHD and PAD were studied in 3267 men 30–59 years of age. An intervention group consisted of 2325 male automobile factory workers and a control group of 942 men of the same age, employees of another LIAZ automobile factory. Because the prevalence and incidence of manifest IHD and PAD in men 30–39 years of age was found to be very low, the male groups of 40–59 years of age were chosen for the first five-year incidence study.

Serono Symposium No. 37, "Vascular Occlusion: Epidemiological, Pathophysiological and Therapeutic Aspects", edited by M. Tesi and J. Dormandy, 1981. Academic Press, London and New York.

The medical examination consisted of family and personal history, physical examination with blood pressure measurement and body weight determination, rest and post-exercise ECG registration, oscillometric pulse-wave measurement in legs, biochemical examination of serum cholesterol and beta-alpha lipo-protein index and urine analysis.

The diagnosis of manifest IHD was based on the occurrence of definite myo-cardial infarction, definite angina pectoris, and sudden death attributed to coronary insufficiency. The diagnosis of manifest PAD was based exclusively on the deve-lopment of intermittent claudication. Asymptomatic peripheral arterial disease discovered by physical findings was not included in this paper. The diagnosis of overt cerebrovascular disease was based on the occurrence of apoplexy.

Subjects with pre-existing IHD, PAD or with definite evidence of a cerebro-vascular accident at initial examination were excluded from the incidence study. After a period of 5 years, 2558 men were re-examined. Total response was 80%.

The medical examination was supplemented by individual conversations dealing with the primary preventive procedures. Every subject received a special booklet titled *Save your heart* with material containing instructions on antiatherogenic dietary regimen, body weight control, increasing physical activity and cessation of smoking. Twice a year, educational seminars with special films were organized in the intervention factory.

RESULTS

The prevalence of IHD and PAD were found to be similar in men 40–59 years of age, working in the intervention factory (4.5% resp. 1.2%) and those working in the control factory (4.2% resp. 1.0%).

The 5-year incidence of IHD in men 40–59 years of age, working in the inter-vention factory was shown to be significantly lower than in men of the same age, working in the control factory (5.8% *vs* 10.5%; $P < 0.01$). The 5-year incidence of PAD in workers of both factories was found to be low, without significant differences (1.5% *vs* 1.2%) (Fig. 1).

These findings were correlated with three major risk factors: hypertension, cigarette smoking and hypercholesterolaemia.

Evaluating the prognostic validity of a single risk factor, we have found that the incidence of IHD was significantly higher in hypertensive subjects and/or in cigarette smokers than in normotensives and/or in non-smokers. These results were shown not only in the control group, but also in the intervention group. However, the occurrence of IHD was found to be substantially lower in the last group. The influence of a single reading of hypercholesterolaemia on the incidence of IHD could not be confirmed in the control nor in the intervention groups. It is interesting that hypertension as a single factor did not play such an important role in the incidence of PAD as in the occurrence of IHD (Fig. 2).

The simultaneous effect of two risk factors on the incidence of IHD was observed in the combination of cigarette smoking and hypertension. The hyper-tensive cigarette smokers have a significantly higher incidence of IHD than the normotensive smokers in both factories. However, it was always lower in the intervention group. The hypertensive cigarette smokers also revealed substan-

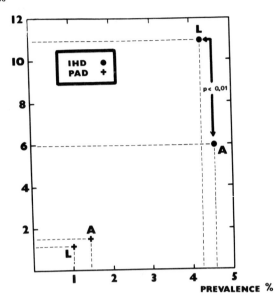

Fig. 1. Prevalence and 5-year incidence of manifest ischemic heart disease (IHD) and peripheral arterial disease (PAD) in men 40–59 years of age, employees of two automobile factories. A = intervention group, L = control group.

	TOTAL		CIGARETTE SMOKING		BLOOD PRESSURE TORR		CHOLESTEROLEMIA mg%	
	▨ A ▦ L		NO	YES	< 160/95	≥ 160/95	< 260	≥ 260
IHD	78	49	24	13	54	36	47	23	31	26	51	32	27	17
PAD	22	6	–	–	22	6	17	4	5	2	10	4	12	2
N	1335	485	610	206	725	279	1103	344	232	141	925	325	410	160

Fig. 2. Five-year incidence of ischemic heart disease (IHD) and peripheral arterial disease (PAD) in men 40–59 years of age in intervention (A) and control (L) factories.

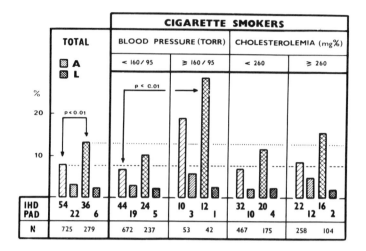

Fig. 3. Five-year incidence of ischemic heart disease (IHD) and peripheral arterial disease (PAD) in men 40–59 years of age in intervention (A) and control (L) factories.

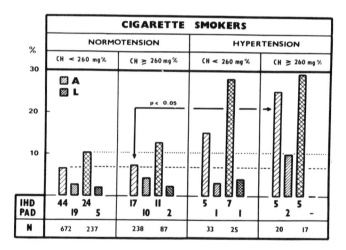

Fig. 4. Five-year incidence of ischemic heart disease (IHD) and peripheral arterial disease (PAD) in men 40–59 years of age in intervention (A) and control (L) factories.

tially higher incidence of PAD than the normotensive smokers, but this was evident in the intervention factory only.

The hypercholesterolaemic cigarette smokers working in the intervention factory also had substantially higher incidences of PAD than the normocholesterolaemic smokers, but it was not observed in the control group (Fig. 3).

The simultaneous effect of three major risk factors on the incidence of IHD and PAD was registered only in workers of the intervention factory. The hypertensive cigarette smokers with hypercholesterolaemia suffered from IHD and PAD more frequently than the hypertensive smokers with lower cholesterol-

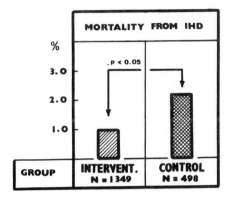

Fig. 5. Five-year mortality from ischemic heart disease (IHD) in intervention and control groups of men 40–59 years of age.

aemia. It is surprising that no case of PAD was observed among hypertensive smokers with hypercholesterolaemia in the control group. The remarkable differences in the 5-year incidence of IHD between the intervention and control factory were evident (Fig. 4).

The effect of multifactorial preventive procedures was also demonstrated in the 5-year mortality of coronary heart disease and cerebrovascular accident. IHD was found to be the cause of death in 12 subjects in the intervention factory and in 11 subjects of the control factory. Cerebrovascular haemorrhage was found to be the cause of death in two workers in the intervention factory, and in two workers in the control factory. The mortality ratio from IHD was proven to be significantly higher in the control group than in the intervention group (2.3% *vs* 0.9%; $P < 0.05$) (Fig. 5).

The influence of multifactorial intervention was further estimated on the incidence of the main risk factors. During the first 5-year period, significant changes occurred in cigarette smoking. The percentage of stop-smokers was found to be significantly higher in the intervention group than in the control group (7.0% *vs* 3.8%; $P < 0.05$). In other words, the frequency of cigarette smokers decreased significantly in the intervention group in comparison with the control group.

Significant changes in body weight, cholesterolaemia and blood pressure were not observed either in the intervention group or in the control group.

CONCLUSIONS

The results of the first 5-year period of the educational cardiovascular prevention programme in the middle-aged male industrial population of North Bohemia have shown that primary prevention of IHD was effective. The 5-year incidence of the disease in workers of the intervention factory was found to be significantly lower than in the control factory.

A decrease of the morbidity of IHD in the intervention group was followed by substantial lowering of mortality from the disease, as compared with the control group. The significant changes of risk factor levels was observed only in cigarette

smokers. A significantly higher number of smokers stopped smoking in the intervention factory than was observed in the control factory.

On the other hand, the 5-year incidence of PAD was found to be low and
similar in workers of both factories. The disease occurred in cigarette smokers
only. Significant changes in blood pressure values and cholesterolaemia were
not observed either in workers of the intervention factory or in workers of the
control factory.

From the prognostic point of view, the combination of hypertension, cigarette
smoking and hypercholesterolaemia revealed the most detrimental effect on
coronary circulation.

REFERENCES

Keys, A. (1970). *Circulation* **XLI**, No. 4. Suppl. No. 1.
Stamler, J. (1978). *Circulation* **58**, No. 1, 3.
Turpeinen, O. (1979). *Circulation* **59**, No. 1, 1.

TAKAYASU'S ARTERITIS — CURRENT STATUS IN JAPAN

Y. Mishima

Department of Surgery, University of Tokyo, Tokyo, Japan

INTRODUCTION

In 1908, Takayasu reported the peculiar ocular manifestation seen in a young female patient with attacks of blindness and syncope. Thereafter, in 1948, Shimizu and Sano described the clinical triad of this disease (including absence of pulsation of radial arteries, arteriovenous anastomosis in the ocular fundi and hypersensitive carotid sinus), as due to an obliterative process of the aortic arch and its main branches, and named the disease "pulseless disease".

Through the recent development of clinical and laboratory studies, the concept of this disease has definitely changed and it has been categorized as "aortitis syndrome" in Japan by Ueda (1963, 1968), because the disease process involves not only the aortic arch and its branches, but also the entire aorta and its branches —sometimes extending into the pulmonary arteries.

Takayasu's arteritis is caused by a non-specific inflammation and affects almost exclusively young females; although in recent years there has been an increasing number of reports of male patients. Almost all authors agree on its prevalence in the Orient.

ETIOLOGY

The exact etiology is still unknown. Although infections, such as syphilis and tuberculosis, were once thought to be related to the development of the disease, they were no longer considered to be etiological factors. In some aspects Takayasu's arteritis is similar to a collagen disease, but there are many discrepancies between

Serono Symposium No. 37, "Vascular Occlusion: Epidemiological, Pathophysiological and Therapeutic Aspects", edited by M. Tesi and J. Dormandy, 1981. Academic Press, London and New York.

them both clinically and pathophysiologically. It was also anticipated that female sex hormones may be related to the development of the disease because of its prevalence among young females. This has also now been denied. The relationship between Takayasu's arteritis and the HLA antigen was investigated in recent years, but has not yet been disclosed.

Nowadays, an auto-immune process, with an artery as the target organ, is highly suspected in Japan. The following findings support the concept that some immunological factors may play a significant role in the development of the disease and many studies have been performed along these lines: an increase of erythrocyte sedimentation rate, especially in the active stage; positive C reactive protein; increased serum $alpha_2$-globulin and gamma-globulin; histologically confirmed inflammation of involved segments; coexistence with collagen disease; and clinical improvement with administration of steroids in the active stage. Itoh (1966) reported that anti-aortic antibodies were frequently detected in the sera of the patients and suggested the possible role of various infections, including streptococcal, viral and tuberculous infections, as one of the trigger mechanisms in antibody production.

PATHOLOGY

From the histological investigation of 76 autopsy cases collected over the last 16 years, Nasu (1977) classified this lesion pathohistologically into three types: granulomatous inflammation type, diffuse productive inflammation type and fibrosis type.

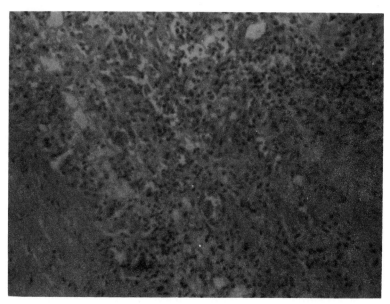

Fig. 1

Granulomatous inflammation type (28%). Granulomata, often accompanied by Langhans' giant cell and foreign body giant cells, are formed with or without the presence of small necrotic foci and microabscesses.

Diffuse productive inflammation type (14%). Diffuse infiltration of lymphocytes and plasma cells along with proliferation of connective tissue and new growth of blood vessels are seen in the media. A few solitary giant cells are found scattered in rare cases (Fig. 1).

Fibrosis type (58%). This type was observed in a large majority of cases and was thought to be the sequela of the inflammatory changes. The severe fibrosis occurred chiefly in the media, due to scar formation following granulomatous and productive inflammation. Fibrosis of the adventitia is thought to be a protective reaction against passive distention due to diminished elasticity of the weakened media. Secondary fibrosis was also detected in the intima and its severity depended mostly on the duration of the disease process.

In the autopsy cases, pulmonary artery involvement was detected in 45%.

From the histological picture and the morphogenesis of the pathological changes, Nasu suggested that the primary cause of the disease may be some sort of infection, even though the organism has not yet been discovered.

PATHOPHYSIOLOGY

The clinical picture of Takayasu's arteritis is extremely variable depending on the distribution of the arterial lesions (Table I). There has not yet been a definite classification of the disease, however we have classified it into three types according to their hemodynamic characteristics (Fig. 2, Table II) (Imada, 1977). Type 1 is the classical pulseless disease, which manifests itself as hypotension of the head and upper extremities. Dizziness, syncope, impaired vision and claudication of the upper extremity are the most common complaints. The type 2 is characterized by the presence of systemic hypertension or hypertension of the upper half of the body, similar to the signs and symptoms due to coarctation of the aorta. Type 3 is a mixed type, in which type 1 and 2 are combined, and is characterized by hypotension of the upper extremity and head, hypertension above the coarctated segment and, less frequently, systemic hypertension. Aortic insufficiency may be associated with Takayasu's arteritis in some cases. Occasionally, aneurysm formation of the involved segments is reported. The pulmonary artery is also not uncommonly involved, although signs and symptoms are rarely obvious.

The triad pointed out by Shimizu and Sano is no longer considered to be representative of the disease. For example, the ischemic change of the ocular fundi reported by Takayasu is not so prominent as was believed, except in cases categorized as having a type 1 lesion.

Erythrocyte sedimentation is accelerated in the majority of cases, especially in the active stage of the disease. An increase in serum $alpha_2$-globulin and gammaglobulin is frequently noticed. C-reactive protein is also frequently positive. These findings result from an active inflammatory process and are helpful for differentiating Takayasu's arteritis from other conditions.

The electrocardiogram frequently reveals evidence of left ventricular hyper-

Table I. Initial symptoms.

Symptoms	Frequency	
Cerebral	873/1351	64.6%
Visual	310/1297	23.9%
Cardiac	742/1344	55.2%
Hypertension	606/1336	45.4%
Pain	492/1292	38.1%
General malaise	885/1324	66.8%

(Inada, Ministry of Health Japan)

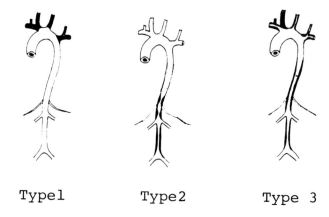

Type 1   Type 2   Type 3

Fig 2. Classification.

Table II. Frequency.

	Cases	Retinal	Blood Pressure	
			Ascending aorta	Abdominal aorta
Type 1	169	↓	normal	normal
Type 2	44	↑	↑	↑ ↓
Type 3	41	↓	↑	↑ ↓
Total	254			

(Inada, Ueno, Mishima)

trophy often associated with changes in ST segment and T wave. They are presumably due to hypertension and/or aortic insufficiency, though a contribution from lesions of the coronary arteries and myocardium is not ruled out. Cardiac enlargement is a common finding on the chest X-ray film. Calcification of the aorta is also seen in some cases (Table III).

Table III. Laboratory findings.

	Frequency	
Accelerated ESR	868/1193	72.8%
Leucocytosis	437/1249	35.0%
Anemia	563/1175	47.9%
Gamma-globulin ↑	483/1008	47.9%
ASLO ↑	155/1067	14.5%
Positive CRP	666/1287	51.7%
Positive RA	108/1185	9.1%
Positive Wa-R	23/1105	2.1%
Positive Tub-R	366/ 532	68.8%
CT ratio ↑	413/1028	40.2%
Calcified aorta	239/1160	20.6%
Abnormal ECG	538/1221	44.1%

(Inada, Ministry of Health Japan)

ARTERIOGRAPHY

Aortography is the most valuable diagnostic examination and should be performed in every suspected case. Total aortography (including all brachio-cephalic

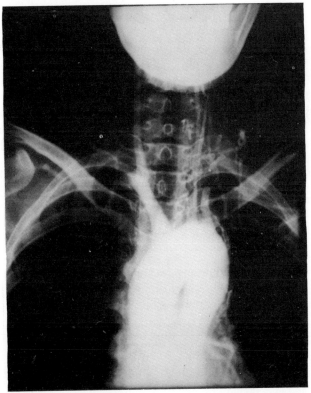

Fig. 3

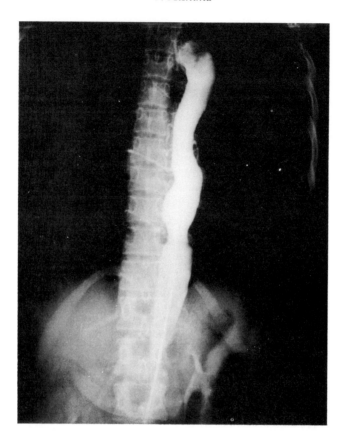

Fig. 4

vessels, the entire aorta and the renal and ilio-femoral arteries) is useful for
delineation of the full extent of the disease, as Laude and Gross (1972) reported.

Usually the involved arteries are revealed by stenosis or obstruction but pre- or
poststenotic dilatation may also be seen. Occasionally, aneurysm formation is
recognized. In type 1, as already stated above, the lesions are located mostly in
the aortic arch and its branches (Fig. 3). The ascending aorta may also be affected,
resulting in aortic insufficiency in some cases. In type 2, the clinical picture simu-
lates coarctation of the aorta, or renovascular hypertension may predominate.
Atypical coarctation affects a long segment usually, most commonly located
just above or below the diaphragm (Fig. 4). In type 3, multiple or widespread
arterial lesions involve the entire aorta and its main branches.

In many cases, lesions of the pulmonary arteries are also detected. They are
also demonstrated by pulmonary scintiscanning.

DIAGNOSIS

There are no pathognomonic symptoms of Takayasu's arteritis. Onset is often
overlooked and may mimic a rheumatic or non-specific illness with acute systemic
symptoms in many cases.

General weakness and fatigue are common, especially in the initial stage of the disease. Usually, after an asymptomatic quiescent stage of variable duration, the inflammatory lesion of the arteries becomes manifest, most commonly in the brachio-cephalic vessels, with pain and tenderness over the neck, shoulder or anterior chest. These pains are presumably vascular in origin.

The complaints most frequently noticed are due to impaired cerebral circulation, such as dizziness, headache and visual disturbances. Ischemic symptoms of the upper extremity, such as numbness, cold sensation and claudication, are also encountered frequently. Dyspnea and palpitation are not uncommon and angina pectoris may occur in some cases.

Careful palpation of bilateral radial arterial pulsation and blood pressure measurement in both arms are useful for the screening of the patients. Depending on the distribution of the lesions, pulsation of carotid artery, aorta and femoral artery may be diminished or absent. Vascular murmurs are also audible over the involved segments of the arteries.

Hypertension is also noteworthy. Hypertension of the upper half of the body suggests coarctation of the descending aorta, while systemic hypertension is the consequence of coarctation in the abdominal aorta and/or renal artery involvement.

X-ray examination often reveals cardiomegaly, with an enlarged and calcified aortic arch.

In some cases, aortography may be helpful to establish the diagnosis.

CLINICAL COURSE AND PROGNOSIS

The natural history of the disease is not yet fully clarified. Prognosis of the patients is greatly influenced by the grade of hypertension. Aortic insufficiency is frequently associated with hypertension and is also related to the prognosis.

Table IV. Causes of death.

Causes	Nasu (autopsy) 1958–1973	Koide 1972–1975
Cardiac failure	18	16
Postop. death	17	5
Cerebral accident	5	8
Infection	4	1
Pulmonary edema	3	0
Aneurysm rupture	2	1
Leukemia	2	0
Renal insufficiency	1	3
Myocardial infarction	1	4
Pulmonary infarction	1	1
Others	4	7
Unknown	18	14
Malignancy	0	6
Sudden death	0	3
Total	76	69

(Inada, Ministry of Health Japan)

The ten-year survival rate after the establishment of the diagnosis is estimated as about 65%. The causes of death in 76 autopsy cases from 1958 to 1973 and in 69 cases epidemiologically studied from 1972 to 1975 are listed in Table IV. Cardiac failure and cerebrovascular accidents due to hypertension were most frequent. The reduction of operative deaths is attributed to improved selection of the patients and recent advances of operative techniques.

TREATMENT

Treatment currently consists of long-term steroid therapy. Subjective symptoms together with abnormal laboratory findings improve rapidly in most cases with administration of steroids, especially in the active stage. Itoh reported that an initial dose of 30 mg of prednisolone per day is usually sufficient, and then the dose is reduced gradually until withdrawal of steroids is achieved. However, long-term administration of a small dose, 5 to 10 mg/day, is often required to maintain the therapeutic effects. Other medical treatment includes control of hypertension, congestive heart failure and angina pectoris, etc.

It is estimated that surgical intervention is mandatory in about 20% of cases. Arterial reconstructive surgery is indicated for severe hypertension, for cerebral ischemia, especially with progressive visual impairment, and for aneurysm with impending rupture (Fig. 5). Aortic valve replacement may be considered in cases of severe aortic insufficiency.

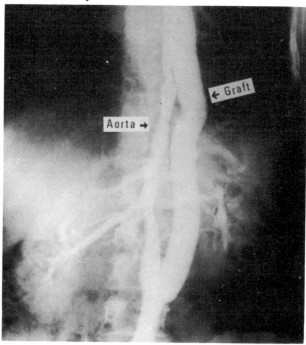

Fig. 5

Of the operative procedures, endarterectomy has been abandoned since 1966 because of the technical difficulty. Bypass procedures with a synthetic graft have taken the place of endarterectomy.

From our own experiences, it is desirable when performing arterial reconstructive surgery to pay special consideration to the hemodynamic changes caused by various degrees of pathologic processes. Determination of the arterial pressures of the various segments, such as the aorta, upper and lower extremities and especially retinal pressure, are the best parameters in case selection for the surgical treatment.

REFERENCES

Cipriano, P. R., Silverman, J. F. and Perlroth, M. G. *et al.* (1977). *Am. J. Cardiol.* **39**, 744.

Inada, K. (1977). *In* "Vascular Lesions Collagen Disease and its Related Conditions." 143–148. University of Tokyo Press, Tokyo.

Ito, I. (1966). *Jap. Circulation J.* **30**, 75.

Laude, A. and Gross, A. (1972). *Am. J. Roentgenol.* **116**, 165.

Nasu, T. (1977). *In* "Vascular Lesions of Collagen Disease and its Related Conditions." 149–160. University of Tokyo Press, Tokyo.

Shimizu, K. and Sano, K. (1951). *J. Neuropathol. Clin. Neurol.* **1**, 37.

Takayasu, M. (1908). *Acta Soc. Ophthalmol. Jap.* **12**, 554.

Ueda, H. (1968). *Jap. Heart J.* **9**, 76.

Ueda, H., Ito, I. and Okada, R. (1963). *Jap. Heart J.* **4**, 224.

THE OCCURRENCE OF ATHEROSCLEROTIC ARTERIOPATHY AND ISCHEMIC HEART DISEASE IN A MALE INDUSTRIAL POPULATION

V. Bazika, Z. Reiniš, J. Pokorný, Vl. Puchmayer, R. Cifkova,
E. Stucklikova and F. Hrabovsky

*Laboratory of Angiology, IVth Medical Clinic, Charles University,
Prague, Czechoslovakia*

In our study we followed up the health conditions in a male industrial population examining 3281 employees in the car industry. We have followed up the age group from 30–59 years (as shown in Table I).

METHOD AND RESULTS

To detect an arterial stenosis or obliteration of the lower extremities we used current clinical methods including palpation and auscultation. The latent form of arteriopathy we detected by the presence of a murmur and a pulse deficiency. The positive findings were verified by arteriography.

Ischemic heart disease (IHD) we classified as latent or manifest.

Latent IHD was diagnosed in men without symptoms when the resting or effort ECG showed specific changes of ischemia evaluated according to the criteria of the Minnesota code.

The manifest form of IHD was classified in this way: (a) angina pectoris; (b) myocardial infarction; (c) myocardial infarction confirmed by autopsy.

The occurrence of peripheral atherosclerotic arteriopathy and IHD rises rapidly with age (Fig. 1). IHD occurs at least 5 to 10 years earlier than peripheral arterio-

Serono Symposium No. 37, "Vascular Occlusion: Epidemiological, Pathophysiological and Therapeutic Aspects", edited by M. Tesi and J. Dormandy, 1981. Academic Press, London and New York.

V. Bazika et al.

Table I.   Age distribution of the men examined.

Age	Number	%	Age	Number	%
30–34	297	9.0	30–39	925	28
35–39	628	19.1			
40–44	938	28.6	40–49	806	55
45–49	868	26.5			
50–54	394	12.0	50–59	550	17
55–59	156	4.8			
Total	3281	100	Total	3281	100

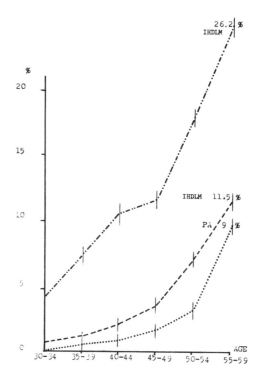

Fig. 1.   Occurrence of peripheral atherosclerotic arteriopathy and ischemic heart disease. PA: peripheral arteriopathy; IHDM: ischemic heart disease manifest; IHDLM: ischemic heart disease latent and manifest.

pathy. The dramatic increase in frequency of IHD at the age of 45 to 59 and by peripheral atherosclerotic arteriopathy at 55 to 59 is very striking.

The frequency of risk factors such as family history, smoking, high blood pressure, high cholesterol level, increased beta/alpha lipoprotein index, obesity, diabetes mellitus and angiosclerosis retinae did not show a significant difference in either group.

However, some risk factors, especially high blood pressure, influence the development of atherosclerotic changes in the coronary artery bed and patients with atherosclerotic arteriopathy in a different way.

Clinically, we detected an arterial stenotic or occlusive process in the lower extremities in 53 men altogether, i.e. 1.6% of observed men. The average age of these workers with atherosclerotic angiopathy was 50.5 years. The youngest of them was 37 and the oldest was 59 years of age.

However, the first complaints which indicated a lesion of the arteries supplying the lower extremities had usually been manifested earlier. On average, the patients had symptoms at the age of 46.6 years, i.e. 3.5 years earlier than the diagnosis was made. The extent of damage to the arteries was variable. Only rarely could we prove a solitary stenosis. Most arteriograms showed polysegmental damage of arteries of variable extent, sometimes with poststenotic dilatation. Occasionally, the occurrence of a latent form of occlusive atherosclerotic angiopathy was revealed. This latent form was found in 4 men when an audible murmur was found. These findings were verified arteriographically. Manifest IHD, including angina pectoris and myocardial infarction was found in 108 men, i.e. 3.3%. The latent form of IHD was present in 273 men, i.e. 8.3%. By ECG examination, we found the latent form of IHD twice as often as the manifest one.

With the help of modern research methods, we tried to detect the early stages of peripheral atherosclerotic arteriopathy, which could not be revealed by conventional methods. We examined a group of 76 men with high risk score. All these probands were bearers of at least three risk indicators such as smoking, high blood pressure, high cholesterol level or increased beta/alpha lipoprotein index. The youngest man was 36 years of age, the oldest one 59. The proband's average age was 50.6 years.

Examining with a plethysmographic method after effort and using Doppler's ultrasound technique we detected 16 men from a group of 76, i.e. 21%, where these research methods indicated poor circulation in the arterial bed of the lower extremities. In all these patients we verified our findings arteriographically (Table II).

For detecting the early forms of coronary insufficiency, we examined 407 clinically healthy men with a negative ECG, but having a high risk score. Risk indicators included a high blood pressure, smoking, a high level of cholesterol in the blood, an increased beta/alpha lipoprotein index, a positive family history, diabetes, obesity and angiosclerosis retinae. There were always at least three risk factors present.

For most of the patients we stopped the bicycle-ergometric loading test when the heart rate reached 160/min, which means an efficiency of maximum oxygen

Table II. Detected latent forms of peripheral atherosclerotic arteriopathy (PA) and ischemic heart disease (IHD) in men with high risk score.

	High risk men	Positive findings
PA	76	16–21%
IHD	407	98–24%

uptake higher than 75%. All who finished the loading test were consequently exceeding the submaximal heart rate according to Anderson. In some cases, the loading test was interrupted before reaching the maximum heart rate. There were several reasons for interruption of bicycle ergometry:

1. a hypertensive reaction, when the value of the blood pressure reached over 230/120 as it did with 21 probands;
2. dyspnoea—the cause was bronchitis and emphysema in seven examined.
3. pain in lower extremities in five examined altogether: two with claudi-cation, one with arthralgia, two with pain of untrained muscles;
4. obesity (after Broca index) 30% over the normal weight. These probands showed fatigue.

The bicycle ergometric loading tests were interrupted by 35 men altogether, i.e. 8.6%.

Changes in the ECG trace after the bicycle-ergometric loading test, indicating coronary insufficiency, occurred in 98 out of 407 probands, i.e. 24%. If we subtract from this number the group of 35 men not completing the loading test, we could suppose that the number of ECG positive findings was even higher.

CONCLUSION

Using auxiliary detection methods, namely plethysmography with a loading test and Doppler's ultrasound method to detect the early forms of peripheral atherosclerotic angiopathy, we showed, in the group of men with a high-risk score, insufficiency of the arterial bed supplying the lower extremities in 21% of examined probands.

The ergometry loading test detected, in a group of men with a high-risk score, 24% with coronary insufficiency. This had not been shown by the conventional research methods. The use of these diagnostic methods in epidemiological studies, as well as during clinical work, helped us to define the diagnosis more precisely and has value in preventive cardiology by revealing the early stages of peripheral and coronary angiopathies.

REFERENCES

Anderson, K. H., Shephard, R. J., Denolin, H., Vyrnauskas, E. and Masironi, R. (1971). In "Fundamentals of Exercise Testing". WHO Geneva.
Bazika, V., Baziková, K., Slabý, A. and Reiniš, Z. (1970). Sborník lékařský. 72, 119–123.
Puchmayer, Vl. and Bazika, V. (1974). Čas. lék. ces. 113, 172–178.
Reiniš, Z., Pokorný, J., Bazika, V., Horáková, D., Tišerová, J. and Reisenauer, R. (1976). Cor Vasa. 18, 129–138.
Schoop, W. and Köhler, H. (1966). Verh. dtsch. Ges. Kreisl. Forsch. 32, 233–237.
Widmer, L. K. (1963). Bibl. cardiol. 13, 67s.

HYPERTENSION AS A POSSIBLE RISK FACTOR IN
ARTERIAL OCCLUSIVE DISEASE

V. Puchmayer, W. Schoop, J. Pokorný, Ellen Jacob, O. Vanderbeke,
Renata Cifkova and J. Fanta

*IVth Medical Clinic, Charles University, Prague, Czechoslovakia, Aggertalklinik,
Engelskirchen, BRD*

From clinical experience, epidemiological studies and experimental reports
several risk factors of arterial occlusive disease are known. We have been interested
in what role hypertension and its combination with other risk factors play in this
disease.

METHODS

A total of 982 men and 30 women suffering from arterial occlusive disease and
a control group of 411 men and 50 women free from any symptoms of such
disease were examined during a period of one year (Table I). All patients of both
groups were thoroughly investigated according to the same criteria: clinically,
angiologically and biochemically. The blood pressure was measured in normotensives twice a week; in hypertensives every day. A systolic pressure of 160–200
Torr (21.3–26.6 kPa) was considered to be slightly raised, above 200 Torr to be
markedly raised. Similarly, a diastolic pressure of 95–105 Torr (12.5–13.8 kPa)
was slightly raised and above 105 Torr to be markedly raised. All data were calculated by means of a computer and the statistical significance was evaluated with a
chi-square test.

Serono Symposium No. 37, "Vascular Occlusion: Epidemiological, Pathophysiological and
Therapeutic Aspects", edited by M. Tesi and J. Dormandy, 1981. Academic Press, London
and New York.

Table I.   Division of patients.

Diagnosis	Number of patients	Age range (years)	Average age (years)
Atherosclerosis obliterans	908	26–71	54.5
Thrombangiitis obliterans	59	27–49	39.5
Uncertain aetiology	15	35–63	53.5
Total	982	26–71	53.6
Vasoneuroses	74		
Varices	152		
Post-phlebitic syndrome	89		
Root ischaemia	27		
Others	69		
Total	411	26–73	52.7
Number of stenoses and occlusions 2863		Arteriographically proven 1436 = 50.1%	

RESULTS

Normal systolic and diastolic blood pressure was found more often in the control groups (Table II). By contrast, increased systolic and normal diastolic pressure was more frequently found in the group with obliterative disease. It was shown on closer analysis that it is a slightly increased systolic pressure of 160-200 Torr which occurs more frequently in obliterative disease. We found these differences, in the over 50 years of age category, in men with claudication for less than one year, from 1 to 5 years and over 5 years. In the group with occlusive disease, both systolic and diastolic pressures were raised, either with slightly increased systolic (160-200) and diastolic (95-105) or a highly elevated systolic (over 200

Table II.   Importance of systolic and diastolic hypertension in AOD.

Number of patients	AOD[a] 982	Controls 411	AO[b] 908
Normal systolic + diastolic BP[c]	488 $P < 0.001$ ◄—	267 ◄— $P < 0.001$ —►	436
Systolic BP 160-200 + normal diastolic BP	169 ◄ $P < 0.001$	36	$P < 0.001$ —► 168
Elevated systolic BP + normal diastolic BP	171 ◄ $P < 0.001$	36	$P < 0.001$ —► 169
Systolic BP > 200 + normal diastolic BP		NS[d]	
Systolic BP 160-200 + diastolic BP 95-105	236 ◄ $P < 0.001$	64	$P < 0.001$ —► 225
Systolic BP > 200 + diastolic BP > 105	21 ◄ $P < 0.05$	3	$P < 0.05$ —► 21
Elevated systolic + diastolic BP	257 ◄ $P < 0.001$	67	$P < 0.001$ —► 246
Elevated diastolic BP + normal systolic BP		NS	
Elevated systolic + diastolic BP	Women		NS
	Thrombangiitis obliterans		NS

[a]AOD = arterial occlusive disease; [b]AO = atherosclerosis obliterans; [c]BP = blood pressure; [d]NS = not significant.

Table III. Statistical significance of hypertension in combinations with other risk factors.

Number of patients	AOD[a] 982	Controls 411	AO[b] 908
H + FH + S	25 ◄— $P < 0.05$	3	$P < 0.025$ —► 24
H + S + LD	64 ◄— $P < 0.025$	13	$P < 0.01$ —► 64
H + S + FH + LD	78 ◄— $P < 0.001$	10	$P < 0.001$ —► 73
H + other combinations		NS[c]	
H as the only risk factor		NS	

[a] AOD = arterial occlusive disease; [b] AO = atherosclerosis obliterans; [c] NS = not significant.
H: Hypertension; S: Smoking; FH: Positive family history; LD: Blood lipids disturbances.

Torr) and diastolic (over 105 Torr). We have found similar significant differences in all age categories of men including the youngest one, i.e. up to 39 years, regardless of the duration of claudication. It is interesting that there were no significant differences between the obliterative and the control groups with the occurrence of an elevated diastolic pressure only, whether slightly (95–105 Torr) or markedly raised (above 105 Torr), if combined with a normal systolic one. No difference in systolic or diastolic hypertension was found in women with occlusive disease or in patients with thrombangiitis obliterans.

We have further investigated whether, in the groups with occlusive disease, systolic or diastolic hypertension occurs more frequently as a single factor or as a combination with other risks. Therefore, we have looked at different combinations of systolic-diastolic hypertension, smoking, positive family history, diabetes, obesity and disorders of lipid metabolism. It has been shown that in the obliteration group, systolic-diastolic hypertension occurred with smoking and either a positive family history or a lipid disorder (Table III). A combination of all four factors was the most significant, even in the youngest age category of men. All other combinations of these factors were insignificant. Likewise, no difference appeared between patients with obliterations and the control ones in the occurrence of hypertension as a single factor. A positive family history and smoking was of great importance as a risk. A disorder in lipid metabolism was already known before the beginning of illness in 5% of hypertensives. In men with obliterative disease, from a total of 494 hypertensives, an increased systolic or diastolic pressure was noted before the onset of disease in 194, i.e. 39.2%. Other hypertensives knew nothing of their claudication difficulties. Patients with obliterative disease and with only slightly increased systolic pressure (160–200 Torr) did, however, know of their elevation of pressure before the beginning of their difficulties in only 10%.

It is hard to decide whether the increased frequency of hypertension in obliterative disease is a sign of general atherosclerosis or whether it makes itself felt as one of the aetiopathogenetic risk factors. Considering the first alternative, one would expect evidence of a more frequent occurrence of a slight systolic hypertension in atherosclerotics. On the other hand, the relatively high occurrence of hypertension before the onset of difficulties, a greater incidence of systolic-diastolic hypertension among even the youngest age categories and, finally, the frequent occurrence of only certain combinations of systolic-diastolic hypertension, smoking, positive history in the family and disorder of lipid metabolism in occlusive disease, points to the second alternative.

CONCLUSION

In total, 982 men and 30 women with occlusive disease, including 908 men with atherosclerosis obliterans and 411 men and 50 women free from any symptoms of such an illness, were investigated. In the control group, normal systolic and diastolic blood pressure occurred significantly more often. By contrast, men with obliterations had systolic hypertension more frequently, particularly up to 200 Torr. They also had increased systolic-diastolic pressure, both slightly and markedly in all age categories including the youngest one. No significant differences in the occurrence of increased diastolic pressure with a normal systolic one were found. In women and in patients with thrombangiitis obliterans, we did not find any significant changes of pressure. Furthermore, we have established that hypertension as a single factor occurred equally as often in controls as in occlusive disease. In the group with occlusive disease, a combination of systolic-diastolic hypertension and smoking together with a positive family history or with a disorder of lipid metabolism occurred significantly more frequently.

REFERENCES

Bazika, V., Puchmayer, V., Reiniš, Z., Pokorný, J., Horáková Dana and Hrabovský, F. (1978). *Časopis lékařů českých* **117**, 38–39, 1214.
Puchmayer, V. and Bazika, V. (1974). *Časopis lékařů českých* **113**, 6, 172.
Widmer, L. K., Da Silva, A. and Madar, G. (1976). *In* "Hyperonie–Risikofaktor in der Angiologie (E. Zeitler, ed) 67–70. G. Witzstrock Verlag, Baden-Baden, Brüseel, Köln.

PREVENTION OF REOCCLUSION IN ARTERIAL RECONSTRUCTIVE SURGERY BY DIPYRIDAMOLE AND ASA

T. Pekka, M. D. Harjola and M. D. Heikki Meurala

Department of Cardiovascular and Thoracic Surgery, University Central Hospital, Helsinki, Finland

INTRODUCTION

The inhibitory effect of dipyridamole (Persantin®, Boehringer Ingelheim) and dipyridamole/acetylsalicyclic acid (ASA) on arterial thromboembolism in connection with artificial heart valve surgery has been confirmed in several clinical trials (Arrants and Hairston, 1972; Harker and Slichter, 1970; Pell, 1975; Sullivan, 1974; Taguchi *et al.*, 1975). It has been shown that dipyridamole alone and in combination with ASA has a beneficial effect in the treatment of chronic coronary heart disease and in coronary bypass surgery (Horwitz *et al.*, 1974; Ritchie and Harker, 1974; Rittenhous and Wu, 1974; Salky and Dugdale, 1973; Sullivan, 1974). There are also experimental studies which confirm the effect of dipyridamole and ASA in arterial reconstructive surgery (Harker *et al.*, 1977; Metke *et al.*, 1978; Oblath *et al.*, 1978). Two clinical studies confirm the antithrombotic effect of dipyridamole and ASA in endarterectomized patients, and in patients with recanalized femoral arteries using the Dotter method (Bollinger *et al.*, 1978; Hess *et al.*, 1978). However, no data have been published on dipyridamole/ASA in connection with arterial reconstructive bypass surgery.

The aim of this clinical trial was to study the antithrombotic effect of dipyridamole and ASA on post-operative arterial occlusions in a prospective controlled series of peripheral vascular reconstructions.

Serono Symposium No. 37, "Vascular Occlusion: Epidemiological, Pathophysiological and Therapeutic Aspects", edited by M. Tesi and J. Dormandy, 1981. Academic Press, London and New York.

MATERIALS AND METHODS

There were 400 consecutive patients randomly allocated into four groups according to the antithrombotic medication given. The antithrombotic medication received in different groups is described in Table I. In 25 patients, the only operative procedure was a high lumbar sympathectomy, therefore they were excluded from this series. During the second trial, more patients were excluded from the series. The remaining 364 patients were subjected to different types of arterial reconstructive operation (Table II). The observation time equalled the post-operative hospitalization time.

Table I. Daily medication given in different groups.

Group I	Dipyridamole 150 mg tid + ASA 0.5 g tid
Group II	Dipyridamole 150 mg tid
Group III	ASA 0.5 g tid
Group IV	Control

Table II. Types of different operative procedures in series of 364 patients subjected to arterial surgery.

Operation	Number of patients
Aorto-cervical	81
Abdominal aortic	139
Abdominal + lower extremity	39
Lower extremity	100
Complex operations	5
Total	364

RESULTS

The random distribution of patients into different groups is presented in Table III. The age and sex distribution in the different groups was equal as was the number of various reconstructive operations performed.

The reocclusion rate seemed to be dependent, not on the type or anatomical site of operation, but mainly on the antithrombotic medication given (Table IV). The reocclusion rate was 24 out of 364 (6.6%). There were no reocclusions in the group receiving both dipyridamole and ASA, six reocclusions in the group receiving dipyridamole or ASA alone, and the number of reocclusions doubled in the control group receiving no antithrombotic medication. The difference between the dipyridamole/ASA group and the control group was statistically highly significant (Table V).

The difference between the dipyridamole group and the control group as well as between the ASA group and the control group was not significant. In only two cases did ASA cause dyspepsia and in two cases a mild rash was verified.

Table III.   Result of randomization in a series of 389 patients.

	D/ASA 99 pts	D 96 pts	ASA 97 pts	Control 97 pts
Sex female/male	1:4.1	1:5.2	1:5.0	1:3.7
Mean age years	57.1	57.5	57.2	57.8
Operation:				
supra-aortal	22	20	20	19
lower extremity major	49	43	48	43
minor	28	33	29	35
Total	99	96	97	97

DISCUSSION

In several clinical trials, dipyridamole and ASA have been shown to have an antithrombotic effect in patients with artificial valves (Arrants and Hairston, 1972; Harker *et al.*, 1977; Pell, 1975; Taguchi *et al.*, 1975). It has also been shown that dipyridamole and ASA have a favourable effect on the patency of coronary bypass grafts (Sullivan, 1974). There are also some experimental studies which prove that dipyridamole and ASA have a statistically significant effect on the platelet survival time in conjunction with arterial prosthetic replacement (Harker *et al.*, 1977). A preventive effect on neointimal fibrous proliferation at the anastomoses of prosthetic vascular grafts and venous grafts has also been proved in animal series (Metke *et al.*, 1978; Oblath *et al.*, 1978). This seems to be the first published clinical trial in which a statistically highly significant effect on the early patency in arterial bypass reconstructions by dipyridamole and ASA medication has been proven.

Using experimental models, Harker and Slichter have shown that dipyridamole has a beneficial effect on platelet survival time (Harker and Slichter, 1970). In the present clinical series, this effect did not alter the reocclusion rate significantly. Dipyridamole and ASA given alone had an equal effect on the reocclusion rate, which was half that in the control group. However, it was not statistically significant. Aspirin inhibits the release reaction, secondary ADP-induced platelet aggregation and adherence to collagen *in vitro* (Harker and Slichter, 1970). Dipyridamole inhibits primary and secondary aggregation induced by ADP-epinephrine and collagen and decreases platelet retention by glass bead columns (Emmons *et al.*, 1965). Dipyridamole also potentiates the effect of prostacyclin on platelets (Hess *et al.*, 1978). Dipyridamole and ASA have a synergistic effect, thus resulting in a clinically effective means of preventing thrombogenesis (Harker and Slichter, 1970).

Preoperative medication has been advocated by some authors (Oblath *et al.*, 1978). However, oral medication started immediately after the operation has been proved in this study to be sufficient to prevent the early reocclusion in arterial reconstructive surgery.

Table IV. Effect of antithrombotic medication on post-operative arterial occlusion rate in series of 364 consecutive arterial reconstructions.

Site of operation	D/ASA		D		ASA		C	
	Patent	Occluded	Patent	Occluded	Patent	Occluded	Patent	Occluded
Supra-aortal	22	0	20	0	16	4	17	2
Lower extremity								
Major operation	49	0	42	1	48	0	37	6
Minor operation	22	0	25	5	22	2	20	4
Total	93	0	87	6	86	6	74	12

Table V.   Difference in reocclusion rate in arterial reconstructions on 364 consecutive patients.

Antithrombotic medication	No. patients	Reocclusions
Dipyridamole/ASA	93	0 $P < 0.001$
Dipyridamole	93	6 NS
ASA	92	6 NS
Controls	86	12
Totals	364	24 (6.6%)

REFERENCES

Arrants, J. E. and Hairston, P. (1972). *Am. Surg.* **38**, 432.

Bollinger, A., Fritschy, J., Torres, C. and Piquerez, M. J. (1978). *Studie Vasa* **70**, 82.

Emmons, P. R., Harrison, M. J. G., Honour, A. J. and Mitchell, J. R. A. (1965). *Lancet* **2**, 603.

Griepp, R. B., Stinson, E. B., Bieber, C. P., Dong, E. Jr. and Shumway, N. E. (1974). "Control of human heart graft arteriosclerosis". Symposium on Antithrombotic Prophylaxis after Coronary Surgery. Helsinki, Finland.

Harker, L. A. and Slichter, S. J. (1970). *New. Engl. J. Med.* **283**, 1302.

Harker, L. A., Slichter, S. J. and Sauvage, L. R. (1977). *Ann. Surg.* **186**, 594.

Hess, H., Mueller-Fassbender, H., Ingrisch, H. and Mietaschk, A. (1978). *Dtsch. med. Wschr.* **103**, 1994.

Horwitz, L. D., Curry, G. C., Parkey, R. W. and Bonte, F. J. (1974). *Circulation* **50**, 560.

Metke, M. P., Lie, J. T., Fuster, V., Josa, M. and Kaye, M. P. (1978). *Am. J. Cardiol.* **41**, 411.

Oblath, R. W., Buckley, F. O. and DeWeese, J. A. (1978). *Am. J. Cardiol.* **41**, 411.

Pell, E. (1975). "Essai clinique controle du dipyridamole dans le traitement preventif des accidents thrombo-emboliques chez les porteurs de protheses valvulai". Theses, Lyon.

Ritchie, J. L. and Harker, L. A. (1974). *Circulation* **50**, Suppl. III, Abstr. 1088.

Rittenhous, E. A. and Wu, K. K. (1974). "Aortocoronary Bypass: Clinical Results and Studies of Platelet Aggregation". Symposium on Antithrombotic Prophylaxis after Coronary Surgery. Helsinki, Finland.

Salky, N. and Dugdale, M. (1973). *Am. J. Cardiol.* **32**, 612.

Sullivan, J. M. (1974). "The Use of Antiplatelet Agents after Cardiac Surgery". Symposium on Antithrombotic Prophylaxis after Coronary Surgery. Helsinki, Finland.

Taguchi, K., Matsumura, H., Washizu, T., Hirao, M., Kato, K., Kato, E., Mochizuki, T., Takamura, K., Mashimo, I., Morifuji, K., Nakagaki, M. and Suma, T. (1975). *J. Cardiov. Surg.* **16**, 8.

THE FREQUENCY OF SYMMETRICAL CAROTID LESIONS

R. London, S. London, M. Epstein, J. Benson,
J. Raines and A. Drexler

Miami Heart Institute, Miami Beach, Florida, USA

The serious effects of carotid obstruction has generated increasing interest in the investigation of asymptomatic carotid bruits, transient ischemic attacks and mild strokes (Gomensoro *et al.*, 1973). In weekly vascular conferences held at our institution, during which individuals are evaluated for surgical or medical therapy, it became apparent that a high percentage of patients had symmetrical lesions of the common or internal carotid vessels on arteriogram — lesions which were often unsuspected clinically. Because the presence and localization of exactly symmetrical disease had not been previously emphasized as significant, we reviewed 100 consecutive arch studies in patients suspected of extracranial vascular pathology.

METHOD

Selection of Cases

Patients with asymptomatic carotid bruits, transient ischemic attacks or mild stokes, who had been referred by their physicians for evaluation, were screened in a non-invasive vascular laboratory. When significant abnormalities of the extracranial vessels were detected by ocular pneumoplethysmography, carotid audiofrequency analysis, cerebral Doppler evaluation and echo-imaging, the patients underwent neurologic evaluation and were then admitted to hospital for arteriograms. This group was considered to have 50% or more stenosis of the affected vessel and comprised 5% of the total number of patients screened.

Serono Symposium No. 37, "Vascular Occlusion: Epidemiological, Pathophysiological and Therapeutic Aspects", edited by M. Tesi and J. Dormandy, 1981. Academic Press, London and New York.

Analysis

The selective arteriograms of 100 consecutive arch studies performed according to the Seldinger technique were reviewed for evidence of symmetrical, bilateral lesions of the common and internal carotid vessels. Charts were reviewed for the risk factors of hypertension, diabetes, hyperlipidemia and smoking, as well as for evidence of associated vascular disease of the heart, aorta and peripheral vessels. Surgical correction and pathology specimens were also reviewed.

RESULTS

In the 100 consecutive cases, evidence of bilateral and symmetrical disease was found in the common carotid and internal carotid vessels in 79 patients (Figs 1-4). Four patients had no vascular disease of the carotid system and were therefore eliminated. Seventeen showed asymmetrical involvement. Endarterectomy was carried out unilaterally in 48 patients and bilaterally in ten for a total of 58 patients. In seven of the latter group, coronary bypass surgery was also performed. One stroke followed surgery but no mortality was experienced in the entire surgical group. The disease, as assessed by arteriogram, surgery and pathologic specimens, was evaluated as to location, extent of the lesion, degree of stenosis, ulceration of or hemorrhage into the plaque and superimposed thrombosis. While

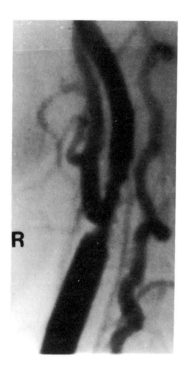 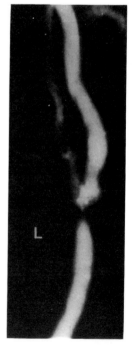

Fig. 1. Symmetrical lesions of both right and left common carotids and internal carotids 1 cm from the origin.

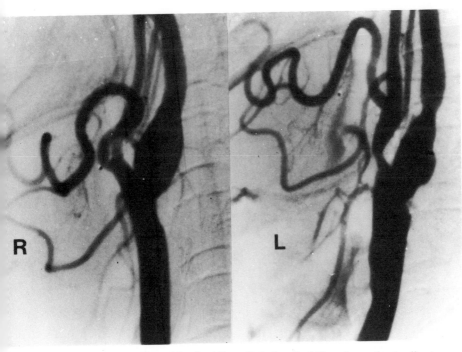

Fig. 2. Large bulbous lesions originating bilaterally below the bifurcation and extending to mid-internal carotids.

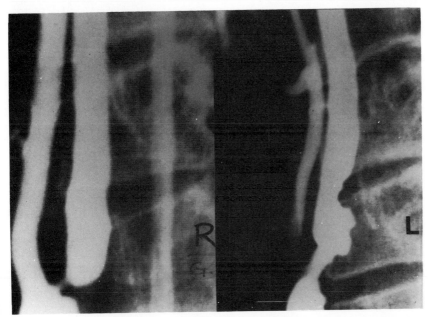

Fig. 3. Bilateral lesions involving bifurcation and extending distally with marked irregularity of wall, particularly on the left. Both surgical specimens showed partially organized thrombi.

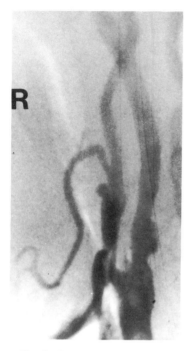 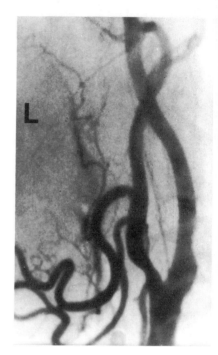

Fig. 4. Symmetrical involvements of the internal carotids distal to bifurcation with ulcerated plaque on right.

Table I. Microscopic pathology of 64 endarterectomy specimens.

Hemorrhage in plaque	26	(40.6%)
Ruptured plaque	9	(14.0%)
Thrombus	27	(42.5%)

the localization of the disease was exact and symmetrical, the degree of stenosis produced by the pathologic process varied considerably (Table I). Thrombosis was found in 27 of 64 surgical specimens and hemorrhage in plaque in 26. Ulceration of the plaque without thrombosis was seen in nine cases.

Generally, the area of bifurcation was the most frequent site of plaque formation; however, in certain cases arterial involvement was in proximity to protruding osteophytes of the cervical vertebrae (Fig. 5). This suggests that in addition to turbulence and jet lesions, local factors may influence the site of predilection.

Table II shows the various risk factors and the association of other significant vascular disease. Transient ischemic attacks or mild strokes were seen in 70 of the 96 patients. Unilateral bruits were detected in 26 and bilateral bruits in 45, suggesting that their absence does not exclude the presence of significant lesions.

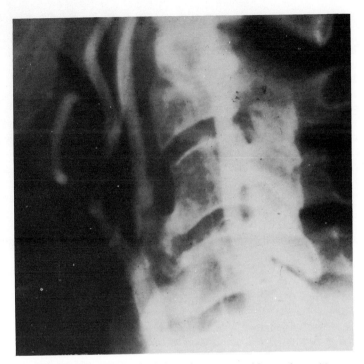

Fig. 5. Shows conformity of vascular lesion of common and internal carotid to protruding osteophyte, suggesting impingement.

Table II. Significant factors in 96 patients with carotid occlusive disease.

Average age	64	(43–80)
Sex — male	62	
Sex — female	34	
Hypertension	52	
Diabetes	25	
Positive family history	27	
Smoking	44	
Hyperlipidemia	54	
Associated vascular disease:		
coronary	59	
peripheral vessels	27	
aorta	8	
Bruits — unilateral	26	
Bruits — bilateral	45	
Transient ischemic attacks or mild strokes	70	

CONCLUSIONS

The finding of bilateral symmetrical lesions in 80% of our cases and the high incidence of thrombus formation in 42.5% of the surgical specimens leads us to suggest the following.

1. The finding of a single asymptomatic bruit, unless proven otherwise, should raise suspicion of significant contralateral symmetrical arterial disease.

2. The definitive diagnosis of unilateral carotid artery disease by non-invasive studies or selective arteriograms and successful unilateral carotid artery surgery may not solve the potentially dangerous problems of bilateral pathology.

3. Arteriograms clearly indicate the degree of stenosis or occlusion but cannot delineate the varied pathology in the lesions. The 42.5% incidence of thrombus formation demonstrated in the surgical specimens was unsuspected on the arteriograms.

4. In order to successfully prevent the complications of progressive vascular disease in the symmetrically paired vessel, our data suggest the need for continuous anticoagulant therapy.

REFERENCE

Gomensoro, J. B., Maslenikov, V., Azambuja, N., Fields, W. S. and Lemak, N. A. (1973). *The Journal of the American Medical Association* **224**, 985.

THE POSSIBILITIES OF SURGICAL TREATMENT IN PATIENTS WITH CEREBROVASCULAR INSUFFICIENCY DUE TO CAROTID LESIONS

P. Fiorani, G. R. Pistolese and V. Faraglia

Department of Vascular Surgery, University of Rome, School of Medicine, Italy

Even after 25 years of carotid artery surgery, this therapy still offers cerebro-vascular patients a better prognosis than medical therapy. However, there are the problems of complications and operative mortality whose extent, according to statistical data, we cannot underestimate. In a recent review concerning this problem, out of a total of 3820 patients there was a mortality of 3.8% with permanent complications in 5.7% (West *et al.*, 1979). These percentages certainly indicate too high a risk for surgery which, in principle, should be prophylactic. These average values come from different and extremely heterogeneous sources; but one may observe that the mortality ranges between 0 and 11% and the compli-cations between 1% and 27%. This mortality stems from the surgical technique, from the selection of patients and from the different ways of dealing with surgical risks.

Carotid artery surgery is safe only when a proper patient selection is made; considering the general conditions and the neurological status at the moment of operation. Selection must also consider the angiographic findings and exclude the risk of cerebral ischemia during clamping. The patient's general condition only rarely represents a contraindication to such operations since, due to their brevity, they are generally well tolerated without problems of anesthesia.

The results of surgical treatment of 224 patients with ischemic cerebrovascular disease are reported. The mean age of these patients was 58 years (47–74) but many operations were carried out on patients older than 70 years. The age, con-sidered from the biological viewpoint, does not represent a strict contraindication

Serono Symposium No. 37, "Vascular Occlusion: Epidemiological, Pathophysiological and Therapeutic Aspects", edited by M. Tesi and J. Dormandy, 1981. Academic Press, London and New York.

to this form of surgery. The same is true for ischemic heart disease. Arterial hypertension and disorders of glucose and lipid metabolism are risk factors in the evolution of the disease, so instead of being contraindications, they may indicate the need for operation.

Another very important risk factor that can be shown by angiography is the extent of the lesion. A long course of the internal carotid artery can make it difficult or impossible to perform endarterectomy. Lesions of vessels arising from the aortic arch or from the circle of Willis can also impair the circulatory compensation during carotid clamping, especially when an occlusion of the anterior communicating vessels is found. Nevertheless, the above-mentioned factors do not change the surgical indications because it is possible to measure the adequacy of the collateral circulation during the operation and therefore to know when brain protection can be assured.

The selection of patients on the basis of their neurological status is based on the evaluation of the early and late effects of surgical therapy (Table I). The ideal patients for carotid artery surgery are those suffering from one or more transient ischemic attacks with complete regression and in whom the angiography shows a carotid artery stenosis on the appropriate side. In these patients surgery is preferred both to avoid transient ischemia and to prevent cerebral infarction: it is possible to get positive results in 80% of these patients. Similarly, good results can be obtained in patients with stabilized neurological deficits and transient ischemia. In these cases, the purpose of the operation is not to cure the neurological deficit but to prevent further ischemic attacks and improve the cerebral perfusion. A good result may be obtained in 65% of these cases. Surgery is thus effective in patients suffering from transient ischemic attacks because it eliminates the source of emboli and the causes of the hemodynamic disturbances. At the same time, the evolution of the stenosis towards complete obstruction of the artery may be avoided.

These considerations encouraged us to extend the surgical indication to patients with asymptomatic carotid lesions or to those affected by chronic low cerebral perfusion: in both these groups of patients, a good result seems to be obtained. The evaluation of surgical therapy in a group of 48 patients followed up for 5 to 10 years after the operation shows that the patients benefited from surgery for many years (Table II). In our experience, the mortality rate during a 1 to 10 year-period is 8% and can be attributed to cerebral ictus in a third of the cases while

Table I. Early results of carotid surgery for CVD (30 days) in 103 consecutive patients seen between 1972 and 1979.

Clinical manifestation	Patients	Improved	Unchanged	Worsened	Death
Asymptomatic	8	–	8 (100%)	–	–
TIA	50	40 (80%)	7 (14%)	2 (4%)	1 (2%)
Completed stroke + TIA	34	22 (65%)	10 (29%)	1 (3%)	1 (3%)
Chronic low perfusion	11	6 (55%)	5 (45%)	–	–
Total	103	68 (66%)	30 (29%)	3 (3%)	2 (2%)

Table II. Late results of carotid surgery for CVD in 48 patients (follow-up 5–10 years).

Clinical manifestation	Patient	Improvement	No change	Worsening	Death
Asymptomatic	2	—	2 (100%)	—	—
TIA	35	28 (81%)	2 (5%)	2 (5%)	3 (9%)
Completed Stroke + TIA	10	7 (70%)	—	—	3 (30%)
Chronic low perfusion	I	I	—	—	
Total	48	36 (75%)	4 (8%)	2 (4%)	6 (13%)

other diseases, such as heart disease or cancer, may be the cause of death in some other patients (Fiorani *et al.*, 1978).

By contrast with past practices, emergency surgical treatment is not indicated in patients with an acute stroke. The results of surgery in these patients are poor, as demonstrated by our results and by those in the literature (Fields, 1979). In our 15 patients, only two patients operated on within 6 h after onset of stroke improved, while three became worse and four died. Thus at the moment, emergency operation can be advised only in selected cases of progressive stroke with mild neurological deficit and without coma, especially if occlusion of the carotid artery has followed endarterectomy or angiography, in patients with known carotid artery stenosis in whom the cervical bruit has disappeared.

At the moment, emergency carotid surgery has more of a prophylactic value in preventing occlusion of the artery and irreversible cerebral lesions. In fact, the natural evolution of an arterial stenosis towards occlusion and its possible effects on the cerebral circulation oblige us to consider a severe stenosis accompanied by TIA especially dangerous if these transient attacks are repeated frequently ("crescendo" TIA). During the last year we operated upon seven such patients and in all the cases the results were good.

The last point to be considered is the surgical risk, namely the possible occurrence of cerebral ischemia during carotid clamping. We do not agree with the routine use of the internal shunt because we think that its application may be a source of complications itself as has been suggested in the more recent literature (Prioleau *et al.*, 1976). Its use must be limited to a very low percentage of cases. The intra-operative monitoring of the cerebral circulation by the use of the intra-arterial 133-Xe technique (Pistolese *et al.*, 1971) allows the identification of patients in whom the internal shunt or other techniques of cerebral protection are the only way of ensuring sufficient brain perfusion during carotid clamping.

The cerebral hemodynamics during carotid surgery of our last 100 consecutive patients showed that in 75% of them (Fig. 1a), the cerebral blood flow during clamping was above the critical level (20–23 ml/100 g/min) (Boysen *et al.*, 1974). In these cases, the operation may be confidently performed, even with prolonged carotid clamping occlusion times, providing that systemic mean arterial blood pressure and pCO_2 are constant. In 25 patients (Fig. 1b), carotid clamping decreased the CBF below the critical level: in these cases, when endarterectomy was impossible in a very short time (a few minutes), the internal shunt was used. In 13 cases,

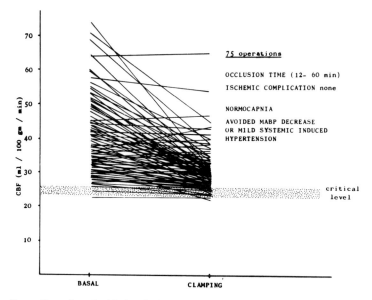

Fig. 1a. Prevention of cerebral ischemia during carotid surgery (100 cases).

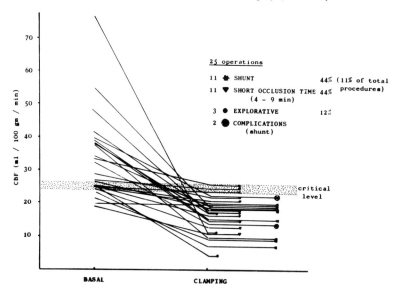

Fig. 1b.

the operation was performed with the application of an internal shunt, but a complication occurred twice.

With our policy, the ischemic complications related to carotid clamping may be reduced. Before 1969, we performed 95 operations and the internal shunt was used in about 30% of cases with a complication rate of 10%. During the last years, the internal shunt was used in 9% of cases and the ischemic complications were correspondingly reduced to 3%. In the last 25 endarterectomies, the internal shunt was never used.

REFERENCES

Boysen, G., Engell, H. C., Pistolese, G. R., Fiorani, P., Agnoli, A. and Lassen, N. (1974). *Circulation* **49**.

Fields, W. S. (1979). *World Journal of Surgery* **3**, 147–154.

Fiorani, P., Pistolese, G. R., Faraglia, V. and Spartera, C. (1978). *Eur. Neurol.* **17** (Suppl. 1), 68–72.

Pistolese, G. R., Citone, G., Faraglia, V., Benedetti-Valentini, F., Pastore, E., Semprebene, L., De Leo, G., Speran, A. V. and Fiorani, P. (1971). *Neurology* **21**, 95–100.

Prioleau, W. H., Aiken, A. F. and Hairston, P. (1976). *Ann. Surg.* 678–683.

West, H., Burton, R., Roon, A. J., Malone, J. M., Godstone, J. and Moore, W. S. (1979). *Stroke* **10**, 117–121.

INDICATIONS AND RESULTS OF SURGICAL TREATMENT IN PATIENTS WITH BILATERAL CAROTID LESIONS

G. R. Pistolese, V. Faraglia, M. Ventura, C. Spartera, C. Fieschi[1],
C. Iadecola[1] and G. Martino

Department of Vascular Surgery, University of Rome, School of Medicine, Italy
[1] *First Clinic for Mental and Nervous Disease, University of Rome, School of Medicine, Italy*

Two main findings may be gleaned from the literature on the results of surgical treatment of patients with bilateral carotid artery lesions: (a) the long-term results were decidedly better in surgically treated patients than in patients treated by medical therapy; (b) the surgical patients showed a high surgical mortality in the early stages.

The data of the Joint Cooperative Study on Ischemic Cerebrovascular Diseases (Fields *et al.*, 1970) show that, surgically treated patients, both with bilateral stenosis and with stenosis and contralateral occlusion, are free of symptoms in higher percentages. But the same data also show that in these patients there is an unacceptably high surgical mortality: in fact 22% of the patients died within a month of surgery and this percentage rises to 28% if the follow-up is extended to 2 months, neurological complications are included (Fields and Lemak, 1976). However, these data are not especially valid in patients with contralateral occlusion because in some patients, the artery operated on was an occluded internal carotid (66%) and, more importantly, because some of these patients were operated on during the acute phase of the neurological deficit. It is now well known that in such circumstances the operation may be followed by cerebral hemorrhage secondary to revascularization of the ischemic brain. In spite of these considerations, the risk of brain ischemia during carotid clamping is noticeable and some surgeons believe that the extensive use of the internal shunt may obviate this

Serono Symposium No. 37, "Vascular Occlusion: Epidemiological, Pathophysiological and Therapeutic Aspects", edited by M. Tesi and J. Dormandy, 1981. Academic Press, London and New York.

problem (Thompson and Talkington, 1976; Javid *et al.*, 1979). This is not the opinion of many surgeons who point out the complications of shunt application (Prioleau *et al.*, 1976).

The aim of this paper is to evaluate the results of the surgical treatment of 45 patients with bilateral carotid artery occlusive lesions, operated on for cerebrovascular insufficiency. None of these patients was operated on in the acute stage of the disease and in patients with contralateral carotid artery occlusion, endarterectomy was performed on the stenotic artery. In the other patients, we first operated on the side of the stenosis appropriate to the symptoms, or the more severe stenosis. Only in a few patients was the selection of the side performed on the pre-operative evaluation of carotid clamping tolerance, on the basis of the angiographic findings, the EEG studies and Doppler examination.

The clinical picture of these patients was TIA in 29 cases (64%), completed stroke and TIA in 22% of the cases, and chronic low cerebral perfusion syndrome in 14% of the cases. No patient was asymptomatic and when the unilateral lesion group of patients was compared to the bilateral lesions group, a higher percentage of the chronic low perfusion syndrome and of the multiple associated diseases were observed in the latter group: 55.5% *vs* 33.8% of the cases. The angiographic findings show that 32 patients exhibited a bilateral carotid artery stenosis and 13 patients had a stenosis and a contralateral carotid artery occlusion. The degree of the stenosis was evaluated on the basis of the combined analysis of the percentage of the lumen reduction judged on the arteriography or at the operation, and after Doppler examination.

In all the patients, the cerebral blood flow during surgery was measured by the intra-arterial 133-Xenon technique (Pistolese *et al.*, 1971) and the results obtained in patients with bilateral lesions were compared to those obtained in patients with unilateral lesions (Fig. 1). In 16 patients (20% of the cases) with unilateral carotid artery stenosis, the CBF during clamping dropped below the level which is considered to be critical (Boysen *et al.*, 1975): the same percentage occurred in the

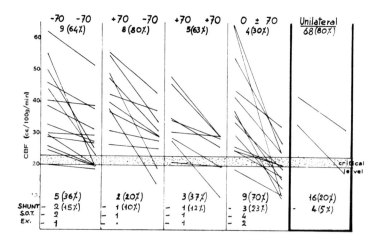

Fig. I. Effect of carotid clamping on CBF in 45 patients.

bilateral group of patients with one carotid artery stenosis greater than 70% of the lumen. The relatively small number with this CBF pattern during clamping may be explained by the existence of the adequate collateral brain supply via the contralateral, although stenotic, carotid artery and vertebro-basilar arteries.

The percentage of the patients in whom the CBF during clamping dropped below the critical level is higher in patients with bilateral stenosis of less than 70% than those with bilateral severe stenosis. Finally, the CBF dropped below the critical level in the great majority of patients with carotid artery stenosis and contralateral occlusion (70% of the cases). In patients with bilateral, though not severe, carotid artery stenosis, the clamping of one of the carotid arteries may suddenly precipitate a crisis with a borderline hemodynamic cerebral supply. The patients with bilateral severe stenosis or with contralateral carotid occlusion, despite a collateral cerebral circulation, do not tolerate carotid clamping. All the patients with CBF during clamping above the critical level were operated on under normocapnia avoiding any decrease of the systemic arterial blood pressure or under mild induced systemic hypertension.

Table I.   Early results of carotid surgery (1–30 days) in 45 patients.

| | | | COMPLICATIONS | | | |
| | | | Intraoper. | | Post-op. | |
	Improv.	Unchang.	Worsen.	Dead	Worsen.	Dead
TIA	22 (76%)	5 (17%)	–	–	2 (7%)	–
Completed St. + TIA	5 (50%)	3 (30%)	1 (10%)	–	–	1 (10%)
Chronic low per s.	3 (50%)	3 (50%)	–	–	–	–
Total	30 (67%)	11 (24%)	1 (2%)	–	2 (5%)	1 (2%)

Table II.   Late results of carotid surgery (3–5 years) in 19 patients.

	Improv.	Unchang.	Worsen.	Dead
TIA Compl. St. + TIA	9 (50%)	3 (17%)	2 (11%)	4 (22%)
Chronic low p.s.	–	1	–	–
Total	9 (48%)	4 (21%)	2 (10%)	4 (21%)

Causes of death		
Stroke 2	Heart disease 1	Cancer 1

The internal shunt was used in 11 patients with lower CBF values during carotid clamping. The internal shunt was necessary in 15% of the patients with bilateral carotid artery lesions while it was used only in 5% of the patients with unilateral carotid artery stenosis. Among the patients with bilateral lesions, those with contralateral carotid occlusion needed the internal shunt in almost a quarter of the cases. In some patients, however, the anatomical position of the carotid plaque allowed us to perform an endarterectomy with a short occlusion time. When the CBF was very low and the application of the internal shunt would be too dangerous, especially in patients with contralateral carotid occlusion, the operation was not performed. In a few patients, an extra-intracranial anastomosis was considered useful in order to increase the total cerebral blood flow before performing endarterectomy.

The early and the long-term results of surgical treatment of these patients are reported in Tables I and II. A good result may be achieved in 91% of such patients, with a complication rate of 9% and a surgical mortality of 2%. However, one ischemic intra-operative complication and three post-operative complications occurred. One patient died because of a myocardial infarction and two became worse: one because of internal carotid artery thrombosis and one because of a contralateral neurological deficit due to systemic hypotension. The long-term results show that the good results at follow-up are quite similar to those obtained in patients with unilateral carotid artery lesions, while the mortality was related to causes other than stroke in many patients.

In conclusion, patients with bilateral carotid artery lesions are higher risk patients. However, the intra-operative CBF studies allow us to ascertain that:

    a.   the poor-risk patients are those with stenosis and contralateral carotid artery occlusion;

    b.   the internal shunt may be selectively but not extensively used;

    c.   it is possible to decrease the operative complications related to cerebral ischemia.

Finally, the long-term results are similar to those obtained in patients with the unilateral carotid artery lesion and in some instances an extra-intracranial anastomosis has been proposed as a "first step" in surgical management of patients with contralateral occlusion.

REFERENCES

Boysen, G., Engell, H. C., Pistolese, G. R., Fiorani, P., Agnoli, A. and Lassen, N. (1974). *Circulation* **49**

Fields, W. S., Maslenikov, V., Meyer, J. S., Hass, W. K., Remington, R. D. and MacDonald, M. (1970). *JAMA* **12**, 1993

Fields, W. S. and Lemak, N. A. (1976). *JAMA* **25**, 2734

Javid, H., Julian, O. C., Dye, W. S., Hunter, J. A., Najafi, H., Goldin, M., Serry, C. and DeLaria, G. A. (1979). *Wld J. Surg.* **3**, 167

Pistolese, G. R., Citone, G., Faraglia, V., Benedetti–Valentini, F., Pastore, E., Semprebene, L., De Leo, G., Speranza, V. and Fiorani, P. (1971). *Neurology* **21**, 95

Prioleau, W. H., Aiken, A. F. and Hairston, P. (1976). *Ann. Surg.* **678**

Thompson, J. E. and Talkington, C. M. (1976). *Ann. Surg.* **184**, 1–15

EPIDEMIOLOGICAL STUDY OF VARICOSE VEINS IN A
WORKING POPULATION OF 512 INDIVIDUALS

J. A. Jiménez Cossio, E. Viver Manresa and A. Rodríguez Mori

Ciudad Sanitaria "La Paz", Madrid, Spain

In certain areas of the world, venous diseases constitute a serious problem resulting in enormous sanitary, social and economic consequences. To date there are few varicose vein epidemiological studies described in the world literature. As well as a bibliographic review, we can consider this as the first study achieved with the help of Spanish industry.

If varicose veins are present in at least 10% of the adult European population, and considering the fact that the Spanish population over 15 years of age in 1975 amounted to 24 581 000 inhabitants, about two and a half million varicose vein patients can be estimated for Spain. This figure amply justifies a more thorough investigation of the problem and an epidemiological study.

The present study was accomplished in Barcelona, during the summer of 1975, on a sampling of employees from a pharmaceutical industry. The sample includes 512 individuals, of which 280 were female and 232 male. The ages ranged from 16 to 75 years (Fig. 1).

METHOD

The criteria we have adopted for the varicose vein classification are similar to those used by Widmer *et al.* (1967) and Rougemont (1973). The three major groups subject to investigation were trunk varicosity of the internal and/or external saphenous veins, reticular varicose veins and hyphenwebs. Considering the entire venous pathology obtained, three diagnostic grades were established. Hyphenwebs and reticular varicose veins represent grade I, severe reticular varicose

Serono Symposium No. 37, "Vascular Occlusion: Epidemiological, Pathophysiological and Therapeutic Aspects", edited by M. Tesi and J. Dormandy, 1981. Academic Press, London and New York.

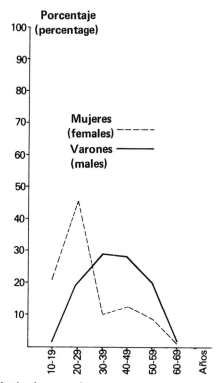

Fig. 1. Sample distribution by sex and age groups.

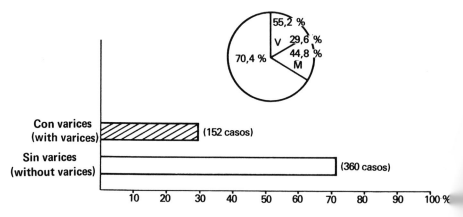

Fig. 2. Varicose vein prevalence in the entire sample.

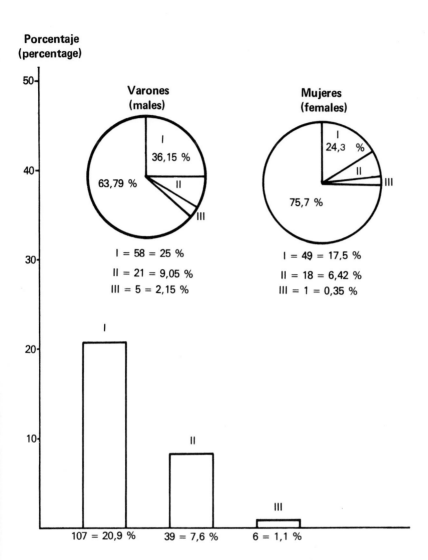

Porcentaje (percentage)

Varones (males)

I = 58 = 25 %
II = 21 = 9,05 %
III = 5 = 2,15 %

Mujeres (females)

I = 49 = 17,5 %
II = 18 = 6,42 %
III = 1 = 0,35 %

107 = 20,9 %   39 = 7,6 %   6 = 1,1 %

Fig. 3. Grade distribution of varicose veins, considering both sexes, and in relation to the whole sample.

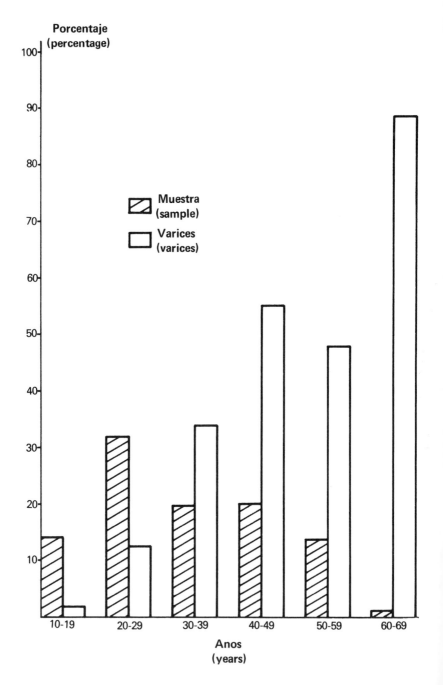

Fig. 4. Varicose vein percentage in each age group, in relation to the entire sample.

Table I. Relationship between symptoms and the existence of varicous veins.

	Right lower limb		Left lower limb	
	F	M	F	M
Presence of varicose veins without symptoms	17.5	22.41	19.28	25.86
Symptoms in the absence of varicose veins	20.36	12.06	20.35	9.91
Varicose veins and symptoms	32.14	13.91	30	20.68

Table II. Osteoarticular abnormalities and their relationship with varicous veins.

Osteoarticular abnormality	Female		Male			
	Number	%	Number	%	With V.	Without V.
Callousness	74	26.4	27	11.6	25.9	74.1
Hallux valgus	44	15.7	12	5.1	50	50
Limitation of hip rotation	3	1.07	1	0.4	50	50
Flat feet	30	10.7	27	11.6	29.9	70.1
Transverse feet	47	16.7	30	12.9	15.5	84.5

veins correspond to grade II and trunk varicosities belong to grade III.

Investigations performed: All individuals were measured, weighed and venous pressure measurements were determined. Physical examination of the venous system was aimed at detecting the presence and location of any kind of lower limb varicose dilatation, as well as oedema, hyperpigmentation, ulcers or chronic venous incompetence. Trendelenburg tests were performed on trunk varicose veins. Osteo-articular abnormalities such as callouses, hallux valgus, flat feet and hip motility were investigated.

Risk factors investigated were: age, sex, marital status, birthplace, way of life, tobacco, obesity, height, number of pregnancies, contraceptive pills, hypertension and lower limb osteoarticular abnormalities.

Data analysis and evaluations: the information from the patient's symptomatic history and physical examination were transcribed to specially conceived forms and subsequently processed by an IBM 370/165 computer with a central unit memory of 128 K and a disc "on-line" memory of 210 MB. It was finally submitted to a complete tabulation.

RESULTS

From the entire population examined, formed by 512 individuals, a diagnosis of varicose veins was established in 152 cases (29.6%) (Fig. 2). Figure 3 indicates the grade distribution of varicose veins in relation to the complete sample, considering both sexes. The greatest frequency of varicose veins belonged to grades I and II in both sexes (20.9% and 7.6% respectively), while grade III constituted only 1.1% of the whole. A slight predominance of left-sided varicose veins (130) compared to the right side (124) was observed. The percentage of varicose veins in each age group in relation to the whole sample is indicated in Fig. 4. Table I represents the relationship between the presence or absence of symptoms and the existence or non-existence of varicose veins, considering both sexes and both lower limbs. The prevalence of osteoarticular abnormalities and their relation to varicose veins is seen in Table II.

The association between investigated risk factors and varicose veins was as follows:

    a.   Birthplace: individuals born in the Catalan region compared to other Spanish regions (female $r = 0.004$, $p = 5.804$; male $r = -0.016$, $p = 19.974$).

    b.   Marital status: married, single or widowhood (female $r = 0.199$, $p = 99.921$; male $r = 0.221$, $p = 99.933$).

    c.   Tobacco (female $r = -0.125$, $p = 96.38$; male $r = -0.113$, $p = 91.64$).

    d.   Contraceptive pills. $r = -0.185$, $p = 99.80$.

    e.   Height (female $r = -0.08$, $p = 82.13$; male $r = 0.088$, $p = 82.101$).

    f.   Weight (female $r = 0.096$, $p = 89.216$; male $r = -0.053$, $p = 58.671$).

    g.   Number of pregnancies. $r = 0.227$, $p = 99.95$.

    h.   Previous history of varicose veins. (female $r = 0.269$, $p = 100$; male $r = 0.06$, $p = 64.74$).

    i.   Hypertension. (female $r = 0.268$, $p = 99.99$; male $r = -0.03$, $p = 35.25$).

DISCUSSION

The prevalence of all grades of varicose veins obtained was 29.6%, which is, significantly, similar to the figures of the four principal varicose vein investigations achieved in European industry (Widmer (1969), Pirnat (1967) Rougemont (1973) and Jimenez Cossío (1978)). This figure amounts to a working population of 8325 individuals, of which 2486 presented varicose veins, corresponding to 29.7%.

The prevalence of varicose veins in men (55.2%) compared to women (44.8%) (1.2:1) is the result of the lack of homogeneity in the female population sample, with a significant peak in the first two decades. The prevalence of varicose veins does not differ in either sex ($\chi^2 = 4.17$; $P < 0.025$) if both sexes are limited theoretically to those above 30 years of age. Considering the population as a whole, the growing prevalence of varicose veins with age is clearly evident, specially in those individuals over 30 years of age ($r = 0.417$, $p = 100\%$). Significantly, the presence of varicose vein symptoms is not always related to the existence of varicosities. When the relationship between the presence or absence of symptoms and the existence or non-existence of varicose veins in both sexes was studied, a greater percentage of symptoms without varicose veins was manifest in the female population. Interestingly, a considerable percentage of osteoarticular abnormalities has been found in the studied population, although a statistical correlation with varicose veins could not be proven.

In the future we will be able to obtain a better and more profound knowledge of the aetiology and possible risk factors that influence varicose diseases by means of new epidemiological studies in which other possible risk factors are considered (nutrition, genetic factors, collagen study, climate etc), and with the incorporation of new non-invasive diagnostic methods.

BIBLIOGRAPHY

Borschberg, E. (1967). "The Prevalence of Varicose Veins in the Lower Extremities." S. Karger Basel, New York.

Cleave, T. L. (1965). *Am. J. Proctol.* **16**, 35.

Cleave, T. L. (1959). *Lancet* **22**, 172.

Da Silva, A., Widmer, L. K., Martin, H., Mall, Th., Glaus, L. and Schneider, M. (1974). *VASA* **2**, 118.

Drury, M. (1965). *Br. med. J.* **2**, 304.

Jiménez Cossio, J. A. (1978). "Epidemiologia y Tratamiento de las Venopatias." Monografia Sandoz, Barcelona.

Jiménez Cossio, J. A., Viver Manresa, E., Rodríguez Mori, A y Oliver, S. (1977). *Medicina Clinica* **8**, 415.

Jiménez Cossio J. A. (1975). *Angiologia* **2**, 97.

Martorell, A. (1974). *'Acta de las reuniones cientificas Instituto Policlinico* **XXVIII**, 41.

Pinto Ribeiro, A. (1977). *Rev. bras. Clin. Terap.* **6**, 117.

Pirnat, L. (1967). *Phlebologie* **2**, 265.

Rougemont, A. (1973). Tesis Doctoral, Lausana.

Widmer, L. K., Plechl, S., Leu, H. J. and Boner. (1967). *Schweiz. med. Wschr.* **97**, 107.

Widmer, L. K., Leu, H. J. and Breil, H. (1967). *Pheboligie* **2**, 257.

Widmer, L. K. (1969). *Therapeutische Umschau* **26**, 185.

PROPHYLAXIS OF DEEP VEIN THROMBOSIS AND PULMONARY EMBOLISM : COMPARISON OF HEPARIN (3 × 5000), HEPARIN (2 × 5000) + DIHYDERGOT AND VENOUS FLOW STIMULATOR — VALUE OF DOPPLER IN SYSTEMATIC DVT DETECTION

G. Moser[1], A. Donath[2] and B. Krahenbühl[3]

[1] *Digestive Surgery Unit,* [2] *Nuclear Division,* [3] *Angiology Unit, Hôpital Cantonal, 1211 Geneva, Switzerland*

INTRODUCTION

Subcutaneous low-dose heparin has been shown to be effective in the prevention of deep vein thrombosis (DVT) following abdominal surgery (Kakkar *et al.* 1969 and 1971; Williams, 1971). However, increased pre-operative bleeding and post-operative hematoma formation have discouraged its widespread use, except in high-risk patients. To avoid these troublesome side-effects it is possible to combine reduced doses of heparin with dihydroergotamine mesylate (DHE) (Hor *et al.*, 1976; Stamatakis *et al.*, 1977), or to use mechanical prophylaxis alone (Hills *et al.*, 1972; Roberts and Cotton, 1974; Sabri *et al.*, 1971) for DVT prevention.

METHOD

In this prospective study carried out over one year, consecutive patients (over 40 years old), admitted for elective abdominal surgery were randomized into three groups and received one of the following prophylactic treatments:

a. *Heparin alone (group 1)*: subcutaneous heparin (5000 U) was given three times a day for six days after operation. The first dose was given 2 h before surgery.

Serono Symposium No. 37, "Vascular Occlusion: Epidemiological, Pathophysiological and Therapeutic Aspects", edited by M. Tesi and J. Dormandy, 1981. Academic Press, London and New York.

b. *Reduced heparin and venoconstricting agent (group 2)*: subcutaneous heparin (5000 U) twice a day was combined with subcutaneous dihydroergotamine mesylate (0.5 mg) for six days. Again, the first dose was given 2 h before operation.

c. *Mechanical prophylaxis (group 3)*: all patients in this group received an instruction leaflet describing exercises (foot flexion, extension and rotation) to be performed for 3 min every half hour during the bedridden period. Intermittent compression boots (Flowtron) were used during the entire operation and for one hour every day for six days after surgery.

Systematic DVT detection was carried out in each patient using both the ^{125}I fibrinogen test and the Doppler technique.

1. ^{125}I fibrinogen tests were performed immediately after surgery (fibrinogen injection 2 h before operation) and repeated every day up to the 7th post-operative day (Kakkar *et al.*, 1970).

2. Doppler detection, by measuring the "venous stop-flow pressure" (VSFP) (Simon and Krahenbühl, 1977) was carried out in each patient. The patient is asked to exhale into a water manometer at increasing pressures. While the lower limb is monitored with a Doppler probe, the minimal thoracic pressure able to disrupt the venous flow constitutes the venous stop-flow pressure which is elevated distal to a DVT (Simon and Krahenbühl, 1977).

Independent examiners, one for fibrinogen scanning and one for the VSFP Doppler test, communicated their findings directly to the trial director. When a DVT was suspected by either method, a phlebogram was performed and standard therapy instigated if positive.

Routine pre-operative work-up in each patient included a chest X-ray and ECG as well as pulmonary ventilation — perfusion scan for pulmonary embolism detection. This scan was repeated on the eighth post-operative day.

RESULTS

There were 289 patients admitted in the trial, of which 62 were excluded for the reasons summarized in Table I. Of the 227 patients completing the study, 75 received heparin alone, 76 received reduced heparin and dihydergot and 76 were submitted to physiotherapy and Flowtron.

Sex, age, weight, predisposing factors and type of operation were comparable in the three groups (Tables II and III).

Seven asymptomatic DVTs were detected and confirmed in group 1, seven in group 2 and five in group 3, giving an incidence of 9.3% ± 3.4 in the first group; 9.2% ± 3.3 in group 2 and 6.6% ± 2.8 in the third. Clinical signs developed later in a total of 4 patients, one in group 1, one in group 2 and two in group 3 (see Table IV).

Of the 19 patients with asymptomatic DVT, 18 had a positive fibrinogen test and four a positive Doppler test. False positives were twice as frequent with the Doppler (six) than with fibrinogen scanning (three); false negatives were also more frequent with the Doppler (fifteen) than with fibrinogen test (one).

The specificity (i.e. the percentage of subjects with a normal test among subjects who did not have a DVT) was 99% for ^{125}I fibrinogen test and 97% for

Table I.   Excluded patients.

Pre-operative pulmonary scan missing	15
Non-functioning ratemeter	14
Delayed surgery	10
Iodine allergy	10
Immediate post-operative death (with no DVT or pulmonary embolism at autopsy)	5
Missing control phlebogram	3
Defective compression boots	2
Transfer to intensive care unit	2
Error in prophylactic treatment	1
Total	62

Table II.   Comparability of groups.

	Group 1	Group 2	Group 3
Number of patients	75	76	76
Female/male	43 / 32	36 / 40	39 / 37
Mean age (years)	58 3/12	59 7/12	59 2/12
Mean weight (kg)	65.1	65.5	61.5
Risk Factors :			
* Previous history of			
superficial phlebitis	2	4	3
DVT	3	3	2
pulmonary embolism	4	1	1
*obesity	11	10	11
cardiac failure	0	1	1
cancer	9	13	10
lower limb varices	25	21	22

VSFP measured with a Doppler method. The sensitivity (i.e. the percentage of patients with a positive test among patients who did have a DVT) was 95% for ^{125}I fibrinogen test and only 21% for VSFP measured by a Doppler method.

Pulmonary ventilation-perfusion scans were positive in one patient in group 1, and three patients in both groups 2 and 3. Of these, one patient in each group presented with clinical signs of pulmonary embolism. Phlebography showed DVT signs in all cases of positive ventilation-perfusion scans except in one case in the last group. This patient presented with atrial fibrillation and having been digitalized, the abnormal pulmonary scan probably represented an endocardial thrombus migration.

Table III.   Type of operations.

	Group 1	Group 2	Group 3
Appendicectomy	2	1	0
Annexectomy	1	0	0
Inguinal hernia	13	14	13
Incisional hernia	2	0	3
Gastro-enteroanastomosis	0	1	1
Gastrectomy (± splenectomy)	5	6	7
HS vagotomy	1	2	0
Cholecystectomy	31	30	37
Bile duct exploration	8	5	8
Biliary diversion (Longmire)	0	0	2
Pancreatectomy	0	3	0
Splenectomy	0	0	1
Colostomy	1	2	1
Colostomy closure	2	2	1
Partial colectomy	5	4	1
Hemicolectomy	2	1	1
Laparotomy	2	5	0
	75	76	76

Table IV.   Incidence of asymptomatic and symptomatic DVT.

	Group 1	Group 2	Group 3	Total
Patients	75	76	76	227
Asymptomatic DVT	6	6	3	15
Symptomatic DVT	1	1	2	4
Total DVT	7	7	5	19
Percent	9.3 ± 3.4	9.2 ± 3.3	6.6 ± 2.8	8.4
Female / male	4/3	2/5	4/1	10/9
Mean age (years)	66 5/12	67 1/12	65 2/12	
Mean weight (kg)	71.1	71.1	67.4	

DISCUSSION

The side-effects of standard heparin DVT prophylaxis have revived interest in other prophylactic measures, in particular those acting against the venostatic component of thrombogenesis (Sagar, 1974; Sagar *et al.*, 1976).

It has been shown that intravenously, dihydroergotamine mesylate (0.5 mg) significantly reduces venous capacitance with negligible effects on arterial resistance (Lange and Echt, 1972; Mellanders and Nordenfelt, 1970), increasing lower limb venous return by 200% (Butterman *et al.*, 1975). In our study, we have combined this agent with reduced doses of subcutaneous heparin without loss of the latter's prophylactic effect, confirming previous studies (Koppenhagen *et al.*, 1977).

Recent reports have demonstrated the value of intermittent compression boots (Coe *et al.*, 1978; Cotton, 1976), showing that even when used on one leg only, the method provided good DVT protection. For maximal protection and avoidance of rebound effects, these boots should be used during surgery and daily in the post-operative period (Coe *et al.*, 1978).

In order to evaluate our results, security belts for proportion have been used according to Clopper and Pearson (1936). The difference between the three groups is not significant. Indeed, in order to demonstrate such a difference between groups 1 and 2 with the same DVT percentage, one would need over 250 000 patients; the risk of having a type II error is thus minimized (Freiman *et al.*, 1978). In order to confirm the hypothesis that Flowtron gives superior prophylaxis, a sample size of a minimum of 522 patients would be needed in each group. For obvious reasons it has not been possible to undertake a study with so many patients.

Our results therefore show that both DHE associated with heparin and mechanical prophylaxis alone are as effective in DVT prevention as the standard heparin regimen. In view of the reduction of heparin-induced complications, intermittent compression boots should be used in most patients, while drug venoconstriction could be combined with reduced heparin doses in those for whom boots are impracticable, in particular orthopedic patients.

It has been reputed that these boots were cumbersome during surgery and that certain patients complained of discomfort related to their use (Saggar *et al.*, 1976). None of the surgeons operating on the patients in the mechanical group complained of their presence and the only patient problem was that of excessive calf sweating, easily reduced by the use of a non-compressive stocking.

The incidence of pulmonary embolism was not statistically different in the three groups. In order to demonstrate a statistical difference with a similar incidence in each group using the binomial distribution, 947 patients would be needed in each group. Therefore, a type II error could be avoided. In our series, there were no deaths due to pulmonary embolism, and at autopsy no DVT or pulmonary embolism were found in the early post-operative deaths. Radioactive fibrinogen scanning confirmed its value in DVT detection.

Several studies (Bollinger *et al.*, 1968; Simon and Krahenbühl, 1977) have reported the value of the Doppler method in detecting femoral and iliac DVT. In the post-operative situation, when DVT is asymptomatic, the sensitivity of the Doppler techniques is very low. We hoped that VSFP would selectively detect DVT threatening to embolize, but out results do not confirm this hope.

ACKNOWLEDGEMENTS

We thank Dr J. R. Scherrer (statistical reviewer and director of the information unit), Professor C. A. Bouvier (director of Haemostasis Unit) and Dr N. Reverdin for their help.

REFERENCES

Bollinger, A., Mahler, F. and de Sepibus, G. (1968). *Dtsch Med. Wschr.* **93**, 2197.

Butterman, G., Theisinger, W., Oechster, H. and Hor, G. (1975). *Dtsch Med. Wschr.* **100**, 2065-2069.

Clark, W. B., Prescolt, R. S., MacGregor, A. B. and Ruckley, C. V. (1974). *Lancet* **2**, 5-7.

Clopper, C. J. and Pearson, E. S. (1936). *Biometrika* **26**, 404-413.

Coe, N. P., Collins, R. E. and Klein, L. (1978). *Surgery* **2**, 230-234.

Cotton, L. T. (1976). *Br. Med. J.* **2**, 1193.

Freiman, J. A., Chalmers, C. and Smith, H. Jr. (1978). *NEJMAG* **249**, 690.

Hills, N. H., Pflug, J. J. and Jeyasingh, K. (1972). *Br. Med. J.* **1**, 131-135.

Hor, G., Buttermann, G., Theisinger, W. M. and Pabst, W. (1976). *Eur. S. Nucl. Med.* **1**, 197-203.

International Multicenter Trial (1975). *Lancet* **2**, 44-51.

Interpreting clinical trials (1978). *Br. Med. J.* 1318.

Kakkar, V. V., Howe, C. T., Flanc, C. and Clarke, M. B. (1969). *Lancet* **2**, 230.

Kakkar, V. V., Nicolaides, A. N., Field, E. S. and Flute, P. T. (1971). *Lancet* **2**, 669-671.

Kakkar, V. V., Nicolaides, A. N., Renney, J. T. G., Friend, J. R. and Clarke, M. B. (1970). *Lancet* **1**, 540.

Koppenhagen, K., Wiechmann, A. and Frey, E. (1977). *Dtsch. Med. Wschr.* **102**, 1374-1378.

Lange, L. and Echt, M. (1972). *Pharmaka. Fortschr. Med.* **90**, 1161-1164.

Mellanders, S. and Nordenfelt, I. (1970). *Clinical Science* **39**, 183-201.

Roberts, V. C. and Cotton, L. T. (1974). *Br. Med. J.* **1**, 358-362.

Sabri, S., Roberts, V. C. and Cotton, L. T. (1971). *Br. Med. J.* **4**, 394.

Sagar, S. (1974). *Br. Med. J.* **2**, 153-154.

Sagar, S., Nairn, D. and Stamatakis, J. D. (1976). *Lancet* **1**, 1151-1154.

Simon, A. C. and Krahenbühl, B. (1977). *Lancet* **1**, 1008-1009.

Stamatakis, J. D., Sagar, S., Lawrence, D. and Kakkar, V. V. (1977). *Br. J. Surg.* **64**, 294.

Williams, H. T. (1971). *Lancet* **2**, 950-952.

PREVENTION OF POST-OPERATIVE DEEP VEIN THROMBOSIS BY SIMULTANEOUS APPLICATION OF AN ANTIPLATELET DRUG AND HEPARIN

H. Vinazzer

Blood Coagulation Laboratory, General Hospital, Linz, Austria

Thromboembolic complications after surgical procedures still represent a certain problem. Though various schemes of prophylaxis are in use, further lowering of the remaining percentage of thromboembolic events without undue increase of side-effects would be desirable. For this reason, an attempt was made to further diminish thrombus formation by simultaneous inhibition of platelet function and of activated plasma clotting factors. For this purpose, a combination of low dose heparin (LDH) and acetylsalicylic acid (ASA) was used.

Prior to a study on surgical patients, the action on the clotting mechanism of this combination was tested in 20 healthy individuals (Loew and Vinazzer, 1974). When the separate and the combined effects of 1500 mg ASA per day and 5000 IU heparin (s.c., b.i.d.) were examined, a very moderate influence of heparin on coagulation and the well-known alterations of platelet functions by ASA were found. Both effects were independent from each other and there was no interaction between the two drugs. The influence of simultaneous application of both drugs on the clotting mechanism was mild enough to permit administration of this combination even prior to surgery.

These tests were followed by a pilot study on 177 surgical cases (Loew *et al.*, 1977). Patients over 40 years of age who had to undergo elective thoracic or abdominal surgery with the exception of appendectomies were included in the study.

Three groups of prophylaxis were formed while a placebo group was not included. The following prophylaxis was given: Group 1: 1500 mg ASA per day and a placebo instead of heparin; Group 2: 5000 IU heparin s.c. b.i.d. and a

Serono Symposium No. 37, "Vascular Occlusion: Epidemiological, Pathophysiological and Therapeutic Aspects", edited by M. Tesi and J. Dormandy, 1981. Academic Press, London and New York.

placebo for ASA; Group 3: 1500 mg ASA per day and 5000 IU heparin s.c., b.i.d. ASA was given intravenously for 3 days and from the 4th day onward by oral administration. Prophylaxis was started on the evening prior to surgery and was maintained for a minimum of 7 days. The trial was double blind. Diagnosis of thrombosis was made by the ^{125}I-fibrinogen method.

The groups were comparable by age, sex, risk factors and type of surgery. The overall incidence of thrombosis was significantly lower in the combined prophylaxis group than in the two other groups. It was of special interest that thrombosis of the thigh could not be detected in the combined prophylaxis group. No significant difference was found between the two other groups.

Though by this study a favourable effect of the combined prophylaxis on the frequency of thrombosis was clearly demonstrated, the number of patients was too low to evaluate possible side-effects and complications. For this reason, an identical study on a considerably larger scale was carried out. Three groups compared to the ones in the pilot study were formed out of a total of 1210 patients. The only difference to the pilot study was the diagnostic approach to thrombosis. Since monitoring with ^{125}I-fibrinogen was technically impossible on this large number of patients, thrombosis was diagnosed by ultrasonic Doppler flow detector. The fact that only thrombosis above the knee could be detected by this method was a necessary compromise.

Since thrombosis of the thigh is more likely to develop serious complications than thrombosis restricted to the calf, the diagnostic disadvantage was not considered to be too great. Moreover, the principal aim of this study was the evaluation of side-effects and complications; the incidence of thromboembolic events was merely additional information.

When statistical analysis was carried out after completion of the study, the following results were obtained. The groups were comparable by age, sex, weight, height as well as by pre- and early post-operative ambulation and by the duration of the hospital stay. They were also comparable by the types of surgery, and there was no significant difference in the incidence of known risk factors.

Out of 1210 cases admitted to the study, 1093 could be completed (Table I). Dropouts were significantly higher in the combined prophylaxis group than in the two other groups. When the reasons for dropouts were compared, there was no significant difference between groups in cases of gastric distress, of allergy,

Table I. Patients admitted, patients completed, and reasons for dropouts.

Group	ASA	LDH	ASA + LDH	p1:3	p2:3
Admitted	404	404	402	0.97	0.97
Completed	365	378	350	0.81	0.14
Dropouts	39	26	52	0.11	0.01
Reasons for Dropouts					
Gastric distress	15	14	15	1.00	0.81
Allergy	2	2	2	1.00	1.00
Haemorrhage	3	3	11	0.01	0.01
Death	17	7	17	1.00	0.12
Discharge	2	0	7	0.14	0.07

Table II. Occurrence of thromboembolic events.

Group	ASA	LDH	ASA + LDH
Completed	365 = 90%	378 = 94%	350 = 87%
DVT (thigh)	14 = 3.9%	9 = 2.4%	1 = 0.3%
PE survived	0	2 = 0.6%	0
PE lethal	1 = 0.3%	1 = 0.3%	0
Combined	15 = 4.1%	12 = 3.2%	1 = 0.3%

P

n.s.   < 0.001

< 0.001

Table III. Causes of death (results of autopsies).

Group	ASA	LDH	ASA + LDH	p1:3	p2:3
Pulmonary embolism	1[a]	1[a]	0	0.52	0.52
Cardiovascular	6	4	8	0.29	0.17
Malignancy	7	3	7	1.00	0.14
Uraemia	1	0	1	1.00	0.52
Peritonitis	1	0	0	0.52	1.00
Pancreatitis	1	0	0	0.52	1.00
Pneumonia	1	0	1	1.00	0.52

[a]Included into the study.

Table IV. Dropouts caused by haemorrhages.

Group	ASA	LDH	ASA + LDH	p1:3	p2:3
Wound haematoma	2	1	7	0.16	0.09
Skin haematoma	0	2	3	0.22	0.41
Haematemesis	1	0	1	1.00	0.52
Combined	3	3	11	0.01	0.01

of preliminary discharge and of death. The number of patients discontinued for haemorrhage was, however, significantly higher in the combined prophylaxis group.

There was no significant difference in the incidence of thrombosis between the ASA and LDH groups. A highly-significant diminution of thrombosis was found in the combined prophylaxis group (Table II) however.

When death occurred during the observation period, autopsies were carried out in all cases (Table III). There was one fatal pulmonary embolism in the ASA group and another one in the LDH group. These two cases were included in the

Table V. Minor side effects and minor bleeding episodes.

Group	ASA	LDH	ASA + LDH	p1:3	p2:3
Gastric distress	55	47	54	0.84	0.53
Impaired healing	47	43	51	0.66	0.47
Minor bleeding					
total frequency	41	30	89	0.001	0.001
Wound haematoma	15	12	33	0.01	0.01
Skin haematoma	22	18	51	0.001	0.001
Epistaxis	1	0	1	1.00	0.52
Gingival bleeding	3	0	3	1.00	0.27
Haematuria	0	0	1	0.52	0.52

study. In all other cases, neither thromboembolism nor bleeding were found and there was no significant difference in the underlying diseases which caused the death of these patients.

When the dropouts for haemorrhagic complications were analysed, wound haematomas were more frequent in the combined prophylaxis group, while other haemorrhagic complications were evenly distributed over the three groups (Table IV). The only two serious haemorrhages which required blood transfusions were two gastric bleedings: one in the ASA group and another one in the combined group. The latter had to be reoperated and arterial bleeding after gastrectomy was found to be the cause of the haemorrhage. All other haemorrhages were not serious, and prophylaxis was discontinued for reasons of safety rather than for blood loss.

When minor side-effects were analysed, small haematomas around sites of injections and minor wound haematomas were significantly more frequent in the combined prophylaxis group (Table V).

As a result of this study, combined prophylaxis with ASA and LDH in the indicated dosage and duration was found to be highly effective to keep post-operative thromboembolism under control. Comparable results were obtained in a pilot study and in a study on a large scale though the diagnostic approach to thrombosis was different. The rate of serious complications and side-effects attributable to prophylaxis was very low. There was a significantly higher occurrence of minor signs of haemorrhagic diathesis in the combined prophylaxis group.

Though the problem of haemorrhage was not serious when the figures obtained were compared to the total number of patients it is realized that the prize for a considerable reduction of thromboembolism was a minor incidence of increased bleeding. Combined prophylaxis in this form was considered to be at the interphase between an optimal thrombosis prophylaxis and an unfavourable effect on the bleeding tendency.

The primary aim of this study was to show that adequate forms of combined prophylaxis can further reduce the incidence of post-operative thromboembolic events. Studies with different combinations of drugs, which are presently in progress, will hopefully further reduce side effects but give equally favourable results with respect to the diminution of post-operative thromboembolism.

REFERENCES

Loew, D. and Vinazzer, H. (1974). *Haemostasis* **3**, 319.
Loew, D., Brücke, P., Simma, W., Vinazzer, H., Dienstl, E. and Boehme, K. (1977). *Thrombosis Research* **11**, 81.

HEPARIN-INDUCED ANTITHROMBIN DECREASE WITH HEPARINIZATION DURING VASCULAR SURGERY

G. Lorenzi, A. Sarcina, L. Gabrielli, G. B. Agus, G. Vercellio,
E. Margstakler and E. Rossi[1]

Institute of Vascular Surgery, University of Milan, Italy
[1] *Blood Transfusion Service, Istituti Clinici di Perfezionamento, Milan, Italy*

INTRODUCTION

Intra-arterial regional heparinization is normally performed during vascular surgery in order to avoid intraluminal thrombosis when arteries are clamped. This surgery is in fact often complicated by thrombosis. The occurrence of an intra- or post-operative hemorrhagic syndrome which is similar to a consumptive coagulopathy is also common.

Recent papers have demonstrated that in the presence of thrombin, heparin reduces antithrombin binding capacity, enhancing the possibility of thrombosis (Marciniak and Gockerman, 1977).

For these reasons we have decided to investigate heparinemia and natural plasma inhibitors in a group of patients who underwent vascular surgery with intra-arterial heparinization.

PATIENTS AND METHODS

Seventeen patients (14 males), aged 35–73 years, with atherosclerotic lesions of the aorto-femoral axis, were submitted to reconstructive vascular surgery (aorto-bi-femoral bypass, aorto-femoral thromboendarterectomy).

During surgery, sodium heparin was administered by intra-arterial infusion

Serono Symposium No. 37, "Vascular Occlusion: Epidemiological, Pathophysiological and Therapeutic Aspects", edited by M. Tesi and J. Dormandy, 1981. Academic Press, London and New York.

G. Lorenzi et al.

(1000-5000 IU). Six patients were also infused with 5 u of fresh frozen plasma.

Blood samples were drawn before surgery, during surgery but before heparin infusion and 15 min, 1, 2, 4 h after heparin infusion.

The following tests were made:

1. antithrombin III—immunochemical assay (Laurell, 1966);
2. antithrombin III—heparin cofactor activity—amidolytic assay with chromogenic substrates (S-2238);
3. anti-Xa activity—amidolytic assay with chromogenic substrates (S-2222);
4. heparin in plasma—amidolytic assay with chromogenic substrates (S-2222).

In a previous step of the study, anti-Xa activity was evaluated by means of a method (Austen, 1975) which depends on circulating heparin.

RESULTS

Figure 1 shows the sequential average values: it is clear that there is a significant correlation between heparinemia, anti-Xa activity and antithrombin III. Coinciding with the heparin level increase, there is a decrease of anti-Xa and antithrombin III, tested by methods not sensitive to circulating heparin.

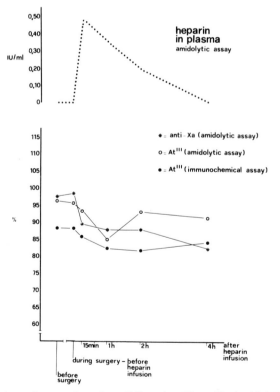

Fig. 1. Comparison of average heparin, anti-Xa and antithrombin (amidolytic and immunochemical assays) levels.

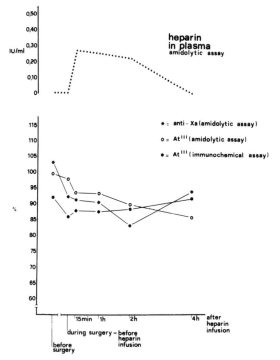

Fig. 2. Comparison of average heparin, anti-XA and antithrombin (amidolytic and immuno-chemical assays) levels.

The decrease of antithrombin III is already present before heparin infusion, but a rapid decrease is evident immediately after heparin administration.

Plasma inhibitor levels in patients treated with intra-operative frozen plasma infusion (Fig. 2), did not show any significant difference in comparison to other patients' levels.

Anti-Xa and antithrombin III, however, decrease more slowly when not treated with plasma. This fact suggests that larger doses of plasma may be of value in preventing inhibitor consumption.

DISCUSSION

According to our results, patients submitted to vascular operations present a decrease of anti-Xa and antithrombin III activity. This decrease is markedly enhanced by intra-arterial infusion of heparin.

Administration of 5 u of frozen fresh plasma during surgery does not seem to be enough to prevent the consumption of plasma inhibitors of coagulation.

In our opinion anti-Xa and antithrombin III levels should be tested in vascular surgical patients in order to prevent thrombosis and hemorrhagic complications more accurately by utilizing tests not sensitive to heparin.

In fact, when a defibrinated plasma method was used for testing anti-Xa in a group of our patients, anti-Xa activity increased in close relationship to the

G. Lorenzi et al.

heparin levels. That occurred because of the pronounced sensitivity of the method to circulating heparin.

REFERENCES

Marciniak, E. and Gockerman, J. P. (1977). *Lancet* 2, 581.
Margstakler, E., Rossi, E., Mondonico, P., Gabrielli, L., Lorenzi, G. and Sarcina, A. (1979). *Thrombosis and Haemostasis* 42, 458.

ANATOMICAL AND CLINICAL CORRELATIONS IN 341 AUTOPSIED CASES OF PULMONARY THROMBOEMBOLISM

R. Collazzo, P. A. Charmet Pietropolli, L. Di Filippo and N. Delendi

*Department of Pathology, Department of Cardiology,
S. Maria degli Angeli Hospital, Pordenone, Italy*

In the past, pulmonary embolism (PE) was considered one of the most important causes of death among in-patients (Dalen and Dexter, 1969; Marion and Binet, 1974; Havig, 1977; Mordeglia *et al.*, 1977; Delgado *et al.*, 1978; Sion and Lopez-Maiano, 1978).

The incidence of PE based on clinical material is underestimated (Coon *et al.*, 1966; Dalen and Dexter, 1969; Havig, 1977; Mordeglia *et al.*, 1977; Ruberti *et al.*, 1978; Sion and Lopez-Maiano, 1978). This is due to the lack of specificity of clinical findings and to the presence of symptoms of one or more associated pathologic conditions.

The incidence of PE is rising (Havig, 1977; Ruberti *et al.*, 1978; Sion and Lopez-Maiano, 1978), probably due to the prolongation of life of the elderly and seriously ill and bedridden patients.

RESULTS

The clinical records and the files of the pathology department of a 1200-bed general hospital were reviewed retrospectively for diagnosis of PE.

PE was identified in 341 of 3574 consecutive autopsies performed between 1975 and 1978 (9.6%). Of these, 331 cases were hospital deaths. They were taken from 3302 autopsies (97.4% of the 3390 were hospital deaths). In the hospital deaths, the incidence of PE was 9.8%. Males were 150 (7.6%) and females were 181 (12.9%); the M/F ratio was 1:1.7. The age range was 10 months to 98 years.

Serono Symposium No. 37, "Vascular Occlusion: Epidemiological, Pathophysiological and Therapeutic Aspects", edited by M. Tesi and J. Dormandy, 1981. Academic Press, London and New York.

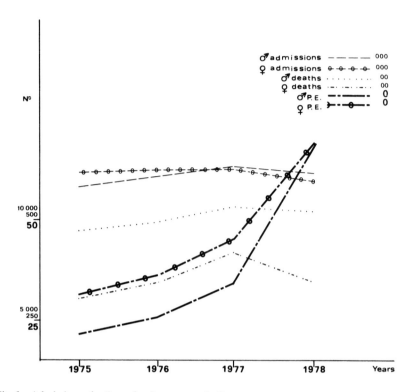

Fig. 1. Admissions, deaths and pulmonary embolism, per sex, per year.

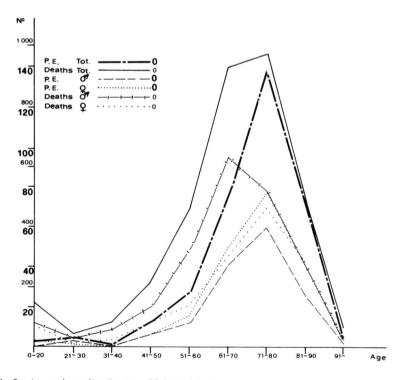

Fig. 2. Age and sex distribution of P.E. and deaths.

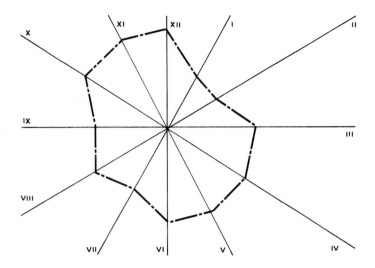

Fig. 3. Distribution of the cases of pulmonary embolism per month.

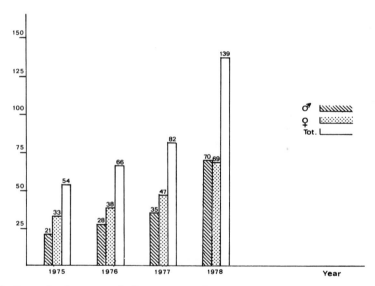

Fig. 4. Cases of pulmonary embolism, per sex and year.

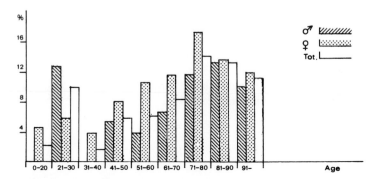

Fig. 5. Incidence of P.E. on the deaths, per age and sex.

The mean age was 71.4 years (68.7 in males, 74.1 in females). The rate of PE was markedly increased in patients more than 70 years old (Figs 2 and 5). The number of PE cases increased progressively from 1975 to 1978 in both sexes (Fig. 4). There was also a rise of the incidence of PE compared with the total number of hospital deaths and admissions (Fig. 1). In most cases (99.1%) PE was, *per se*, lethal (90.6%) or significantly contributed to death (8.5%). It was usually located in both lungs (67.7%). Monolateral PE (31.4%) was more prevalent in the right lung (22.9%). Only few cases of infarcts without PE were found (0.9%) and infarcts were found only in 16.7% of the cases (61.4% monolateral). Phlebothrombosis was associated with PE in 54.5% of the cases, especially in the ileo-femoral veins (92.7%).

No difference was found in the incidence of PE between deaths in medical *vs* surgical departments (9.7% and 9.9%) with the same distribution in both sexes. There was no meaningful association of PE with different seasons (Fig. 3). In the ABO blood groups, group O seems to be the most affected with a ratio O/A 1.6 (in the general Italian population: 1.1). PE does not seem to be correlated with obesity, whereas cachexia was present in 150 cases. Duration of bed rest, particularly more than 14 days, was significantly associated with PE (79.7%). Cerebrovascular and post-operative conditions were the most frequent acute underlying diseases. Pancreatic neoplasm accounts for 9.5% of malignancies in the PE group with malignancies. In the general population, this neoplasm had an incidence of 1.3%. The most common clinical symptoms were dyspnea, tachycardia and cyanosis. Significant was the incidence of fever (39.1%). Of the deaths, 69.3% occurred within 1 h of the onset of symptoms. Chest X-ray was normal in 53.6% of 237 cases before the onset of PE and diagnostic only in 52.8% of the 36 cases in which it was performed during acute PE. The ECG before PE was altered in 227 of 282 patients. The most frequent findings were atrial fibrillo-flutter and left ventricular hypertrophy. ECG performed during acute PE was diagnostic in 72.7% of 77 cases.

CONCLUSIONS

In our cases, the incidence of PE appears to be clearly increasing in hospital patients and deaths. The most affected patients were female, in accordance with Pequignot *et al.* (1978). The most affected age group were patients over 70 years where PE was almost always lethal. Infarcts were rare, possibly because severe PE was present in our cases with short survival time from the onset of symptoms. Thrombosis usually affected the ileo-femoral veins in accordance with Mavor (1967).

No meaningful correlation was found with the different seasons or medical *vs* surgical departments. Bed rest and possibly blood group O and pancreatic cancer are to be considered as risk factors for PE. The main symptoms of PE were dyspnea, tachycardia, cyanosis and fever (UPET, 1973). X-ray and ECG findings were important but not diagnostic.

In our cases, clinical diagnosis was positive only in 18.4% of 331 hospital cases. PE did not figure in the 12 chief clinical causes of death, while at autopsy it turned out to be the first and most important cause of death among our hospital patients.

REFERENCES

Coon, W. W. (1976). *Surgery, Gynecology & Obstetrics* **143**, 385.

Dalen, J. E. and Dexter, L. (1969). *Journal of American Medical Association* **207**, 1505.

Delgado, I. F., Cruz, S. O. and Herrera, E. L. (1978). *Archivos del Instituto de Cardiologia de Mexico* **48**, 871.

Havig, O. (1977). *Acta chirurgica Scandinavica* Suppl. 478, 1–120.

Marion, P. and Binet, J. P. (1974). *In* "Monographies de l'Association Française de Chirurgie, 76° Congrès de Chirurgie" 1–150. Masson & Cie, eds.

Mavor, G. E. and Galloway, J. M. (1967). *Lancet* **1**, 871.

Mordeglia, F., Gandulla, L., Bertorello, M., O'Flaherty, E. and Gil, M. (1977). *Medicina (Buenos Aires)* **37**, Suppl. 2, 112.

Pequignot, H., Morin, Y., Comet, M. and Lafore-Richard, M. (1978). *Semaine des Hopitaux de Paris* **54**, 381.

Ruberti, V., Odeno, A., Giordanengo, F. and Miani, S. (1978). *Minerva Medica* **69**, 1785.

Sion, A. and Lopez-Maiano, V. (1978). *Respiration* **35**, 181

EPIDEMIOLOGICAL STUDY OF PERIPHERAL ARTERIAL DISEASES BY MEANS OF THE COMPUTER*

G. C. Bracale[1], P. Gauthier[1], R. Federico[1], P. Del Rosso[1], M. Bracale[2],
P. Albertini[2] and G. Gullo[2]

[1] *Cattedra di Chirurgia Vascolare, Clinica Chirurgica, II Facoltà de Medicina e Chirurgia, via Pansini n.5, 80131 Napoli, Italy*
[2] *Cattedra di Applicazioni di Elettronica, Istituto Elettrotecnico, Facoltà di Ingegneria, via Claudio n.21, 80125 Napoli, Italy*

INTRODUCTION

Over the past two decades, computers have been increasingly a focus for research on the clinical decision-making process. Over the next two decades computers undoubtedly will play an important role in all fields of medicine.

At present, the communication of medical information is often a critical element in the practice of high-quality medical care. Traditional recording practices rely almost completely on a manual record folder where physician notes are handwritten or dictated and merged with laboratory data. This system has the inherent problems of incomplete data and occasional unavailability of the medical record resulting from different physicians recording data at different places and at different times. Even when the medical record is available, poor organization and frequent illegibility may make retrieving the desired information a laborious and time-consuming task. It is usually necessary to record much redundant data in order to provide the necessary information for patient care, scheduling, billing and management reports. Quality of care studies and clinical investigation research which depend on the aggregation of data from a large number of individual patient records are particularly cumbersome and require the expenditure of many hours of manual searching.

*This work was supported by National Council of Research, Rome.

Serono Symposium No. 37, "Vascular Occlusion: Epidemiological, Pathophysiological and Therapeutic Aspects", edited by M. Tesi and J. Dormandy, 1981. Academic Press, London and New York.

Therefore automation of medical record keeping and the development of a computer-based patient databank are two of the most important fields of the application of computers in medicine.

Databank analysis systems have valuable capabilities to offer the individual clinical decision-maker. Furthermore, medical computing research recognizes the potential value of large databanks in supporting many of the other decision-making processes. There are several important additional issues regarding databank systems:

1. Data acquisition remains a major problem. Many systems have avoided direct physician-computer interaction but have then been faced with the expense and errors of transcription. For these reasons, it is important to implement direct contact between the physician and medical personnel.

2. Analysis of data in the system can be complicated by missing values that frequently occur, outstanding values and poor reproducibility of data with time and between physicians.

Conversely, the system can itself be used to identify questionable values of tests or observations. Normally the patient-clinician dialogue employs two types of data. The first is data expressed by the patient or the clinician. The second is data directly obtained from the patient by the clinician.

The distinction is valuable, since data which are expressed pass through a complex series of intellectual and emotional "filters" and are thereby subject to distortion. Therefore, it is extremely important to avoid all the causes of distortion.

Particularly, data obtained directly from the patient by the clinician do not pass through the patient's intellectual and emotional filters, although they do pass through the clinician's. Directly obtained data include some aspects of the physical examination, and those diagnostic laboratory tests not requiring the co-operation of the patient for their measured values.

3. The decision aids provided tend to emphasize patient management rather than diagnosis.

From all the above mentioned criteria, an interdisciplinary group of medical doctors and bioengineers defined a computer-based medical information system for a vascular surgery department (Gestione Cartella Clinica Vascolare: GE.CA. CLI.V.).

Despite the general objectives previously mentioned, the main goal in design has been to collect the data from patients of the vascular Surgery Department of the Surgery Clinic at the 2nd Faculty of Medicine of Naples University, for implementing statistical analysis to help manage the follow-up of all vascular patients. In the following part, the main characteristics of GE.CA.CLI.V. are summarized.

DATA MANAGEMENT CHARACTERISTICS OF GE.CA.CLI.V.

The GE.CA.CLI.V. is divided into the following five sections.

1. The patient's collected identification information, personal and family medical histories.

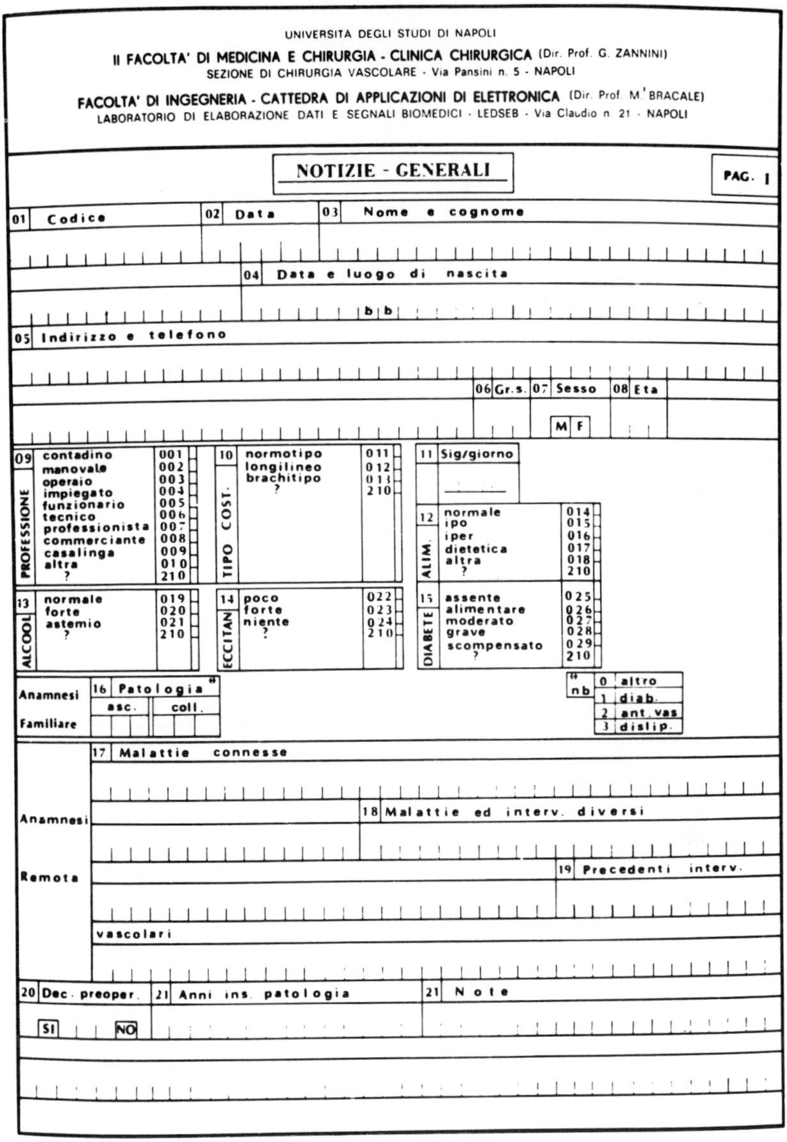
UNIVERSITA DEGLI STUDI DI NAPOLI

II FACOLTA' DI MEDICINA E CHIRURGIA - CLINICA CHIRURGICA (Dir. Prof. G. ZANNINI)

SEZIONE DI CHIRURGIA VASCOLARE - Via Pansini n. 5 - NAPOLI

FACOLTA' DI INGEGNERIA - CATTEDRA DI APPLICAZIONI DI ELETTRONICA (Dir. Prof. M. BRACALE)

LABORATORIO DI ELABORAZIONE DATI E SEGNALI BIOMEDICI - LEDSEB - Via Claudio n. 21 - NAPOLI

NOTIZIE - GENERALI PAG. 1

01 Codice | 02 Data | 03 Nome e cognome

04 Data e luogo di nascita b b

05 Indirizzo e telefono

06 Gr. s. | 07 Sesso M F | 08 Eta

09 PROFESSIONE: contadino 001, manovale 002, operaio 003, impiegato 004, funzionario 005, tecnico 006, professionista 007, commerciante 008, casalinga 009, altra 010, ? 210

10 TIPO COST.: normotipo 011, longilineo 012, brachitipo 013, ? 210

11 Sig/giorno

12 ALIM.: normale 014, ipo 015, iper 016, dietetica 017, altra 018, ? 210

13 ALCOOL: normale 019, forte 020, astemio 021, ? 210

14 ECCITAN: poco 022, forte 023, niente 024, ? 210

15 DIABETE: assente 025, alimentare 026, moderato 027, grave 028, scompensato 029, ? 210

Anamnesi Familiare: 16 Patologia # asc. coll.

nb: 0 altro, 1 diab., 2 ant. vas, 3 dislip.

Anamnesi Remota: 17 Malattie connesse; 18 Malattie ed interv. diversi; 19 Precedenti interv. vascolari

20 Dec. preoper. SI NO | 21 Anni ins. patologia | 21 Note

Fig. 1. Page one of medical record.

2. Data obtained directly from the patient by the clinician. All this information is particularly oriented to vascular areas. Some of this direct data include aspects of the physical examination.
3. Data directly obtained by diagnostic laboratories.
4. Technical information about previous and recent surgical operations.
5. The results of these operations in the short-and long-term. For collecting all

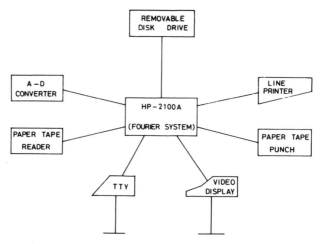

Fig. 2. Layout of a computer system.

Table I. Diagram of statistical incidence.

Table IA. Alcohol Consumption.

normal	✱✱	317	76.39%
high	✱✱✱✱✱✱	42	10.12%
abstain	✱✱✱✱✱✱✱✱	56	13.49%

Total patients	415
Total patients not classified	27
Total patients	442
Scale: ✱ = 6.34	

Table IB. Cigarettes a day.

0-10	✱✱✱✱✱✱✱✱✱✱✱✱✱✱✱✱✱✱✱✱✱✱✱✱✱✱✱	71	20.52%
10-20	✱✱✱	135	39.01%
20-30	✱✱✱✱✱✱✱✱✱✱✱✱✱✱✱✱✱✱✱✱✱✱✱✱✱✱	67	19.36%
30-40	✱✱✱✱✱✱✱✱✱✱✱✱✱✱✱✱✱✱✱	51	14.74%
40-50	✱✱✱✱	10	2.89%
50-60	✱✱✱✱✱	12	3.46%

Total patients	346
Total patients not classified	113
Total patients	459
Scale: ✱ = 2.50	

Table IC. Age.

Range	Bar	Count	Percent
0–10	—	1	0.23%
10–20	*	3	0.68%
20–30	****	10	2.27%
30–40	*****	14	3.17%
40–50	*************************	67	15.19%
50–60	**	124	28.12%
60–70	**	145	32.88%
70–80	*************************	69	15.65%
80–90	***	8	1.81%

Total patients	441	
Total patients not classified	12	
Total patients	453	

Scale: *= 2.60

Table ID. Years since onset of disease.

Years	Bar	Count	Percent
1	**********************************	72	17.95%
1	**	82	20.45%
2	*****************************	62	15.46%
3	********************	43	10.72%
4	************	27	6.73%
5	******************	19	4.74%
6	*****	11	2.74%
7	****	9	2.24%
8	*******	14	3.49%
9	*	2	0.50%
10	*************	26	6.48%
11	*	1	0.25%
12	***	7	1.74%
13	*	2	0.50%
14	*	1	0.25%
15	****	9	2.24%
16	*	1	0.25%
17	=	0	0.00%
18	*	1	0.25%
19	=	0	0.00%
20	****	8	1.99%
20	**	4	1.00%

Total patients	401	
Total patients not classified	20	
Total patients	421	

Scale   * = 2.00

Table IE. Subjective symptoms.

Paresthesia **************	56	11.89%
Slight claudication**************	50	10.62%
Moderate claudication********************************	114	24.20%
Severe claudication******************	70	14.86%
Pain at rest**175		37.15%
None **	6	1.27%
Total patients	471	
Total patients not classified	15	
Total patients	486	
Scale: * = 3.50		

Table IF. Profession.

Farmer**************************	50	13.48%
Construction worker****************	31	8.36%
Civil Servant**	96	25.88%
Technician***	89	23.99%
Professional******	4	1.08%
Merchant*********	6	1.62%
Domestic*******************	13	3.50%
Labourer***	52	14.02%
Clerk ***********************************	18	4.85%
Other ******	12	3.23%
Total patients	371	
Total patients not classified	71	
Total patients	442	
Scale * = 1.92		

this information, a medical record document has been prepared which can be filled in by non-specialized personnel. An example of the first page of this document is shown in Fig. 1. Each patient is identified by a code which permits storage in the information system.

The data are memorized and computed through a Hewlett-Packard 2100 supported by different input-output devices as reported in Fig. 2.

At present, the following procedures are available:

a. data entry in a conventional way through an alphanumeric visual display unit;

b. data entry through a photoreader or a teletyping system;

c. print-out of the complete medical document or of a part of it;

d. erasing of previous records;

e. correction of previous records;

f.   statistical information for internal and external uses (at the hospital, in the town, in the region, etc.);

g.   print-out of histograms with percentage of incidence.

In Table I A–F some examples of these histograms are given.

CONCLUSIONS AND RECOMMENDATIONS

It would be naive to believe that any computer-based information system is completely general-purpose or will completely meet the needs of every similar medical department.

In addition, there is always a cost and efficiency trade off between a system that is specially designed for a well-defined set of needs and a system designed to have sufficient flexibility to support a broad range of functions and provide a great variety of local options.

The dominant objective in the GE.CA.CLI.V. is to provide a system general enough to meet the information processing needs of other similar departments without requiring excessive programming modifications at each local site.

We believe that there is a widespread need for an information system that supports both administrative and medical needs in vascular departments, not only for research and the follow-up of the patients, but mainly for obtaining statistical information.

We also believe that an information system which meets these needs could be strongly supported by regional government. In addition, we hope that the basic design strategy we have chosen (also for further implementation) provides the system capability that can evolve to meet the diverse requirements for national co-operation.

SECTION II
PATHOPHYSIOLOGY

BLOOD COAGULATION AND FIBRINOLYSIS AS REGULATORS IN DISEASES OF ARTERIES AND VEINS

T. Astrup

Gaubius Institute, Leiden, The Netherlands and the University Centre of South Jutland, Esbjerg, Denmark

Damage to the vessel wall brings cellular components in contact with the humoral system of the circulating blood. This initiates processes of haemostasis, wound healing and tissue repair. Platelets aggregate at the site of injury and release compounds initiating activation of the intrinsic blood coagulation system. The damaged cells possess thromboplastic activity and activate the extrinsic coagulation system. Ultimately, both reactions lead to the formation of thrombin, which converts the circulating fibrinogen to fibrin, which in turn solidifies the haemostatic plug already formed by the aggregating platelets. Inhibitory agents, in particular antithrombin-III, regulate the formation of fibrin by binding to thrombin or to intermediary active compounds.

The fibrin deposit then provides the fabric on which fibroblasts and other participating cells migrate and proliferate. At this stage it is necessary to distinguish between two different lines of development. In physiological repair, where there is little tissue destruction and little or no inflammatory reaction, few leucocytes migrate to the area of injury, and those attracted to the area will disappear again leaving the fibrin deposit mostly untouched. The resolution of the fibrin deposit is, in this case, brought about by activation of the humoral fibrinolytic system. If there is an inflammatory reaction, which may be caused by a microbial infection or by necrotic material released from the damaged cells, large numbers of leucocytes will be attracted to the area, and enzymes released from these will contribute to the resolution of the fibrin. Ultimately, the return to a normal situation depends upon a complete resolution of the fibrin deposit.

Serono Symposium No. 37, "Vascular Occlusion: Epidemiological, Pathophysiological and Therapeutic Aspects", edited by M. Tesi and J. Dormandy, 1981. Academic Press, London and New York.

In the process of wound healing, the migration and proliferation of fibroblasts and the growth of capillaries first form a granulation tissue with high fibrinolytic activity (Kwaan and Astrup, 1964). Subsequently, during tissue repair, the blood vessels regress and fibrous tissue devoid of fibrinolytic activity is formed.

Obviously, this sequence of repair can be interrupted and changed at many stages. A delayed haemostasis leads to increased extravasation and deposition of fibrin, resulting in the formation of excessive amounts of fibrous tissue. An example, typical of this situation, is seen in the crippling of injured joints in haemophilic patients previously discussed (Astrup and Brakman, 1975). The specific location is due to the absence in the joint tissues of tissue thromboplastin. This prevents a rapid formation of thrombin by activation of the extrinsic coagulation system, so that clot formation depends solely on the intrinsic system which is deficient in haemophilia. In addition, the fibrinolytic activity is low in the tissues of the joint, so that resolution of the fibrin deposits is delayed, resulting in excessive formation of granulation tissue rich in fibrinolytically-active vessels. These are easily disrupted by the physical trauma caused by the movements of the joints, thus giving rise to new episodes of bleeding with a formation of new deposits of fibrin, in this way continuing the pathological process. To break the continuation of this sequence, the surgical removal of the pathologically changed synovial membrane has been introduced and good results have been reported (Storti and Ascari, 1975). Increased fibrinolysis can be treated with inhibitory agents, such as EACA, but this is a weak inhibitor, which probably has a relatively low effect on local fibrinolysis caused by cell bound activators. This explains the variable results reported on the effect of EACA in haemophilia, where the major defect is the impaired clot formation.

In contrast to the joint, the brain is rich in thromboplastin. Haemostasis in injuries to such tissues is therefore rapid. It was previously reported that intracranial haemorrhage is rare in haemophilia (Aggeler and Lucia, 1944), well in agreement with the high content of tissue thromboplastin. However, newer surveys have reported on several instances of cerebral or spinal cord haemorrhage in the haemophilic patient (van Trotsenburg, 1975; Eyster et al., 1978). The extremely high fibrinolytic activity of the meninges provides an explanation for the occurrence of such bleedings, in particular because the meninges are poor in thromboplastic activity. Whenever a lesion occurs in the highly-vascularized sheets of the brain or spinal cord, this occurs in an area low in thromboplastic activity and high in fibrinolytic activity (Moltke, 1958; Glas and Astrup, 1970; Tovi, 1973a). Only when the injury spreads to the brain tissue proper is the potent effect of the tissue thromboplastin brought into the picture. An increase in the frequency of haemorrhage in normal and haemophilic people should therefore occur only following mild damage in which only the meninges, but not the brain tissue as such is effected. The situation then resembles that in the joint, except that the synovial membrane is low in fibrinolytic activity while the activity of the meninges is high. This also explains why adequate primary haemostasis after surgical intervention to the brain is often followed, after a period of time, by secondary haemorrhage. This is most probably caused by the resolution of the fibrin deposits due to high fibrinolytic activity of the meninges, and it may be reduced by the administration of inhibitors (Tovi et al., 1972; Tovi, 1973b; Sengupta et al., 1976; Filizolo et al., 1978).

The high fibrinolytic activity of the vessels of the meninges is seen particularly well in sections of the spinal cord (Smokovitis and Astrup, 1978). The pia mater has considerably higher fibrinolytic activity than the dura mater, but the granulation tissue developed from the dura and forming an outer membrane around a subdural haematoma contains highly fibrinolytic vessels, which may cause continued bleeding into the haematoma (Ito *et al.*, 1976). There are several examples of the physiological development and involution of vascularized connective tissue with high fibrinolytic activity, such as during the formation of the capsule of the lens (Pandolfi, 1967a) or following closure of the ductus arteriosus (Glas-Greenwalt *et al.*, 1972). The high fibrinolytic activity of the meninges of the brain, which may be increased further when granulation tissue is formed during a process of tissue repair, explains why the administration of urokinase to patients with cerebral infarction with the intention of resolving the thrombus and restoring blood circulation to the affected areas has led to disappointing results with haemorrhagic complications (Hanaway *et al.*, 1976).

Since Todd's histochemical studies (Todd, 1959) is it known that vascular fibrinolytic activity is caused by a plasminogen activator in the endothelial cells. The activity is most pronounced in the adventitia and in the endothelium of veins. The arterial endothelium of man is mostly inactive, but there are exceptions. Thus, the endothelium of the central retinal artery is frequently highly fibrinolytic (Pandolfi, 1967b). Also marked fibrinolytic activity of the endothelium of the large arteries has been reported in a case of aspergillosis (Pelczar *et al.*, 1972) or in cases of sudden death, vasogenic shock or cirrhosis of the liver (Noordhoek Hegt, 1976). In part, this might be due to a loss of an inhibitor of fibrinolysis present in the smooth muscle cells of the normal media (Noordhoek Hegt, 1977). Increased fibrinolytic activity is seen in the adventitia behind arteriosclerotic lesions as an indication of a repair process in response to vascular injury (Astrup and Coccheri, 1962). A possible role of the presence of an inhibitor in the repair of vascular injuries is suggested by the susceptibility of cattle to "high mountain disease" and the presence of large amounts of an inhibitor of fibrinolysis in their lungs, resulting in a delayed resolution of the fibrin and a prolongation of the repair process (Astrup *et al.*, 1968).

The deposition of fibrin in the lungs is influenced by the thromboplastic activity and fibrinolytic activity in the tissues of the lung. Different animal species vary in this respect, explaining differences in their response to injuries (Astrup *et al.*, 1970). All the blood circulating in the organism passes through the lungs, which serve as a filter for particles, including strands of fibrin formed in the vascular system. Accumulation of these particles of fibrin leads to the microembolism syndrome (Saldeen, 1976), which may develop into the general syndrome of disseminated intravascular coagulation (DIC), especially if inhibitors of fibrinolysis are present in the blood, ultimately continuing into a consumption coagulopathy (Lasch *et al.*, 1967).

Susceptibility to thrombosis may also result from a deficiency in the blood of inhibitors of the coagulation system, such as antithrombin-III. The administration of heparin is a common mode of treatment, in order to delay the formation of fibrin, but its use in the treatment of AT-III deficient patients is under debate because heparin may increase the turnover of AT-III and thus aggravate an existing deficiency (Marciniak and Gockerman, 1977). However, subcutaneously administered heparin has been given to AT-III deficient patients for prolonged periods (Brandt and Stenbjerg, 1979) and there are indications that subcutaneous heparin induces a state of sustained anticoagulant effect (Brandt, 1979), which may be beneficial.

The term "disseminated intravascular coagulation" was first introduced in order to describe the pathogenic process in abruptio placentae (Schneider, 1951). The haemorrhagic obstetrical complications continue to represent an important class of DIC, possibly related to the high content of thromboplastin in the placenta and the high fibrinolytic activity of the uterine tissue. Toxaemia of pregnancy (pre-eclampsia) may represent an earlier stage of DIC, in which there is consumption of platelets, but only small changes in the levels of other factors of the coagulation system. However, degradation products of fibrin (or fibrinogen) may be present in the circulating blood, indicating an increased digestion of fibrin (or fibrinogen) and suggesting an activation of the fibrinolytic system (Bonnar et al., 1971). A recent report describes a case of toxaemia of pregnancy in which the administration of acetylsalicylic acid (aspirin) normalized the decreased platelet number (Goodlin et al., 1978). This observation was recently confirmed in a report which also described a correction of the raised levels in serum of fibrin degradation products and uric acid (Jespersen, 1979).

The resolution of fibrin deposits, also influenced by circulating inhibitors of the fibrinolytic system and pathological states, following deviations in the levels of natural inhibitors in blood, have been described, but it is not possible on this occasion to discuss this in detail. A previous review might be helpful (Astrup, 1979).

REFERENCES

Astrup, T. (1979). Fibrinolysis and tissue repair in the lungs. In "The Microembolism Syndrome" (T. Saldeen, ed.), 45. Almqvist and Wiksell, Stockholm.

Astrup, T. and Brakman, P. (1975). Tissue repair and vascular disease in haemophilia. In "Handbook of Hemophilia" (K. M. Brinkhous and H. C. Hemker, eds), 285. Excerpta Medica, Amsterdam.

Astrup, T. and Coccheri, S. (1962). Nature 193, 182.

Aggeler, P. M. and Lucia, S. P. (1944). J. nerv. mental. Dis. 99, 475.

Astrup, T., Glas, P. and Kok, P. (1968). Proc. Soc. Exp. Biol. Med. 127, 373.

Astrup, T., Glas, P. and Kok, P. (1970). Lab. Invest. 22, 381.

Bonnar, J., McNicol, G. P. and Douglas, A. S. (1971). Br. Med. J. 2, 12.

Brandt, P. (1979). Observations during the treatment of antithrombin-III deficient women with heparin and antithrombin concentrate during pregnancy and parturition. (Submitted for publication).

Brandt, P. and Stenbjerg, S. (1979). Lancet 1, 100.

Eyster, M. E. et al. (1978). Blood 51, 1179.

Filizzolo, E., D'Angelo, V., Collice, M., Ferrara, M., Donati, M. B. and Porta, M. (1978). Eur. Neurol. 17, 43.

Glas, P. and Astrup, T. (1970). Am. J. Physiol. 219, 1140.

Glas-Greenwalt, P., Strand, C. and Astrup, T. (1972). Experientia 28, 448.

Goodlin, R. C., Haesslein, H. O. and Flemming, J. (1978). Lancet 2, 51.

Hanaway, J., Torack, R., Fletcher, A. P. and Landau, W. M. (1976). Stroke 7, 143.

Ito, H., Yamamoto, S., Komai, T. and Mizukoshi, H. (1976). *J. Neurosurg.* **45**, 26.
Jespersen, J. (1979). Disseminated intravascular coagulation in toxaemia of pregnancy. Correction of the decreased platelet counts and raised levels of serum uric acid and fibrin (ogen) degradation products by aspirin. (Submitted for publication).
Kwaan, H. C. and Astrup, T. (1964). *J. Path. Bact.* **87**, 409.
Lasch, H. G., Heene, D. L., Huth, K. and Sandritter, W. (1967). *Am. J. Cardiol.* **20**, 381.
Marciniak, E. and Gockerman, J. P. (1977). *Lancet* **2**, 581.
Moltke, P. (1958). *Prac. Soc. Exp. Biol. Med.* **98**, 377.
Noordhoek Hegt, V. (1976). *Haemostasis* **5**, 355.
Noordhoek Hegt, V. (1977). *Thromb. Res.* **10**, 121.
Pandolfi, M. (1967a). *Arch. Ophthalmol.* **78**, 512.
Pandolfi, M. (1967b). *Am. J. Ophthalmol.* **63**, 428.
Pelczar, M. E. , Glas-Greenwalt, P. and Astrup, T. (1972). *Chest* **61**, 394.
Saldeen, T. (1976). *Microvasc. Res.* **11**, 227.
Schneider, C. L. (1951). *Surg. Gynec. Obstet.* **92**, 27.
Sengupta, R. P., So, S. C. and Villarejo-Ortega, F. J. (1976). *J. Neurosurgery* **44**, 479.
Smokovitis, A. and Astrup, T. (1978). *J. Neurosurg.* **48**, 1008.
Storti, E. and Ascari, E. (1975). Long-term evaluation of synovectomy in the treatment of recurrent hemophilic hemarthosis. *In* "Handbook of Hemophilia".
(K. M. Brinkhous and H. C. Hemker, eds), 735. Excerpta Medica, Amsterdam.
Todd, A. S. (1959). *J. Pathol. Bact.* **78**, 281.
Tovi, D. (1973a). *Acta. Neurologica Scand.* **49**, 152.
Tovi, D. (1973b). *Acta. Neurol. Scand.* **49**, 163.
Tovi, D., Nilsson, I. M. and Thulin, C. A. (1972). *Acta. Neurol. Scand.* **48**, 393.
van Trotsenburg, L. (1975). Neurological complications of haemophilia. *In* "Handbook of Hemophilia" (K. M. Brinkhous and H. C. Hemker, eds), 389. Excerpta Medica, Amsterdam.

THE ROLE OF SUBENDOTHELIAL AND MEDIAL FIBRINOID IN THE FORMATION OF ATHEROSCLEROTIC LESIONS

H. Jellinek

2nd Department of Pathology, Semmelweis Medical University, Budapest, Hungary

The two forms of development of arteriosclerosis — hyalinosis and the cellular plaque — were experimentally studied.

The artificial systems used to produce vessel damage experimentally in rats were: renal hypertension; hypoxia produced by double ligature on the infrarenal part of the aorta; painting the abdominal aorta with concentrated hydrochloric acid and feeding on a high-cholesterol diet.

To detect increased permeability we have developed the colloidal iron tracer method. The animals were given a single dose of colloidal iron intravenously (Ferrlecit, Nattermann, Köln) and sacrificed one hour later. The appearance of iron in the vessel wall was detected by staining with Prussian-blue. In the vessels of the controls no iron was ever detectable with this method.

After hypoxia of one hour's duration, iron accumulation was demonstrable in the endothelium and the subendothelial space by the Prussian-blue reaction. The chemical determination of iron content also revealed a maximum value at 36 h. After 10 days only occasional endothelial cells were stained by the Prussian-blue reaction. Similar changes were seen in hypertensive animals where colloidal iron accumulated in the subendothelial space and the media. Staining with hydrochloric acid resulted in necrosis of the vessel wall. One hour after acid staining, there was colloidal iron present in the subendothelial space and after 48 h the whole vessel wall exhibited Prussian-blue positivity as a sign of increased permeability. In experiments on animals fed on a high-cholesterol diet, lipid deposition in the vessel wall was detectable by Sudan-III staining only after 3 weeks. Neverthe-

Serono Symposium No. 37, "Vascular Occlusion: Epidemiological, Pathophysiological and Therapeutic Aspects", edited by M. Tesi and J. Dormandy, 1981. Academic Press, London and New York.

less, the permeability disturbance began after 10 days, as revealed by the Prussian-blue positivity of the endothelial cells.

The increased permeability results in light-microscopic change after some time. Increase of plasma inhibition results in its accumulation in the subendothelial space. This material stains red with azan and black with Mallory's phosphotungstic acid stain and is designated further as a subendothelial fibrinoid. In this phase electron microscopic examination first reveals the subendothelial accumulation of some floccular matter and later the formation of Fibrin of 220 Å periodicity. The amount of this material increases parallel to the persistence of the nosogenic influence. The longer the duration of the damage is, the more fibrin will precipitate. This and some other plasma components form crystalline aggregates occasionally exhibiting a 2200 Å periodicity. Later these crystalline aggregates condense to larger bodies and ultimately fill the total subendothelial space. The periodicity in their structure may occasionally be preserved.

At this stage the material begins to stain blue with azan. In contrast to its original red staining, the blue is typical for fibrinoid. Under the electron microscope the blue staining material appears as a homogenous mass filling the subendothelial space between the endothelium and the elastica. In this phase there are also lipid materials appearing in the hyalinaceous mass.

The plasma imbibition later extends also to the media. This causes enlargement of the space between the smooth muscle cells and the fibrous elements. The plasma also enters into the smooth muscle cells. This results in oedematous degeneration and circumscript local necroses. Ultimately fibrin also makes an appearance within the cells. In this phase, the cells die and the debris and the plasma mix together to produce the medial fibrinoid.

The necrotic cells are replaced by the proliferation of healthy cells in the neighbourhood. Depending on the extent of the damage, the proliferation may be semilunar or circular. In the intercellular space, new elastic fibres are formed from the GAG produced by the cells. The fibres may appear in multiple layers. In larger muscular vessels stained by acid, the proliferation is particularly visible since practically a total elastico-muscular restitution occurs.

On the surface of the proliferate, the development of a new endothelial layer is demonstrable by electron microscopy. In the medial part, new smooth muscle cells and basal membrane-like material appear and new elastica is produced. These phenomena are best demonstrated in acid-stained muscular vessels. The analogy with small vessel changes in hypertension is conspicuous.

In the cells in the proliferation zone, after a prolonged period, the electron microscope reveals the presence of lipid droplets in the endothelium and myeline figures in the medial smooth muscle cells and lipids. After more than 200 days apatite crystals also appear. In certain cases, the subendothelial fibrinoid is ingested by the phagocytes and fibrinoid is replaced by a plaque consisting of smooth muscle cells covered by endothelium. The disturbed transport of plasma through the vessel wall leads, through plasma accumulation and fibrin precipitation, to the development of hyalinaceous or cellular atherosclerotic plaques.

BIBLIOGRAPHY

Elemer, G., Kerenyi, T. and Jellinek, H. (1975). *Path. Europ.* **10**, 123–128.
Hüttner, I., Jellinek, H. and Kerenyi, T. (1968). *Exp. Molec. Path.* **9**, 309–321.

Jellinek, H., Nagy, Z., Hüttner, I., Balint, A., Kocze, A. and Kerenyi, T. (1969). *Br. J. Exp. Path.* **50**, 13–16.
Jellinek, H. (1970). *Angiology* **21**, 691–699.
Jellinek, H. (1970). *Angiology* **21**, 636–646.
Jellinek, H. (1975). "Arterial Lesions and Arteriosclerosis." Akademial Kiado, Budapest.
Jellinek, H., Hüttner, I. and More, R. H. (1977). *Exp. Molec. Path.* **26**, 401–414.
Kerenyi, T., Jellinek, H., Hüttner, I., Goracz, G. and Konyar, Eva (1966). *Acta Morph. Acad. Sci. Hung.* **14**, 175–182.
Kerenyi, T., Hüttner, I. and Jellinek, H. (1966). *Ztsch.f.Mikr.-anat. Forsch.* **74**, 121–131.
Kerenyi, T. and Jellinek, H. (1972). *Exp. Molec. Path.* **17**, 1–5.
Veress, B., Kocze, A. and Jellinek, H. (1969). *Br.J.Exp.Path.* **50**, 600–604.

CIRCULATING IMMUNE COMPLEXES IN CORONARY
ARTERIOPATHY

S. Gerö, Eva Szondy, G. Füst, Zsuzsa Mezei, Judit Székely and J. Fehér

Arteriosclerosis Research Group of the Ministry of Health, Budapest, Hungary

INTRODUCTION

Several hypotheses have been proposed about the pathological mechanisms of the primary lesions leading to the development of arteriosclerosis. Many articles, among them previous findings of our research group, (Gerö *et al.*, 1959; Szigeti *et al.*, 1960; Scebat *et al.*, 1966) have demonstrated that immunological processes can also influence the evolution of the arteriosclerotic lesions.

In our previous work, we demonstrated antibodies and cell-mediated immune response against aortic antigens (Gerö *et al.*, 1975; Horváth *et al.*, 1978) in arteriosclerotic patients. We detected circulating immune complexes (CIC) in the sera of these patients as well.

In our present work, we examined the changes of the concentration of CIC in patients with myocardial infarction. To this end three methods were used, the complement consumption test, the Clq-solubility test described by Johnson *et al.* (1975) and the polyethylene glycol (PEG)-precipitation test, described by Haskova *et al.* (1978).

CIRCULATING IMMUNE COMPLEXES IN MYOCARDIAL INFARCTION

In the first part of our series of investigations, the sera of 45 patients with myocardial infarction were studied using the complement consumption and the Clq-solubility test. In 24 cases, negative results were obtained during the whole

Serono Symposium No. 37, "Vascular Occlusion: Epidemiological, Pathophysiological and Therapeutic Aspects", edited by M. Tesi and J. Dormandy, 1981. Academic Press, London and New York.

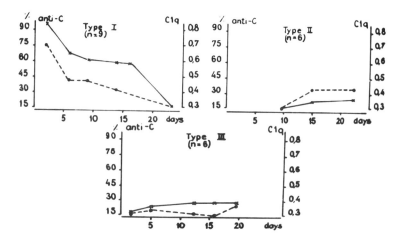

Fig. 1. Quantitative changes in the level of CIC in myocardial infarction. x —— x: Complement consumption test (anti-C); ● - - - - ●: Clq-solubility test (Clq).

Table I. Immune complexes in myocardial infarction.

	First day	First week	Second and third week
Negative	14	3	5
Detected with 1 test	14	14	20
Detected with 2 tests	8	15	11
Detected with 3 tests	1	5	1
Positive total	23 (63%)	34 (91%)	32 (86%)

Table II. Positive results in at least one serum sample in myocardial infarction.

Subendocardial No. = 16			Transmural No. = 21		
First day	First week	Second and third week	First day	First week	Second and third week
11 (69%)	15 (94%)	14 (87%)	12 (57%)	19 (93%)	18 (87%)

period of study and positive results found in 21 patients' sera (Füst *et al.*, 1978). In the quantitative changes of CIC, three types could be observed (Fig. 1). In type I, immune complexes could be detected in the first days after the infarction then, after a gradual decrease, the results became negative. In type II, the immune complexes appeared by the second to third week and their quantity did not change until the end of the observation period. In type III immune complexes could be detected during the whole period of the study. One can assume that in type I immune complexes played a causative role in the pathogenesis of the disease, whereas type II may be an indicator of a subclinical Dressler syndrome.

    In the second part of our studies the concentration of CIC was examined using three tests (the two tests mentioned above and the PEG-precipiation test) in 37

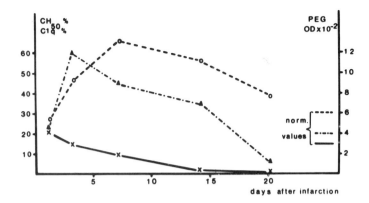

Fig. 2. Quantitative changes in the level of CIC in patient P.J. x——x: Complement consumption test (CH$_{50}$); o——o. Clq-solubility test (Clq); ▲----▲: Polyethylene glycol precipitation test (PEG).

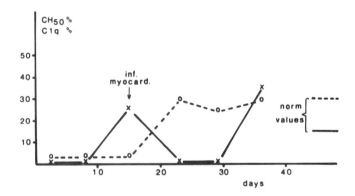

Fig. 3. Quantitative changes in the level of CIC in patient D.M. x——x: Complement consumption test (CH$_{50}$); o- - -o: Clq solubility test (Clq).

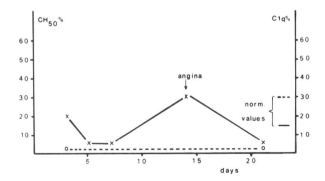

Fig. 4. Quantitative changes in the level of CIC in patient A.S. x——x: Complement consumption test (CH$_{50}$); o- - -o: Clq solubility test (Clq).

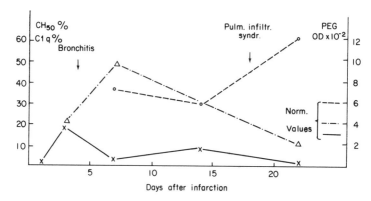

Fig. 5. Quantitative changes in the level of CIC in patient H.I. x———x: Complement consumption test (CH_{50}); o- - -o: Clq solubility test (Clq); Δ-.-Δ: Polyethylene glycol precipitation test (PEG).

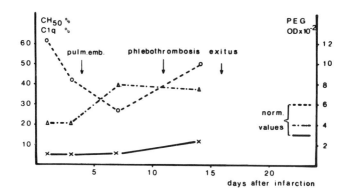

Fig. 6. Quantitative changes in the level of CIC in patient M.F. x———x: Complement consumption test (CH_{50}); o- - -o: Clq solubility test (Clq); Δ-.-Δ: Polyethylene glycol precipitation test (PEG).

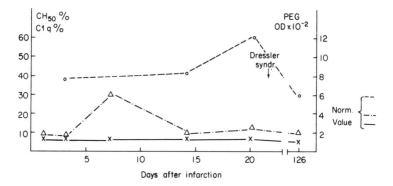

Fig. 7. Quantitative changes in the level of CIC in patient B.A. x———x: Complement consumption test (CH_{50}); o- - -o: Clq-solubility test (Clq); Δ-.-Δ: Polyethylene glycol precipitation test (PEG).

patients. The incidence of CIC in the patients' sera was studied on the first day, the first week and on the 2nd and 3rd weeks. In Table I, it can be seen that on the first day, CIC could be detected in 63% of the cases. The incidence of CIC increased during further serum samplings performed in the first week. We found CIC in 91% of the patients investigated. In the samples taken in the second and third weeks of the disease, CIC could be detected in 86% of the patients.

The correlation of the severity of the disease and the occurrence of CIC was studied in 16 patients with subendocardial infarction and in 21 patients with transmural infarction. Table II demonstrates that no significant difference was found between the two groups, indicating that the presence of CIC does not depend on the severity of the disease. Next some individual cases will be presented.

In patient P.J. (Fig. 2) during the first week CIC could be demonstrated with all the three methods mentioned above. After a gradual fall by the third week, only the Clq-solubility test remained positive.

The patient D.M. (Fig. 3) was hospitalized with an attack of angina pectoris. No CIC could be detected in her sera. In the second week, her condition worsened and on the fifteenth day myocardial infarction was diagnosed. Parallel with the onset of the infarction the complement consumption test and, some days later, the Clq-solubility test also became positive.

Patient A.S. (Fig. 4) with ischaemic heart disease, had a severe attack of angina on the fourteenth day after his admission to the hospital. This attack was associated with a sharp increase in the level of the CIC detected by the Clq-solubility test.

With the following cases we should like to demonstrate that a positive reaction can occur not only with myocardial infarction itself but also be caused by fever, pneumonia, or other complications.

In patient H.I. (Fig. 5) on the fourth day after the onset of the infarction, acute bronchitis was diagnosed. On the eighteenth day, the signs of a right-side pulmonary infiltration syndrome developed. Both the beginning of the acute bronchitis and the onset of the pulmonary complication were associated with an increase in the quantity of CIC.

In Fig. 6 we demonstrate a fatal case (patient M.F.). On the fourth day after the infarction the signs of pulmonary embolism were present and on the eleventh day deep vein thrombosis developed. Both complications were followed by an increase in the quantity of CIC.

In the sera of patient B.A. (Fig. 7) during the first week the PEG precipitation test was positive and on the fourteenth day it reached the normal values. The complement consumption test was negative and the Clq-solubility test remained positive during the whole observation time. In the third week an increase of the concentration of CIC could be detected by the PEG-precipitation method and on the twenty-first day, the clinical signs of a Dressler syndrome were present.

Summarizing, it has been shown that the changes in the quantity of CIC in myocardial infarction are frequently associated with the clinical course of the disease.

IMMUNE COMPLEXES IN EXPERIMENTAL ARTERIOSCLEROSIS

In our previous investigations (Szondy *et al.*, 1978), the occurrence of CIC could be demonstrated in cholesterol-fed rabbits as well. It was also shown that the con-

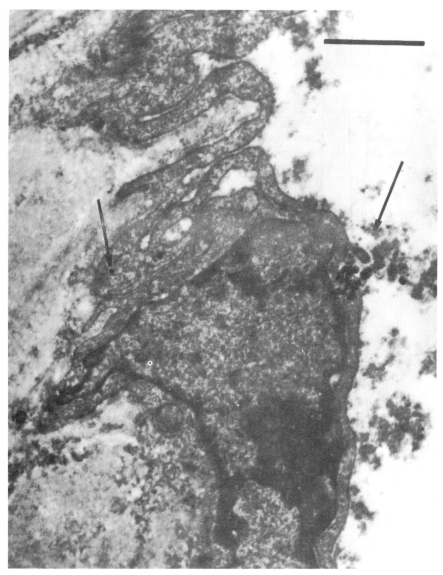

Fig. 8. Immune-electromicroscopic pattern of aortic intima incubated with ferritin-labelled anti-IgG. The surface of the endothelial cells with IgG containing electrondense substances demonstrated in the cytoplasm (arrows).

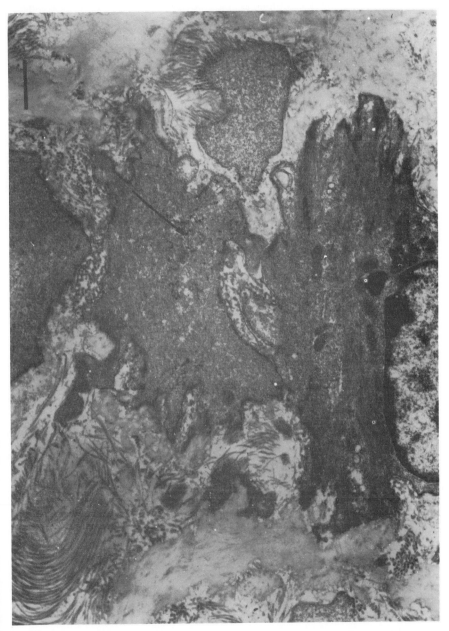

Fig. 9. Immune-electromicroscopic pattern of aortic media incubated with ferritin-labelled anti-IgG. Between the elastic and collagen fibres are destroyed smooth muscle cells. Electron-dense bodies containing IgG (arrow) can be seen.

centration of the immune complexes could be influenced by an anti-lipidaemic (clofibrate) and an anti-atherosclerotic (pyridinol carbamate) drug.

In our further studies, we attempted to detect immune complexes in the aortic intima of cholesterol-fed animals by an immuno-electronmicroscopic method. Using ferritin-labelled anti-IgG immune serum, an increased quantity of IgG, presumably due to the presence of immune complexes could be demonstrated in the endothelial cells (Fig. 8) and in the subendothelial cells (Fig. 9) of the intima of the cholesterol-fed animals.

Our results, obtained by various immunological methods both in human and experimental animals, support the view that immunological processes play a role in the pathology of arteriosclerosis.

REFERENCES

Füst. G., Szondy, E., Székely, J. and Gerö, S. (1978). *Atherosclerosis* **29**, 181.
Gerö, S., Gergely, J., Jakab, L., Székely, J., Virág, S., Farkas, K. and Czuppon, A. (1959). *Lancet* **2**, 6.
Gerö, S., Székely, J., Szondy, E. and Seregélyi, E. (1975). *Arterial Wall* 3/2, 89.
Haskova, V., Kaslik, J., Riha, J., Matl, I. and Rovensky, J. (1978). *Z. Immun.-Forsch.* **154**, 399.
Horváth, M., Alföldi, P., Ónodi, K. and Braun, E. (1978). *Arterial Wall* 4/2, 89.
Johnson, A. J., Mowbray, J. F. and Porter, K. A. (1975). *Lancet* **1**, 762.
Scebaṭ, L., Renais, N., Groult, N., Iris, L. and Lenègre, J. (1966). *Rev. Franc, d'Et. Clin. Biol.* **11**, 388.
Szigeti, J., Ormos, J., Jákó, J. and Tószegi, A. (1960). *Acta Allergologica*, Suppl. VII, 74.
Szondy, E., Horváth, M., Füst, G., Link, E., Fehér, J. and Gerö, S. (1978). *Atherosclerosis* **31**, 251.

REGRESSION OF ATHEROSCLEROSIS: SOME TISSUE REACTIONS

C. W. M. Adams, Y. H. Abdulla and O. B. Bayliss High

Department of Pathology, Guy's Hospital Medical School, London, UK

Consideration of the mechanisms for the regression of atherosclerotic lesions, particularly the removal of lipid, suggests at least three possible mechanisms:

a. breakdown of lipid by enzymatic activity;
b. removal of lipid by phagocytosis and cell transport;
c. the action of plasma lipoproteins as transport vessels.

ENZYMATIC ACTIVITY

Triglycerides and phospholipids are relatively minor constituents of established atherosclerotic lesions (Smith and Slater, 1973). In this case, the arterial wall is equipped with its own phospholipases and triglyceride lipases (Zemplenyi, 1968) which presumably catabolize these lipids. However, cholesterol is not readily degraded into water soluble compounds by tissues, apart from the liver. Thus, cholesterol would tend to accumulate in the atherosclerotic lesion, in contrast to the presumed continued degradation of the phospholipids and triglycerides.

CELL TRANSPORT AND PHAGOCYTOSIS

The cellular response in the early stages of human atherosclerosis seems to be mainly a proliferation of smooth muscle cells. Although such cells may be filled with lipid, it is difficult to see how they could remove it from the arterial wall,

Serono Symposium No. 37, "Vascular Occlusion: Epidemiological, Pathophysiological and Therapeutic Aspects", edited by M. Tesi and J. Dormandy, 1981. Academic Press, London and New York.

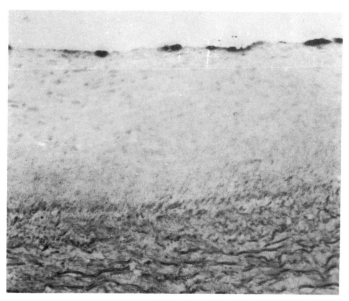

Fig. 1. Subendothelial accumulation of monocytes, but no penetration into the depth of an avascular human aortic atherosclerotic lesion (grade II). Cytochrome oxidase method (× 120).

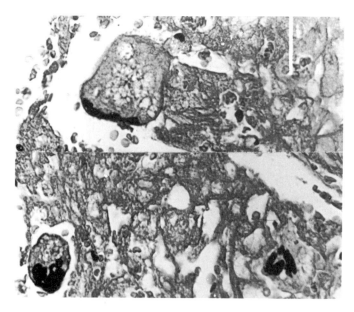

Fig. 2. Giant cells (fused macrophages) in the depth of a capillarized human aortic atherosclerotic lesion (grade III). Haematoxylin and eosin (× 300).

as they are not migratory phagocytic cells. The most effective phagocytic cell in the body is the mononuclear phagocyte (reticuloendothelial system), but the blood representative of this series—the monocyte—does not seem to penetrate deeply into the human atherosclerotic plaque (Fig. 1; Adams *et al.*, 1975; Adams and Bayliss, 1976; Geer and Haust, 1972). This restriction on the penetration of monocytes into the depths of the atherosclerotic plaque may be a result of the avascularity of the lesion, in that capillaries are required to allow monocytes to enter. During tissue repair, capillary formation (granulation) is known to precede the appearance of macrophages and the onset of fibroblastic activity (Payling Wright, 1950).

Advanced human atherosclerotic (grade III) plaques do show considerable capillarization and this is accompanied by the appearance of macrophages and even giant cells (Fig. 2) within such lesions (Bayliss-High and Adams, 1980). It is uncertain to what extent macrophage and giant cell formation results in resorption of lipid and regression of atherosclerosis. However, a reduction of lipid staining has been noticed in the region of macrophage and giant cell infiltration in advanced human atherosclerosis (Adams and Bayliss, 1976; Bayliss-High and Adams, 1980).

LIPOPROTEIN TRANSPORT

In contrast to the cellular mechanisms discussed above, another potential mechanism for lipid removal from atherosclerosis is transport out of the lesions

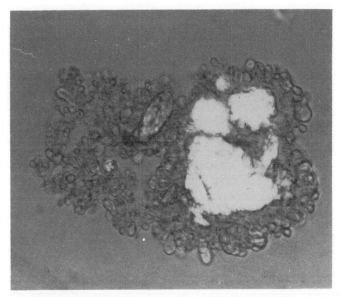

Fig. 3. Giant micelles (liposomes) forming over the surface of a cholesterol crystal exposed to a human high density lipoprotein (~ 4 mg/ml), partly polarized light (X 300).

by the action of lipoprotein vehicles. It seems accepted that low density lipoprotein, and perhaps very low density lipoprotein, are mainly responsible for
transporting cholesterol into tissues, while high-density lipoprotein (HDL) is
concerned with the removal of cholesterol out of tissues (Bondjers and Björkerud,
1974; Stein *et al.*, 1975). It has been suggested that the removal of cholesterol by
HDL from tissue membranes is effected by a sort of shuttle within the HDL
molecule, with phospholipid donating fatty acid through the action of LCAT
to form esterified cholesterol from the free cholesterol taken up from the tissues
(Glomsett, 1968). However, we have found that HDL forms lipid micelles from
cholesterol crystals *in vitro* (Fig. 3), and such micelles contain four times as
much cholesterol as does the HDL molecule when fully loaded with cholesterol
(Adams and Abdulla, 1979; Abdulla and Adams, 1979). This action of HDL is
increased more by the addition of Lipostabil (EPL; Natterman, Koln). This effect
of Lipostabil seems to depend both on the phospholipid and the bile salt in the
drug preparation: each by itself is ineffective in enhancing micelle formation.

The foregoing observations suggest that HDL may act both by removing cholesterol from membrane and by forming soluble micelles with crystalline
cholesterol in the tissues (for example, the atherosclerotic plaque etc.). It is
uncertain to what extent this micelle-formation is of importance *in vivo*. However, histological sections of human atherosclerosis exposed to HDL do show
areas of budding consistent with the formation of lipid micelles (Fig. 4). Thus,
HDL may play a part in the regression of the atherosclerotic lesion by forming
micelles or liposomes over the surface of cholesterol crystals within the plaque.

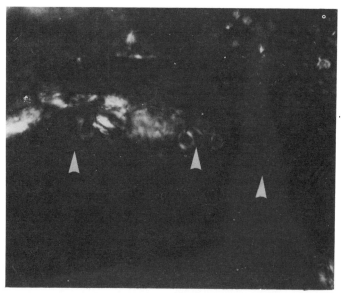

Fig. 4.   Liposomes (arrows) forming over the surface of cholesterol crystals in a section of a
human aortic atherosclerotic plaque. Section exposed to human HDL for 1 h, partly polarized
light, (× 300).

REFERENCES

Abdulla, Y. H. and Adams, C. W. M. (1978). *Atherosclerosis* **31**, 473–480.
Adams, C. W. M. and Abdulla, Y. H. (1978). *Atherosclerosis* **31** 465–471.
Adams, C. W. M. and Bayliss, O. B. (1976). *Br. J. exp. Path.* **57**, 30–36.
Adams, C. W. M., Bayliss, O. B. and Turner, D. R. (1975). *J. Pathol.* **116**, 225–238.
Bayliss-High, O. B. and Adams, C. W. M. (1980). *Atherosclerosis* (in press).
Bondjers, G. and Björkerud, S. (1974). *Artery* **1**, 3–9.
Geer, J. C. and Haust, M. D. (1972). Smooth muscle cells in atherosclerosis: Monographs or Atherosclerosis. No. 2. Karger, Basel.
Glomsett, J. A. (1968). *J. Lipid Res.* **9**, 155–167.
Payling Wright, G. (1950). "An Introduction to Pathology." Longmans Green, London.
Smith, E. B. and Slater, R. S. (1973). *In* "Atherogenesis Initiating Factors." (R. Porter and J. Knight, ed.) NS. 12, pp. 39–62. CIBA Foundation Symposium.
Stein, Y., Glangeaud, M. C., Fainaru, M. and Stein, O. (1975). *Biochim. Biophys. Acta* **380**, 106–118.
Zemplenyi, T. (1968). "Enzyme Biochemistry of the Arterial Wall." Lloyd Luke, London.

CLINICAL SIGNIFICANCE OF ERYTHROCYTE DEFORMABILITY

J. A. Dormandy, A. J. Dodds, P. N. Matthews and P. T. Flute

St James's and St George's Hospitals, London, UK

Ever since Leuwenhoek first looked down his primitive microscope over two centuries ago and described the flow of red cells in a living circulation, we have been aware that the red cells must deform in order to negotiate the microcirculation. The characteristic regular biconcave shape of the red cell we see on a microscope slide is virtually never found in the microcirculation where the cells have to squeeze through capillaries much smaller than the undeformed red cell. Although the principal function of the blood is to flow, it is only in the last few years that haematologists or clinicians have begun to pay attention to the ability of individual red cells to flow through capillaries. The problem has to some extent been methodological: how to clinically measure the ability of red cells to deform. There can be two fundamentally opposite approaches to this problem, illustrated by Scott-Blair's description of the two types of rheologists:

> "Practical rheologists who observe what cannot be explained and theoretical rheologists who explain what cannot be observed."

Our approach has been the practical and clinical one.

OUR TECHNIQUE FOR MEASURING RED CELL DEFORMABILITY

Our method is based on measuring the ability of red cells to pass through a Nucleopore filter of 5 μ in diameter pore size. Figure 1 outlines the procedure which involves the withdrawal of 10 ml of venous blood without occlusion, anticoagulated with solid lithium heparin. Following centrifugation, the plasma is

Serono Symposium No. 37, "Vascular Occlusion: Epidemiological, Pathophysiological and Therapeutic Aspects", edited by M. Tesi and J. Dormandy, 1981. Academic Press, London and New York.

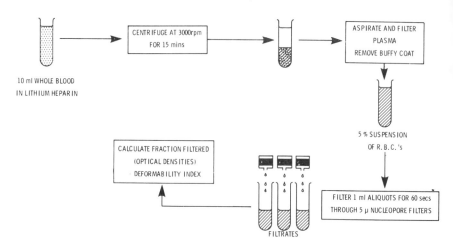

Fig. 1.   Diagram summarizing our filtration technique for measuring red cell deformability.

Table I.   Filtration technique for assessing red cell deformability (Dodds and Dormandy, 1979).

Advantages

Simple and cheap. Therefore clinically practical.
Eliminates possible effects of WBC (approximately 99%) and platelets (approximately 90%).
Independent of haematocrit.
Reproducible. (Coefficient of variation of result on same sample 2.5%.)
Low shear stresses. Therefore probably more physiological.
Low haematocrit appropriate for microcirculation and minimizes effect of aggregation.
Can be correlated with clinical states.

Disadvantages

Measurements have to be carried out soon (within 2 h after withdrawal).
Uncontrolled environment.
Batch to batch variation in filters.

removed, leaving the buffy coat. Any platelet aggregates or white cells remaining in the plasma are removed by filtration through a Micropore or 3 μ Nucleopore filter. The red cells are then resuspended in the plasma at a concentration of 5%. One millilitre aliquots of the suspension are then filtered through a 5 μ Nucleopore filter under gravity and the result is expressed as the fraction of red cells filtered in the first minute. This is termed the deformability index. At least three measurements are made on the same sample, using a new filter each time. Table I summarizes some of the advantages and disadvantages of this technique.

Despite the elimination of the white cells and platelets, the results obtained

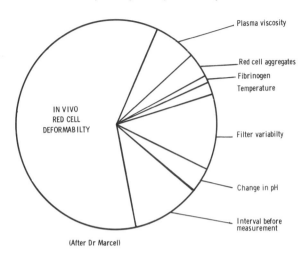

Plasma viscosity

Red cell aggregates
Fibrinogen
Temperature

IN VIVO
RED CELL
DEFORMABILTY

Filter variabilty

Change in pH

Interval before
measurement

(After Dr Marcel)

Fig. 2. Hypothetical diagram suggesting the relative importance of the various factors influencing the results obtained with our filtration technique.

are almost certainly dependent on a number of extraneous factors, variables other than red cell deformability. Figure 2 represents diagrammatically the probable contribution of these various factors to the deformability index obtained using this technique.

The clinical validity of these measurements is based on two types of evidence: the finding of abnormal values in diseases associated with impaired tissue perfusion and the demonstration of abnormal red cell deformability as a significant prognostic risk factor in some of these conditions.

CLINICAL CONDITIONS ASSOCIATED WITH REDUCED RED CELL DEFORMABILITY

Ischaemic Disease of the Legs

A reduced red cell deformability in an unselected group of patients with ischaemic legs was originally reported by us in 1976 (Reid *et al.*) and has since been confirmed by other workers (Drummond *et al.*, 1979). The main interest of the original work was that the abnormality in the red cells appeared to have a prognostic significance; patients who subsequently required an amputation had a much lower deformability index than those who did not (Fig. 3).

Following Surgery

In a recent study, we found that patients' red cells became consistently more rigid after all forms of surgery. The effect begins at the time of operation, reaches

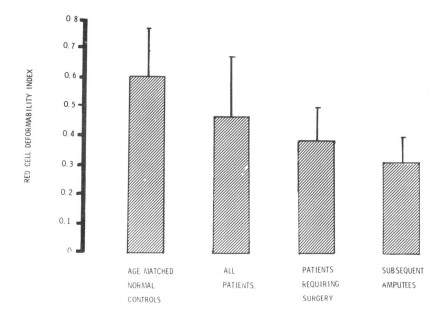

Fig. 3. Mean (and s.d.) of a group of patients with ischaemia of the legs relating it to their subsequent progress and also a normal control group.

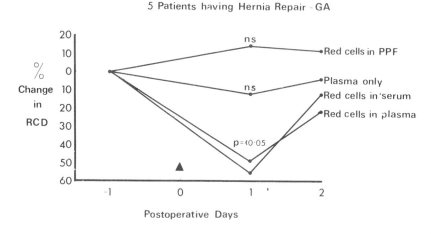

Fig. 4. Deformability index following hernia operations comparing the changes found when the red cells were suspended in their own plasma, their own serum and plasma protein fraction (PPF). The change in the flow rate of the plasma alone is also shown.

a maximum between 24 and 48 h and returns to normal in the subsequent 5 to 10 days. Rather surprisingly, the magnitude of the change in red cell deformability was the same whether the operation was a major arterial reconstruction, varicose vein stripping or repair of a hernia. Nor was it influenced by the intravenous fluids administered, not even when several units of stored blood were used. By comparing hernia repairs performed under general or epidural anaesthesia, the post-operative red cell rigidity was shown not to be due to the anaesthetic agents used.

Although the timing of these changes may suggest a possible connection with the development of post-operative venous thrombosis, the principal interest of these studies so far arose from experiments where the rigid post-operative red cells were resuspended in different solutions other than plasma. The results are illustrated in Fig. 4. The fact that the decreased filterability of the red cells was the same in native plasma and serum, but was abolished when resuspended in plasma protein fraction, strongly suggests that it is principally a plasma factor which altered the deformability of the red cells in this situation. (The plasma alone filtered at a constant rate and therefore the change in the red cell-plasma suspension was not simply due to a change in plasma viscosity.)

Diabetes Mellitus

Abnormalities in red cell deformability in this disease, originally described using our technique (Barnes, 1977), showed an abnormality particularly marked in diabetics with retinopathy. Similar findings have since then been reported by Juhan (1979), who also showed that the use of an artificial pancreas reversed these changes. No prognostic significance has yet been attributed to red cell deformability in diabetes; a particularly difficult disease to quantify in terms of progression.

Myocardial Infarction

Possibly the most interesting clinical finding of abnormal red cell deformability has been in a recent, as yet unpublished, study of 43 patients with myocardial infarction. Full haemorheological studies including whole blood viscosity, plasma

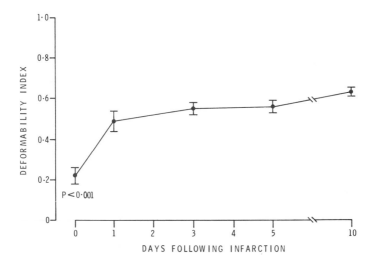

Fig. 5. Changes in the deformability index (mean and s.e.) following myocardial infarction in a group of 43 patients.

J. A. Dormandy et al.

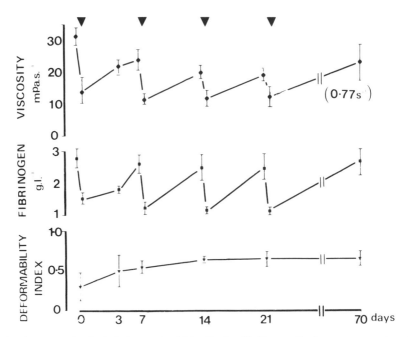

Fig. 6. Haemorheological changes in eight patients with Raynaud's phenomenon undergoing a course of four plasma exchanges.

Table II. Deformability index (± s.e.) immediately after a myocardial infarction in relation to patients' subsequent progress.

			Significance of difference
Pulmonary oedema	n = 11	0.22 ± 0.07	*P* < 0.01
No oedema	n = 27	0.47 ± 0.05	
Cardiogenic shock	n = 5	0.11 ± 0.04	*P* < 0.02
No shock	n = 34	0.44 ± 0.05	

viscosity and fibrinogen were carried out as soon as possible after admission (day 0) and on days 1, 3, 5, 10 and 42. These changes have been described previously and were not found to have any great prognostic significance. The changes in red cell deformability shown in Fig. 5 had not previously been described and were of considerable clinical interest.

Table II shows the striking prognostic significance of the initial deformability index (day 0) in relation to the progress of the patient in terms of the development of pulmonary oedema or cardiogenic shock. The initial red cell deformability of the patients who subsequently developed these complications was significantly lower than that of the patients who did not get complications. Three patients died in this series and in two of these cases, the red cells immediately after the infarct would not pass the filter at all (deformability index of 0).

These results suggest the hypothesis that for some reason ischaemic or infarcted tissue makes the red cells more rigid (supported by the findings in ischaemia of the legs mentioned earlier), but that the change in red cell deformability then plays a critical part in determining the outcome in the marginal ischaemic tissue surrounding the infarct. If the red cells are very rigid, a vicious cycle develops with extension of the area of necrosis, which may lead to death in an ever-increasing spiral. Alternatively, if the decrease in red cell deformability is relatively mild, the marginal area of ischaemia recovers. On the basis of this hypothesis, therapy following an infarct should be directed at minimizing the abnormality in red cell deformability.

POSSIBLE THERAPY FOR IMPROVING RED CELL DEFORMABILITY

The remaining question to be answered is whether reversing or preventing abnormal red cell rigidity in any of the conditions where this has been described would produce a clinical improvement. Unfortunately, for the moment we do not have any definitely proven, effective and certain pharmacological technique for improving red cell deformability.

Plasma Exchange

Plasma exchange is a mechanical technique which has been found to improve markedly the abnormal red cell deformability which we have found in patients with Raynaud's phenomenon (Dodds *et al.*, 1979). Figure 6 shows all the haemo-rheological changes during and for 50 days after a course of four plasma exchanges. Although there is a slight overall decrease in plasma fibrinogen and whole blood viscosity at low shear rate, the most marked change is the improvement in red cell deformability. These changes were accompanied by a subjective and objective improvement in the patients' clinical condition. While the initial improvement in the red cell deformability may be explained by the removal of a plasma factor, the persistence of this improvement (and of the clinical improvement) so long after the last exchange transfusion is difficult to explain.

Pharmacological Treatment

In the field of pharmacological therapy evidence of a beneficial effect on the deformability of red cells has been presented in connection with three drugs: pentoxyfylline, flunarizine and isoxsuprine. These early reports still remain to be confirmed and correlated with objective clinical criteria. This is a rapidly expanding area and possibly the most promising approach available in the near future for the management of many types of ischaemic lesions.

REFERENCES

Barnes, A. J., Locke, P., Scudder, P. R., Dormandy, T. L., Dormandy, J. A. and Slack, J. (1977). *Lancet* 2, 789.
Dodds, A. J., O'Reilly, M. J. G., Yates, C. J., Flute, P. T., Cotton, L. T. and Dormandy, J. A. (1979). *Brit. Med. J.* (To be published.)

Drummond, M. M., Lowe, G. D. O., Belch, J. J. F., Forbes, C. D. and Barbanel,
J. C. (1979). *Thromb. Haemost.* **42**, 106.
Juhan, I., Buonocorem, M., Vovan, L., Durand, F., Calas, M. F., Moulin, J. P. and
Vague, P. (1979). "Proceedings of IVth Congres Francais d'Hematologie".
(To be published.)
Reid, H. L., Dormandy, J. A., Barnes, A. J., Lock, P. J. and Dormandy, T. L.
(1976). *Lancet* **1**, 666.

ON THE MEANING OF BLOOD HYPERVISCOSITY IN VASCULAR DISEASE

T. Di Perri

Istituto di Patologia Speciale Medica e Metodologia Clinica dell'Università di Siena, Italy

According to the first definition of Newton, the viscosity of the fluid may be evaluated by the ratio between shear stress (shearing force per unit area) and shear rate (velocity gradient). In the so-called Newtonian fluid, the viscosity is not dependent on the shear rate changes, while in the non-Newtonian fluid, every change leads to a change of viscosity. Blood is a non-Newtonian fluid.

The viscosity of blood increases as the shear rate decreases and this is due mainly to increased aggregation of red cells at lower shear rates. Blood viscosity assayed *in vitro* is not the viscosity operating *in vivo* in each segment of the circulatory tree. Many variants influence the behaviour of viscosity. Some of them are dependent on the composition of the blood and others on the dynamic influences which regulate the blood streaming inside the vessels. The first group includes: haematocrit (the so-called internal viscosity of erythrocyte), the number of white cells and platelets and the fibrinogen and protein concentration. In the second group, the geometry and the size of the vessels, the rate of the flow and the pulsatility of the flow play an effective role on the distribution of the cellular elements along the longitudinal axis of the stream, thus influencing the rate and the stress of the shearing forces.

The change of one of the constituents regulating viscosity of the blood may cause the development of the so-called primary hyperviscosity syndrome. In this group are the hyperfibrinogenic conditions, macroglobulinic diseases, the polycythaemias and red blood cell diseases, since many haemolytic diseases show a permanent increase of blood viscosity which in turn, may be plasma or celldependent. In these syndromes, the increased blood viscosity impairs the flow

Serono Symposium No. 37, "Vascular Occlusion: Epidemiological, Pathophysiological and Therapeutic Aspects", edited by M. Tesi and J. Dormandy, 1981. Academic Press, London and New York.

in the small vessels, decreasing its velocity until blockage of narrow capillaries occurs. Thus, the cause of the blood hyperviscosity and the mechanism of peripheral vascular insufficiency appear easily identifiable in terms of cause and effect.

A mixture of clinical situations with hypothetical common backgrounds may show an inconstant increase of blood viscosity, and are collected under the definition of secondary hyperviscosity syndromes. The increase of blood viscosity is not due to a primary change of a determinant variant, but to a secondary variant dependent on the influence of extrahaematic factors. The possibility of the rapid reversibility of the increased viscosity might be the key to unify these syndromes even if the mechanisms are not known.

There is corroborating evidence that blood viscosity is increased in vascular disorders leading to regional ischaemia, such as cerebral, coronary or peripheral artery occlusive disease (Dormandy, 1970; Dintenfass, 1976; Schmidt-Schoenbein, 1976; Di Perri et al., 1977). In our experience, blood viscosity assayed *in vitro* is higher in the patients with an occlusive vascular disease than in control subjects. Moreover, the increase of the viscosity is higher in the patients with acute circulatory impairment than in chronic vascular patients.

In acute conditions, such as cerebral or myocardial infarction, the clinical onset of the disease is accompanied by a rapid increase of viscosity which will slowly decrease during the recovery period to a steady level which is normally higher than the so-called normal level.

The question arises whether the presence of elevated blood viscosity in the patient with occlusive vascular disease may be considered in anyway correlated with the disease itself; if yes, which of the regulating factors might be operating as the determining mechanism? Moreover, since the vascular impairment is generally regional, the relationship between the finding of increased blood viscosity in the systemic circulation and the regional disease must be investigated in order to assume some dependence between the two classes of phenomena.

With regard to the first question, a correlation between the clinical picture of the disease and the modifications of the blood viscosity has been found, in the sense that the rapid worsening of the regional circulation was always accompanied by an abrupt increase of the whole blood viscosity. In our experience, the most impressive example is the spontaneous anginal attack of the coronary patient. The onset of the pain is followed by a rapid increase of the viscosity of the venous blood. The amount of the increase of blood viscosity is very marked, increasing to 50% or more of the basal value. The end of the pain, either spontaneous or pharmacologically induced, is then followed by the return of the viscosity to the starting level. Consequently, the development of the myocardial ischaemic attack appears closely related to the marked increase of blood viscosity. The possibility that the increase of the blood viscosity might precede the anginal crisis has also been postulated, but not proven.

Moreover, a statistically significant increase of blood viscosity was observed in coronary patients after an exercise test which was followed by the typical electrocardiographic changes of ischaemia and by the appearance of precordial pain. Also, in patients with peripheral occlusive arterial disease, the walking test leading to the appearance of claudication was followed by a reversible increase of blood viscosity, while a strenuous exercise test in a control group of normal subjects did not show any change of blood viscosity.

These findings lent support to a relationship between the acute ischaemic process and the increase of blood viscosity, since only in the patients with an impaired regional circulation was the increase of the physical work followed by an increase of blood viscosity. The regional ischaemia due to the impaired metabolic balance, dependent on the reduced blood flow may be considered as the pathway leading to the increase of blood viscosity. Even if it is theoretically possible that a primary increase of blood viscosity induces ischaemia (Dormandy, 1970; Dintenfass, 1976), in our opinion the increase of blood viscosity in the patients with vascular disease appears to be the effect of the ischaemic process.

Some other information can be obtained by analysing the changes of the determinant factors of viscosity. In chronic vascular disease patients, the increase of blood viscosity appears related to a significant increase of haematocrit only in the patients with peripheral arterial occlusive disease. Neither in chronic coronary patients nor in peripheral arterial occlusive disease patients was plasma fibrinogen increased in a significant amount. In acute circulatory disease, haematocrit was significantly increased only in myocardial infarct.

The acute exercise-dependent increase of blood viscosity was not related to significant changes of haematocrit or of fibrinogen concentration. On the basis of these findings the possibility that several apparently different mechanisms may operate in chronic and acute states of circulatory disorders can be proposed.

The dependence of the increased blood viscosity on regional ischaemia appears supported by the investigation carried in our laboratory on the difference of viscosity values between the arterial and the venous blood of the same region. In the normal subject, the viscosity of the arterial blood is scarcely higher than the viscosity of the arterial blood of the same vascular area. In the patient with vascular disease, the regional arterio-venous difference of the blood viscosity appears higher than in the normal subject when measured in the affected region (Forconi *et al.* 1980). Moreover, this difference increases after exercise. These observations suggested that the increase of the blood viscosity is generated in the post-arterial vessels and probably in the microcirculatory tree. The increase of the viscosity might be due to the circulatory alterations at this level: thus, the flow decreases and the secondary metabolic imbalance can be regarded as the causal factor.

According to these findings, the cause of the increased viscosity in vascular disease seems to be due to some change in the red blood cells, leading to an increase of aggregability or to a decrease of deformability. The role of the haematocrit and fibrinogen concentration can be considered additional and dependent upon alterations of vessel permeability and on associated inflammation. The increase of erythrocyte aggregability may influence the blood flow in the large vessels by producing some change in the laminar and radial movement of the blood. The decrease of deformability will change the blood flow in small vessels and in the capillaries with an internal diameter which is less than the diameter of the erythrocytes.

These findings seem to agree with the theory proposed by Schmidt-Schoenbein (1976) on the role of blood viscosity, considered as a whole, in regulating blood flow. In normal conditions, the peripheral blood flow is mainly regulated by a metabolic mechanism:ischaemia induces the liberation of vasodilator mediators acting on the muscular cells of the distribution vessels by a rapid negative feed-back. In organic vascular disease this metabolic pathway is generally insufficient to cancel ischaemia: in this case the persistence of a low flow is followed by an increase of the aggregability and by a decrease of deformability of the red blood cells and consequently by an increase of blood viscosity. A positive feed-back leads to a progressive decrease of the blood flow thus inducing a progressive and self-maintaining deterioration of the microcirculation. According to this hypothesis, the blood outflow of the ischaemic region shows a marked hyperviscosity which is diluted to lower values when the blood is mixed in bigger vessels. Thus, the blood taken from the general circulation has a higher viscosity value than that of the control mean but probably lower than that of the blood taken directly from the ischaemic area.

In conclusion, from the pathophysiological point of view, the increase of blood viscosity in vascular patients must be interpreted as a change due to the progression of ischaemia, which results from the circulatory imbalance. On the other hand, it must be remembered that blood hyperviscosity can be regarded as a determinant variable of a positive feed-back which progressively lowers the circulation rate. Thus we can assign a double meaning to blood hyperviscosity in vascular disease. First, it is a sign of an impending ischaemic episode and therefore it can be considered a "risk factor". However, it is not a risk factor of developing vascular disease but of ischaemia, since hyperviscosity is associated with the onset of the ischaemic process. The second meaning concerns the role of blood hyperviscosity as a factor in a self-recruiting mechanism of the ischaemia.

REFERENCES

Ditensass, L. (1976). "Blood Microerheology. Viscosity Factors in Blood Flow, Ischaemia and Thrombosis." Butterworths, London.
Di Perri, T. (1979). *Angiology* 30, 480.
Di Perri, T., Forconi, S., Guerrini, M., Rossi, C. and Pecchi, S. (1977). *Bollettino della Società* Italiana di Cardiologia 22, 1138.
Dormandy, J. A. (1970). *Annals of the Royal College of Surgeons of England* 47, 211.
Forconi, S., Biasi, G., Guerrini, M., Ravelli, P., Rossi, C., Fenozzig and Pecchi, S. (1980). *Journal of Cardiovascular Surgery* (In press.)
Schmidt-Schoenbein, H. (1976). *In* "International Review of Physiology. Cardiovascular Physiology." (A. C. Guyton and A. V. Cowley, eds) Vol. 9, p. 1. University Park Press, Baltimore.

STUDY ON RED CELL FILTERABILITY AND 2-3 DPG AMONG DIABETIC PATIENTS WITH AND WITHOUT ARTERIOPATHY

C. Le Devehat, A. Lemoine, B. Cirette, M. Ramet and E. Roux

*Centre de Diabétologie et des Maladies de la Nutrition, C. H. Nevers,
Pougues les Eaux, France*

INTRODUCTION

Weed and La Celle's (1969) works have underlined the tight link that exists between the mechanical behaviour of the red cell membrane and its metabolism. The existence of spectrin within the erythrocyte membrane plays a prominent role. La Celle's work (1973) has shown that a decrease of the old erythrocyte deformability occurs due to a metabolic alteration, an erythrocyte ATP decrease (1.1 ± 0.2 mm/l for 1.6 ± 0.3 mm/l in the young red cells) and a decreased 2-3 DPG level (4.5 ± 0.7 mm/l for 5.4 ± 0.6 mm/l).

The ATP/Ca^{++} ratio is five times less in the old red cells than in the young ones. These results permit us to postulate that metabolic exhaustion is one of the more likely mechanisms in the alteration of the red cell filterability. Weed and La Celle's observations (1969) about the influence of pH and oxygen partial pressure on the deformability suggest that hypoxia and acidosis, conditions seen in diabetes mellitus, make it an interesting study model. Chanutin and Curnish (1967), Benesch and Benesch (1967) as well as Ditzel (1972) have shown that the haemoglobin affinity for oxygen is related to the intraerythrocyte level of the organic phosphates, mainly to the 2-3 DPG level but also to the ATP level. The structural modification of the microcirculation of diabetic subjects that appears at the very beginning of the illness, causes a relative state of hypoxia. The result of acute hypoxia, proven by various authors, is first a vasodilatation and increase in 2-3 DPG, which allows a better transport and release of oxygen.

Serono Symposium No. 37, "Vascular Occlusion: Epidemiological, Pathophysiological and Therapeutic Aspects", edited by M. Tesi and J. Dormany, 1981. Academic Press, London and New York.

Kanter *et al.* (1975) have shown that diabetic subjects with arterial disorders have an increase of 2-3 DPG level. The same patients, with or without arterial disorders, also have an alteration of the erythrocyte filterability. This study has been made to try to determine the relationship between the "tissue hypoxia indicators" (2-3 DPG and red cell filterability) for a diabetic subject suffering from different stages of peripheral arterial disorders. The existence of a tissue hypoxia due either to a micro- or macro-angiopathy or to a metabolic deficiency has been considered as an aetiological factor in the development of the lesions.

MATERIALS AND METHODS

To study the 2-3 DPG variations, erythrocyte red cell filterability variations and the possible relation between these two parameters, we have studied:

GROUP A. a reference group of 34 subjects (23 women and 11 men) aged from 20 to 50 years old, non-smokers, none obese, without any personal or family history of diabetes mellitus, any medical treatment and exempt from any arterial signs.

GROUP B. 23 insulin dependent and non-insulin dependent subjects without any perceptible arterial abnormality, without any coronary history, with a normal ECG and with no peripheral neuropathy.

GROUP C. 30 insulin dependent and non-insulin dependent subjects suffering from a very severe acute lower limb arteriopathy.

The erythrocyte red cell filterability was measured on whole blood, according to Reid *et al.* (1976). The samplings and the measurements have always been made by the same technicians and at the same hour.

Filters The filtering membrane is made of polycarbonate with 5 μ pores. Each membrane has an average of 4×10^5 pores per cm^2 (Nucleopore corporation 7035 Commerce Circle Neasanton CA 94566 USA). The thickness of the membrane is 10 μ. The variation percentage of the pores is of 5.5%. For this study, we used the same batch of filters (54 A8 A29).

Results The uncorrected results represent the time of filtration in seconds of 1 ml of blood. To make interpretation easier, we give the result as a flow: 1/TFE × 10^3. TFE means the time (in seconds) of filtration of 1 ml of blood. The erythrocyte 2-3 DPG level is measured according to Ericson and Verdier's (1972) enzymatic method. The statistical analysis has been made by Student's *t* test.

RESULTS

2-3 DPG Level

All the previous work about the non-acidotic diabetic's erythrocyte 2-3 DPG level report varying results (Fig. 1). Alberti *et al.* (1972) finds a similar 2-3 DPG level when comparing normal and diabetic subjects. Ditzel and Standl (1975) consider that, for a newly-diagnosed diabetic, the 2-3 DPG level is higher than for non-diabetic subjects. They found it much higher for a non-keto-acidotic

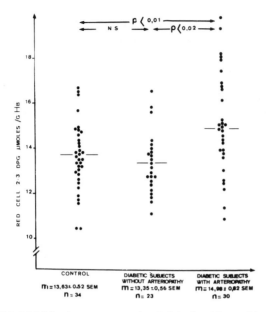

Fig. 1. Red cell 2-3 DPG levels among normal and diabetic subjects with and without arteriopathy.

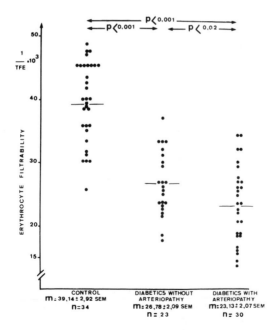

Fig. 2. Erythrocyte filtrability among normal and diabetic subjects with and without arteriopathy.

ambulatory diabetic subject. These differences are related to the metabolic activity and insulin activity when the sample is drawn, without any relationship to the blood glucose level (Ditzel, 1979). Figure 1 shows that diabetic subjects without arteriopathy have a 2-3 DPG level which is slightly lower than that of the normal subject, although this difference is not significant. These results agree with Alberti *et al.* (1972) and Kanter *et al.* (1975). In contrast, the 2-3 DPG level for a diabetic subject suffering from a severe arteriopathy is significantly higher than the levels in Group A and Group B.

Red Cell Filterability

Our results confirm those of various authors with a reduction of the filterability which is significant between Groups A, B and C (*P* varying from 0.02 to 0.001): normal subjects, 39.14 ± 2.92 s.e.; diabetic subjects without arteriopathy: 26.78 ± 2.09 s.e.; and diabetic subjects with a severe arteriopathy: 25.13 ± 2.07 s.e. (Fig. 2).

2-3 DPG and Red Cell Filterability

The study of the correlation between the 2-3 DPG level and the filterability shows a close positive correlation between these two parameters. We notice a parallel variation of the 2-3 DPG level and the filterability. These results agree with those of others. For a normal subject, it seems that the filterability is dependent mostly on the red cell ATP but also on the 2-3 DPG level (Fig. 3). Among group B the correlation between the 2-3 DPG level and the filterability is still very close. Here we find the 2-3 DPG compensation as part of a situation

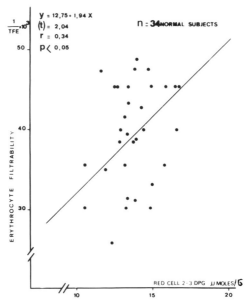

Fig. 3. Correlation between increment in red cell 2-3 DPG and increment of erythrocyte filtrability (control group).

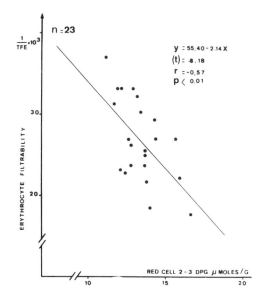

Fig. 4. Correlation between levels of red cell 2–3 DPG and erythrocyte filtrability (diabetic patients without arteriopathy).

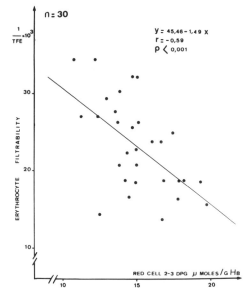

Fig. 5. Correlation between levels of red cell 2–3 DPG and erythrocyte filtrability (diabetic patients with arteriopathy).

of relative hypoxia. The relationship between the 2–3 DPG level and the filterability is reversed in this group of diabetics: a decreased filterability corresponds to an increased erythrocyte 2–3 DPG level. Among group C, we can see the same correlation between the 2-3 DPG level and the filterability as in group B although the significance is more distinct (P 0.001) (Figs 4 and 5).

DISCUSSION AND CONCLUSION

Various works have shown that red cell filterability is directly related to the actin-spectrin system, which is regulated by the ATP level. 2-3 DPG disorders effect the red cell membrane characteristics as well as the haemoglobin level.

Our results show an important increase of the 2-3 DPG level among diabetic subjects with a severe arteriopathy. In the same way, the 2-3 DPG level decreases in diabetics without arteriopathy. We also notice a significant decrease of the filterability among these two groups. Chanutin and Curnish (1967), Benesch and Benesch (1967), Kanter *et al.* (1975) and Ditzel (1975) have shown that the Rapoport Luebering's pathway is a compensative metabolic mechanism to hypoxia. An alteration of this metabolic system carries very important consequences for the red cell. Red cell filterability is certainly partly under the influence of some metabolic phenomena. In diabetes mellitus, haemoglobin A_{ic} or a poorly-regulated insulin control produces a 2-3 DPG decrease, first by a structural modification, but also by an important decrease of the organic phosphates which are necessary for 2-3 DPG synthesis and ATP production. These red cell alterations modify the red cell viscosity and also the available energy in the form of ATP. Among group C, the increased 2-3 DPG produces a decreased filterability and this can be explained as a physiological adjustment to chronic or acute hypoxia. The work of Asakura *et al.* (1968) agrees with these conclusions and they note that red cell glycolysis is stimulated by hypoxia. Diabetic's red cell seems to be characterized by a metabolic degradation, producing changes mainly in the oxygen transport capacity but also in its filterability. These metabolic modifications are noticeable as soon as the illness is diagnosed. This state produces more flexible red cells due to an increased 2-3 DPG level. The 2-3 DPG transitory decreases could be due to inappropriate insulin control. An optimum metabolic regulation of blood glucose or of the red cells glycolysis produces a decreased haemoglobin A_{ic} level, and increased 2-3 DPG and ATP levels. These factors improve the oxygen releasing capacity and the red cell filterability as well.

REFERENCES

Alberti, K. G. M. M., Emerson Pauline, M., Darley, J. H. and Hockaday, T. D. R. (1972). *Lancet* 843.
Asakura, T., Soto, Y., Minakami, S. and Yochikawa, H. (1966). *J. Biochem.* **59**, 524
Benesch, R. and Benesch, R. E. (1967). *Biochem. Biophys. Res. Commun.* **26**, 162.
Chanutin, A. and Curnish, R. R. (1967). *Arch. Biochem. Biophys.* **121**, 96.
Ditzel, J. (1972). *Lancet* 721-723.
Ditzel, J. (1979). *J. A. D.* 47
Ditzel, J. and Standl, E. (1975). *Acta med. Scand.* **578**, 59.
Ericson, A. and Verdier. (1972). *Scand. J. Clin. Lab. Inv.* **29**, 85.
Kanter, Y., Samuel Bessman, P. and Alice Bessman, N. (1975). *Diabetes* **24**, 8, 724.

La Celle, P. L., Kirkpatrick, F. H. and Udkow, M. (1973). *In* "Recent Advances in Membrane and Metabolic Research." 49. (E. Gerlach ed) G. Thieme Verlag.

Reid, H. L., Barnes, A. J., Lock, P. J., Dormandy, J. A. and Dormandy, T. L. (1976). *J. Clin. Path.* **29**, (9), 855.

Weed, R. I., La Celle, P. L. *et al.* (1969). *J. Clin. Invest.* **48**, 795

Yoshikawa, H. and Minakami, S. (1968). *Folia Hemato.* **89**, 357.

THE ASSOCIATION OF PLASMA FIBRINOGEN WITH ARTERIAL DISEASE

G. D. O. Lowe, M. M. Drummond, C. D. Forbes and C. R. M. Prentice

University Department of Medicine, Royal Infirmary, Glasgow, UK

Many studies have been published showing that persons with clinical manifestations of occlusive arterial disease (coronary, cerebral or peripheral) have higher plasma fibrinogen levels than control subjects. Some prospective studies have suggested that increased fibrinogen levels may also predict clinical complications (Hamer *et al.*, 1973; Dormandy *et al.*, 1973). Dormandy (1978) has suggested that increased fibrinogen may promote clinical manifestations of arterial disease by increasing blood viscosity and hence reducing blood flow.

If the raised fibrinogen levels promote arterial events by increasing blood viscosity or through other mechanisms, then therapeutic reduction of fibrinogen levels is an attractive concept. However, increased fibrinogen levels may be a result or "marker" of arterial disease. Alternatively, the association of fibrinogen and arterial disease may be coincidental, in that each is associated with other factors. With this possibility in mind, we have related plasma viscosity and blood viscosity to some established "risk factors" for arterial events.

MATERIALS AND METHODS

Fibrinogen was measured in citrated plasma by a thrombin time method. Plasma viscosity was measured at 37°C in a BSM3 capillary viscometer. Blood viscosity was measured at 37°C, shear rate 100 s^{-1}, in a rotational viscometer and corrected to a standard haematocrit of 0.45. Differences in means were compared using Student t test.

Serono Symposium No. 37, "Vascular Occlusion: Epidemiological, Pathophysiological and Therapeutic Aspects", edited by M. Tesi and J. Dormany, 1981. Academic Press, London and New York.

RESULTS

In all our studies, we found correlations between fibrinogen, plasma viscosity and blood viscosity ($r > 0.38, P < 0.02$). Table I shows the relationship of the blood variables to selected risk factors.

Age. In a group of 90 healthy men aged 16-80 years, fibrinogen and viscosity were significantly higher in those aged 45 or more, compared with those under 45 years.

Cigarette Smoking. Within the same group, cigarette smokers had higher levels of fibrinogen and viscosity than non-smokers.

Oestrogen Use. Within a group of 50 healthy women, age 18-30, fibrinogen and viscosity were significantly higher in subjects who had been taking oestrogen-containing oral contraceptives for at least 3 months, compared with women who had never taken oestrogens.

Diabetes. Fibrinogen and viscosity were increased in 38 male diabetics aged 16-50 years, compared with matched non-diabetics.

Table I. Fibrinogen and viscosity related to risk factors.

Group	Number	Plasma Fibrinogen g/I	Plasma Viscosity cP	Blood Viscosity cP
Age under 45	45	2.46	1.36	6.70
Age 45 or over	45	3.11	1.42	6.88
		***	*	*
Smokers	45	3.01	1.41	6.88
Non-smokers	45	2.56	1.37	6.69
		***	*	*
Oestrogen users	25	2.71	1.39	6.84
Non-users	25	2.31	1.35	6.57
		*	*	*
Diabetics	38	3.17	1.41	7.13
Non-diabetics	38	2.54	1.34	6.78
		***	**	**
High cholesterol	21	3.51	—	—
Normal cholesterol	21	2.47	—	—
		**		
Coronary stenosis:				
2 or 3 vessel	26	3.19	1.42	6.97
0 or 1 vessel	24	2.76	1.39	6.72
Controls	25	2.70	1.38	6.75
		*		*

$*P < 0.05; ** P < 0.01; *** P < 0.001$; cP = centipoise.

Hypercholesterolaemia. Plasma fibrinogen was higher in 21 patients with primary Type II hyperlipoproteinaemia, aged 16–55 years, compared with matched controls with normal cholesterol levels.

Extent of Coronary Artery Stenosis. Within a group of 50 men, aged 30–55 years, undergoing coronary arteriography for the assessment of chest pain, fibrinogen and blood viscosity were higher in those with stenosis (lumen occlusion of at least 50%) of 2 or 3 major coronary arteries, compared with either those with stenosis of 0 or 1 coronary vessels or compared with control subjects without chest pain. Plasma viscosity was also increased in this group, but the difference was not statistically significant ($P > 0.05$).

DISCUSSION

Our results are supported by epidemiological studies of unselected populations which have also found significant associations of plasma fibrinogen with age and smoking (Meade *et al.*, 1979), use of oral contraceptives (Meade *et al.*, 1976), and hyperglycaemia and hypercholesterolaemia (Korsan-Bengtsen *et al.*, 1972), as well as other risk factors such as hypertension (Korsan-Bengtsen *et al.*, 1972) and obesity (Meade *et al.*, 1979). In addition, we have shown that the elevations of fibrinogen are sufficient to increase plasma viscosity and blood viscosity (measured at the arterial shear rate of 100 s^{-1}). We must therefore ask the question, is the association of fibrinogen and viscosity with arterial disease a coincidence, resulting from mutual association with these "risk factors"? We have also shown a relation between fibrinogen and viscosity on the one hand, and the extent of coronary artery disease on the other. Is this relationship cause, consequence or coincidence? Do the subjects with extensive coronary artery disease have high fibrinogen because of multiple, additive associations with other risk factors?

Whatever the explanation for the association of fibrinogen with arterial disease, increased fibrinogen levels may play a part in promoting clinical events arising from ischaemia. Increased blood viscosity may be the critical determinant of blood flow in some circumstances, and the association of blood viscosity with extensive arterial stenosis may then be a dangerous combination. While there is little evidence that increased blood viscosity promotes atherogenesis, the concept that plasma fibrinogen infiltrates the arterial wall and contributes to vessel wall lesions has recently received some support (Smith *et al.*, 1976). *In vitro* experiments have associated increasing plasma fibrinogen with increasing platelet adhesion to collagen (Lyman *et al.*, 1971) and increasing deposition of platelets and fibrin in thrombi (Schultz *et al.*, 1978). If these relationships apply *in vivo*, then hyperfibrinogenaemia may play a role in clinical events arising from thrombus formation. Platelet aggregates may play a role in sudden coronary death and transient cerebral ischaemic attacks: we have recently described an association between plasma fibrinogen and platelet aggregates measured by a formalin fixation method (Lowe *et al.*, 1979).

In conclusion, there is evidence for an association of plasma fibrinogen and blood viscosity with arterial disease. We must keep in mind several explanations for this relationship. There are also several mechanisms by which increased fibrinogen may promote ischaemia.

ACKNOWLEDGEMENTS

We thank Dr J. C. Barbenel, Dr W. G. Manderson, Dr A. C. McCuish, Professor T. D. V. Lawrie, Dr A. R. Lorimer and Dr I. Hutton for their help in these studies.

REFERENCES

Dormandy, J. A. (1978). *In* "International Conference on Atherosclerosis" (L. A. Carlson, R. Paoletti, C. R. Sirtori and G. Weber, eds) 409–416, Raven Press, New York.
Dormandy, J. A., Hou.e, E., Khattab, A. M., Arrowsmith, D. E. and Dormandy, T. L. (1973). *Br. Med. J.* 4, 581.
Hamer, H. D., Ashton, F. and Meynell, M. J. (1973). *Br. J. Surg.* 60, 386.
Korsan-Bengtsen, K., Wilhelmsen, L. and Tibblin, G. (1972). *Thrombosis et Diathesis Haemorrhagica* 28, 99.
Lowe, G. D. O., Reavey, M. M., Johnston, R. V., Forbes, C. D. and Prentice, C. R. M. (1979). *Thromb. Res.* 14, 377.
Lyman, B., Rosenberg, L. and Karpatkin, S. (1971). *J. Clin. Invest.* 50, 1854.
Meade, T. W., Brozovic, M., Charkrabarti, R., Howarth, D. J., North, W. R. S. and Stirling, Y. (1976). *Br. J. Haemat.* 34, 353.
Meade, T. W., Chakrabarti, R., Haines, A. P., North, W. R. S. and Stirling, Y. (1979). *Br. Med. J.* 1, 153.
Schultz, J. S., Ciarkowski, A. A., Lindenauer, S. M. and Penner, J. A. (1978). *Trans. Am. Soc. Artif. Intern. Org.* 24, 565.
Smith, E. B., Alexander, K. M. and Massie, I. B. (1976). *Atherosclerosis* 23, 19.

VARIATIONS IN VISCOSITY AND HbA_{1c} IN PATIENTS WITH DIABETIC MICROANGIOPATHY

P. Pola, L. Savi, M. Grilli and R. Flore

Department of Internal Medicine and the Center for the Study, Prophylaxis and Therapy of Angiopathies, Catholic University of the Sacred Heart, Rome, Italy

The outstanding advances achieved in the knowledge of hemoglobins allows us to discuss them with greater clarity in terms of molecular biology, structure and physiopathology. The recent findings about glycosylated hemoglobins, apart from their fascinating theoretical outlooks, have stimulated the development of a new and interesting study, extremely important from many clinical and social points of view.

After the sixth month of life, three physiological types of hemoglobins can be found: A, A_2, F (Cerami and Koenig, 1978), which comprise respectively 90, 2.5, 0.5% of total hemoglobin (Bunn *et al.*, 1978); they differ in their polypeptide chains, whose synthesis is controlled by different genes. In the adult, several secondary types of hemoglobin are found, A_{1a}, A_{1b}, A_{1c}, which are defined by specific electrophoretic and chromatographic features (Allen *et al.*, 1958); these hemoglobins account respectively for 1.6, 0.8, 4% of the total Hb value.

Among the secondary hemoglobins, HbA_{1c} is surely the most important, not only because it represents the major fraction (Bunn *et al.*, 1976), but because its value rises significantly in experimental and clinical diabetes mellitus (Koenig and Cerami, 1975; Rahbar, 1968; Trivelli *et al.*, 1971). In physiological conditions, HbA_{1c} is synthetized (Holmquist and Schroeder, 1965) by means of condensation of a molecule of HbA with a molecule of glucose, through a slow progressive and irreversible process (Bunn *et al.*, 1976; Koenig and Cerami, 1975) lasting the whole lifetime of the erythrocyte, i.e. 120 days (Bunn *et al.*, 1978). Therefore, HbA_{1c} concentration is constantly lower in the younger red blood cells if compared with the older ones. This Hb is produced by a post-synthetic modification of HbA,

Serono Symposium No. 37, "Vascular Occlusion: Epidemiological, Pathophysiological and Therapeutic Aspects", edited by M. Tesi and J. Dormany, 1981. Academic Press, London and New York.

since a molecule of glucose links to the terminal amino group of the valine of the beta chain (Bunn *et al.*, 1976).

Recently, two forms of HbA_{1a} have been identified, HbA_{1a_1} and HbA_{1a_2}; HbA_{1a_1} is marked by a fructose-1.6-DP connected to valine, while HbA_{1a_2} attaches a glucose-6-P (Cole *et al.*, 1977; McDonald *et al.*, 1978). Our knowledge about the synthesis of HbA_{1c} is still incomplete, and recent views suggest a non-enzymatic addition of glucose to HbA or a dephosphorylation of a compound of G-6-P and HbA_{1a_2}. The first contention is supported by the very slow synthesis of the molecule and by the fact that HbA_{1c} levels are higher in diabetes, while G-6-P is normal. This may prove that apart from an enzymatic glycosylation of proteins, which plays a major role in maintaining the integrity of cell membranes and helping the protein secretion in the extracellular space, a non-enzymatic glycosylation of proteins can also occur (Bunn *et al.*, 1978).

Human Hb is involved in this kind of reaction: Hb glycosylation is independent from genetic control (Tattersal *et al.*, 1975) and directly correlated to the intra-erythrocytic content of glucose per unit of time (Bunn *et al.*, 1976). In fact, several experimental works have suggested that plasma glucose level is the fundamental factor regulating intraerythrocytic synthesis of HbA_{1c} (Bunn *et al.*, 1976; Fitzgibbons *et al.*, 1976; Gonen *et al.*, 1977; Graf and Porte, 1977; Welch and Boucher, 1978).

It is evident that poorly controlled diabetes is associated with an excessive rate of synthesis of HbA_{1c}, which appears to be strictly correlated with the degree of metabolic imbalance (Koenig *et al.*, 1976). This phenomenon occurs because in diabetes, glucose metabolism is shifted towards insulin-independent pathways, which causes an increase in glycoprotein synthesis, in particular an increase in glycosylated hemoglobins. This is why in uncontrolled diabetes high levels of HbA_{1c} are observed.

HbA_{1c} hardly reacts with 2-3 DPG (Bunn and Brihel, 1970), and therefore it has an increased O_2 affinity if compared with HbA, while its capacity to release O_2 to peripheral tissues decreases. Therefore, the reduction of tissue oxygenation in diabetes could be explained partly by high levels of HbA_{1c} (Ditzel *et al.*, 1973).

In physiological conditions, hypoxia is counteracted by an increase of 2-3 DPG; such a compensatory mechanism is upset by high levels of HbA_{1c}. 2-3 DPG attaches to the beta chain of hemoglobin, increasing oxygen release. But since, in diabetic patients, the terminal amino-group of this chain is occupied by glucose, attachment of 2-3 DPG becomes impossible (Holmquist and Schroeder, 1966). Thus the increased biosynthesis of HbA_{1c} in diabetes seems to be directly involved in the etiopathogenesis of the microangiopathy, because it affects the processes of transport and release of O_2 to peripheral tissues and presumably leads to an increased thickness of the basement membrane.

From the above considerations, we assume that the evaluation of Hb-glycosylation may represent a very important parameter in clinical practice, since it could detect successive variations of blood glucose level (Gonen *et al.*, 1977), give information about the effectiveness of the treatment (Graf and Porte, 1977) and the onset of complications. There is no general agreement about the association of diabetes without vascular complications and blood hyperviscosity (Cogan *et al.*, 1961; Dintenfass, 1964; Ditzel, 1968; McMillan, 1974; Zöller and Gross, 1976), while such increase in viscosity is commonly assumed when microangiopathy is evident.

Several biochemical considerations suggest that humoral and rheological abnormalities can lead to hyperviscosity even when angiopathy is not detectable. Such abnormalities consist of alterations in serum protein concentration and molecular structure and in abnormal rheological features of the erythrocytes (Schmid-Schönbein and Wells, 1969; Marchesi and Steers, 1968; Weed *et al.*, 1969). The latter phenomenon has always been easily detected in diabetes, and it has been attributed to variations in aggregating property and deformability due to biochemical alterations, such as ketoacidosis (Ditzel, 1959; Little *et al.*, 1974; Volger *et al.*, 1975), abnormal level of free fatty acids, dehydration, all strictly related to the metabolic inbalance of the patients.

Erythrocytes are the blood fraction which mostly influences blood viscosity; their aggregating capacity relies upon an interaction between their surface and plasma proteins such as globulins, lipoproteins, fibrinogen, etc. On the other hand, red cells deformability is influenced by: (1) osmolarity of the medium; (2) pH; (3) composition of the erythrocyte membrane (Nakao, 1974; Weed *et al.*, 1969). The molecular basis of the regulation of their deformability lies in the intra-erythrocytic content of ATP, Ca^{++}, Mg^{++} (Weed *et al.*, 1969), which act by influencing the sol-gel transformation of "spectrin", a fibrillar protein (Marchesi and Steers, 1969). A decreased concentration of ATP provokes increased rigidity of the membrane of red blood cells and thus a reduction of flexibility (Nakao *et al.*, 1960). Among the intrinsic factors which regulate the internal viscosity of erythrocytes, the content, the type and the state of the hemoglobin play an important role. Mean cytoplasmatic concentration of Hb is 33%; if it could exist as a pure solution, Hb would have a viscosity 10 000 times greater than blood viscosity (Dintenfass, 1964). The plasticity of red blood cells is therefore assured by the crystal-like suspension of hemoglobin. Hb molecules are arranged in a peculiar fashion, so that little variations of intra-erythrocytic concentration provoke remarkable changes in viscosity (Schmid-Schönbein and Wells, 1969).

The type of Hb itself plays an important role in determining the viscosity of erythrocytes: as a matter of fact, all hemoglobinopathies are associated with increased internal viscosity of red cells, due to alteration of the cell membrane (Charache *et al.*, 1967; Murphy, 1968; Weed, 1970; Weis, 1965). There are many reasons to suggest that variations in hemoglobin are associated with an appreciable alteration in viscosity. This could occur in diabetes mellitus, where the content of HbA_{1c} is significantly increased. In fact, the structural features and the biological properties we have just discussed strongly suggest a direct influence of this hemoglobin upon the complex mechanisms regulating blood viscosity. Therefore, the aim of the present study was to investigate the correlation between HbA_{1c} and blood viscosity.

MATERIAL AND METHODS

We examined 20 male diabetic patients aged between 40 and 75 years. Ten of them had vascular disease stage II and III, according to the Fontaine classification; 10 of them were affected by adult type diabetes mellitus, dating from a maximum of 20 years to a minimum of 5 years, but they had no sign of angiopathy. These patients were admitted in a state of metabolic decompensation, and were treated with oral anti-diabetic drugs or insulin and suitable diet. In each patient, several periodic controls were performed for serum glucose profile, fractionated glyco-suria, HbA_1, hematocrit value and blood viscosity. Such controls were repeated at 10-day intervals for a period of 30–60 days.

Blood viscosity was evaluated by means of a Wells Brookfield LTV viscometer (Microcone plate viscometer); the 1.5 ml sample was kept at $37°C$ by a thermo-static pump (Colora mod.N3). We utilized the following shear rates: 230, 115, 46, 23, 11.5 s^{-1}. Reading of each sample took place after about 1 min of stabilization at a shear rate of 230 s^{-1}.

Blood viscosity and HbA_1 samples were drawn under fasting conditions, by means of heparinized syringes. We considered HbA_1 level as an index of diabetic control: HbA_1 was determined by a rapid and repeatable method (Gonen *et al.*, 1977).

HbA_1 is a cumulative fraction of HbA, which includes secondary components such as $HbA_{1a+b+c+d}$. While HbA_{1a} and HbA_{1b} levels are quantitatively constant, both in diabetic patients (2–3%) and in non-diabetic (1–2%); HbA_{1c} is highly variable (Kynock and Lehmann, 1977; Trivelli *et al.*, 1971). Thus, we assumed that the values obtained by our methodology would be indicative mainly of HbA_{1c}.

We utilized 100 ml of heparinized blood plus 500 ml of hemolysing agent (polyoxyethylene ether in aqueous solution), in order to hemolyse red blood cells and obtain hemoglobin. A 100 ml of hemolysate was introduced into a disposable chromatographic column, filled with a cation-exchange resin, weakly acid, and kept at room temperature. Fifteen minutes later, 10 ml of developing-eluting reagent were added to the column (buffer phosphate pH 6.7; 0.065% KCN), in order to separate the fast hemoglobin from the slow hemoglobin. Fast hemoglobin, eluted from the column directly into counting vials, and total Hb, prepared with 20 ml of hemolysate plus 10 ml of developing-eluting reagent, were measured by means of a spectrophotometer at 415 nm, versus blank vials containing eluting reagent only.

A percentage of HbA_1 was obtained by calculating the ratio between the optical density of HbA_1 and the optical density of total Hb, multiplied by 5. The result was multiplied by 100.

$$\frac{HbA_1 \text{ fraction (OD)}}{5 \times \text{total Hb (OD)}} \times 100 = \% \, HbA_1.$$

Hematocrit values were measured by means of Hemalog 8 Technicon.

RESULTS AND CONCLUSIONS

Table I shows the mean values of maximum and minimum levels of HbA_1, blood viscosity and hematocrit, the mean values of their difference and the percentage variations, in the group of diabetic patients without vascular disease. Statistical significance was verified by Student's *t* test on coupled data. A correlation between the decrease of HbA_1 levels and the decrease of blood viscosity is shown, while hematocrit does not significantly change.

A similar trend can be found in Table II, which describes the group of diabetic patients affected by angiopathy. In both groups of patients, the significance of blood viscosity is higher when shear rates are lower.

Table I. Diabetic subjects without angiopathy.

| | HbA$_1$ % | \multicolumn{5}{c}{Blood viscosity cp s^{-1}} | PCV % |
		230	115	46	23	11.5	
Average maximum values	12.77	4.76	5.57	6.97	9.02	10.47	38.4
Average minimum values	9.01	4.42	5.15	6.1	7.23	8.39	40.2
Average variations	− 3.76	−0.34	−0.42	− 0.87	− 1.79	− 2.08	+1.84
Percentage variations	−29.44	−7.14	−7.54	−12.48	−19.84	−19.86	+4.78
P	< 0.001	< 0.20	< 0.20	< 0.05	< 0.02	< 0.005	<0.60

Table II. Diabetic subjects without angiopathy.

| | HbA$_1$ % | \multicolumn{5}{c}{Blood viscosity cp s^{-1}} | PCV % |
		230	115	46	23	11.5	
Average maximum values	13.41	4.8	5.43	6.46	7.54	9.54	39.2
Average minimum values	9.21	4.35	4.83	5.5	6.41	7.8	38.6
Average variations	− 4.2	−0.45	− 0.6	− 0.96	− 1.13	− 1.73	− 0.6
Percentage variations	−31.3	−9.37	−11.04	−14.86	−14.98	−18.13	− 1.53
P	< 0.001	< 0.20	< 0.10	< 0.05	< 0.05	< 0.01	< 0.90

In Figs 1 and 2, in order to make the results clearer, the same data are related in diagrams. It is evident that HbA$_1$ values in both groups decrease in compensated diabetic patients, and that HbA$_1$ correlates significantly with blood viscosity at lower shear rates. In fact when HbA$_1$ values are higher, blood viscosity is higher, and vice versa.

In conclusion, our present preliminary results pointed out the presence of high blood viscosity even in diabetic patients without angiopathy. There is no universal agreement on this matter, since some authors think that blood viscosity is higher only when angiopathy is evident. Furthermore, we think that blood viscosity in the same group correlates with the degree of control of the diabetes and with HbA$_{1c}$ levels. Similar behavior was observed in the group of diabetic patients with angiopathy, so that no clear differences could be found between the two groups when referring to the chosen parameters.

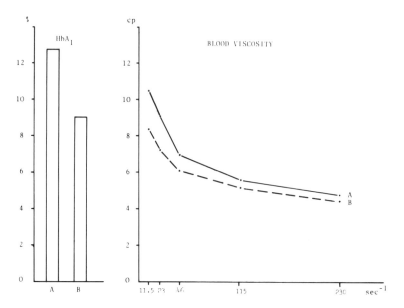

Fig. 1. Diabetic subjects without angiopathy. A: average maximum values; B: average minimum values.

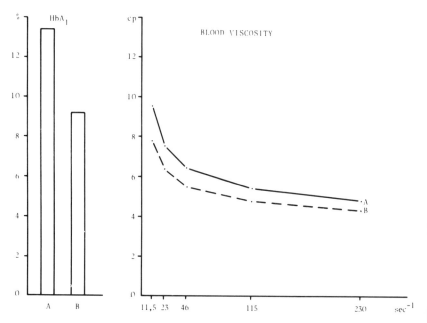

Fig. 2. Diabetic subjects with angiopathy. A: average maximum values; B: average minimum values.

We suggest that HbA_{1c} may have a direct influence on blood viscosity. In uncontrolled diabetes, when a high rate of synthesis of HbA_{1c} occurs, qualitative and quantitative alterations of the normal intra-erythrocytic content of Hb take place, so that the internal red cell viscosity increases. This contention is furthermore supported by the fact that blood viscosity is higher when shear rates are lower, i.e. when red blood cells play the major role in determining viscosity.

The increased viscosity due to excess biosynthesis of HbA_{1c} can actually be explained as the result of different processes:

a. alteration of the endothelium due to hypoxia, since HbA_{1c} is less capable of releasing O_2;

b. decreased flexibility of the erythrocyte membrane and subsequent decreased deformability of red cells;

c. increase in total RBC count as a compensatory reaction to the decreased peripheral release of oxygen (though the present study we could not observe any significant change in hematocrit values).

Therefore, we suggest that strict control of blood glucose level may have an effective role in preventing high blood viscosity, blocking the chain of events which leads to increased synthesis of glycoproteins; as a result, excessive synthesis of glycosylated Hb would be avoided and the rheologic and nutritional abnormalities related to this Hb would be prevented.

REFERENCES

Allen, D. V., Schroeder, W. B. and Balog, J. (1958). *J. Am. Chem. Soc.* **80**, 1628.
Bunn, H. F. and Brihel, R. W. (1970). *J. Clin. Invest.* **49**, 1088.
Bunn, H. F., Gabbay, K. H. and Gallop, P. M. (1978). *Science* **200**, 21.
Bunn, H. F., Haney, D. N., Kamin, S., Gabbay, K. H. and Gallop, P. M. (1976). *J. Clin. Invest.* **57**, 1652.
Cerami, A. and Koenig, R. (1978). *Br. J. Haematol.* **38**, 1.
Charache, S., Conley, C. L., Wangh, D. F., Ugoretz, R. J. and Spurrel, J. (1967). *J. Clin. Invest.* **46**, 1795.
Cogan, D. G., Merola, L. and Laibson, P. R. (1961). *Diabetes* **10**, 393.
Cole, R. A., Bunn, H. F. and Scheldner, J. S. (1977). *Diabetes* **1** (Suppl.) 392.
Dintenfass, L. (1964). *Acta Haemat.* **32**, 299.
Ditzel, J. (1959). *Acta Med. Scand.* **164b**, 43.
Ditzel, J. (1968). *Dan. Med. Bull.* **15**, 49.
Ditzel, J., Andersen, H. and Dangaard Peters, N. (1973). *Lancet* **2**, 1034.
Fitzgibbons, J. F., Koler, R. D. and Jones, R. T. (1976). *J. Clin. Invest.* **58**, 820.
Gonen, R., Rubinstein, A. H., Rochman, A., Tanega, S. P. and Horwith, D. L. (1977). *Lancet* **2**, 734.
Graf, R. and Porte, D. (1977). *Diabetes* **26** Suppl. I.
Holmquist, W. R. and Schroeder, W. A. (1965). *Biochemistry* **5**, 2504.
Holmquist, W. R. and Schroeder, W. A. (1966). *Biochemistry* **5**, 2489.
Koenig, R. J. and Cerami, A. (1975). *Proc. Natn. Acad. Sci. U.S.A.* **72**, 3687.
Koenig, R. J., Aranjo, D. C. and Cerami, A. (1976). *Diabetes* **25**, 1.
Kynock, P. A. M. and Lehmann, H. (1977). *Lancet* **2**, 16.

Little, H. L., Sacks, A. H. and Zweng, H. C. (1974). *XXII Congr. Int. d'Ophtalmologie* Paris.
Marchesi, V. T. and Steers, E. Jr. (1968). *Science* 159, 203.
McDonald, M. J., Shapiro, R., Bleichman, M., Solway, J. and Bunn, H. F. (1978). *J. Biol. Chem.* 253, 2327.
McMillan, D. E. (1970). *Diabetologie* 6, 597.
McMillan, D. E. (1974). *J. Clin. Invest.* 53, 1071.
Murphy, J. R. (1968). *J. Clin. Invest.* 47, 1483.
Nakao, M. (1974). *Verlag Urban* (H. Yoshikawa and S. M. Rapaport eds.) pp. 35–54 Schwarzenberg, München.
Nakao, M., Nakao, T. and Yamazoe, S. (1960). *Nature* 187, 945.
Rahbar, S. (1968). *Clin. Chim. Acta* 22, 296.
Schmid-Schönbein, H. and Wells, R. (1969). *Pflüger's Arch.* 307, 59.
Tattersal, R. B., Pyche, D. A., Ranney, H. M. and Bruckheimer, S. M. (1975). *New Engl. J. Med.* 293, 1171.
Trivelli, L. A., Ranney, H. M. and Lai, N. T. (1971). *New Engl. J. Med.* 284, 353.
Volger, E., Schmid-Schönlein, H., Von Gosen, J., Klose, H. J. and Kline, K. A. (1975). *Pflüger's Arch.* 354, 319.
Weed, R. I., Le Celle, P. L. and Merrill, E. W. (1969). *J. Clin. Invest.* 48, 795.
Weed, R. I. (1970). *Am. J. Med.* 49, 147.
Weis, L. (1965). *J. Cell Biol.* 26, 735.
Welch, S. G. and Boucher, B. J. (1978). *Diabetologie* 14, 209.
Zöller, H. and Gross, W. (1976). *Münch. Med. Wschr.* 118, 493.

EFFECT OF POLYUNSATURATED PHOSPHATIDYLCHOLINE INFUSION ON DEFORMABILITY AND LIPID COMPOSITION OF ERYTHROCYTES

G. Salvioli and A. Mambrini

Institute of Clinical Medicine, University of Modena, Modena, Italy

A reduced red cell (RC) deformability causes impairment of blood flow through the microcirculation where the capillary channels are frequently half the diameter of the individual erythrocytes. RC deformability may be evaluated using a filtration technique through micropore membranes (Gregersen *et al.*, 1973) by which means structural and functional integrity of RC membrane may be examined (Evans and LaCelle, 1975). RC deformability depends on (a) the biconcave shape of the erythrocytes, which in turn depends on a high ratio of surface area to volume, measurably by means of osmotic fragility; (b) the properties of haemoglobin and RC content of calcium and ATP; (c) the structure of RC membranes (the cholesterol/phospholipid (C/PL) molar ratio is an important determinant of membrane fluidity as well as the number of unsaturated double bonds within the phospholipid acyl chain) (Bruckdorfer *et al.*, 1969). A selective increase of cholesterol and/or a reduction of polyunsaturated fatty acids in RC membranes occurs together with a low fluidity and an abnormality in cell contour (Cooper *et al.*, 1972; Salvioli *et al.*, 1978). Phosphatidylcholine (PC) is concentrated in the external leaflet of the RC membrane and exchanges with PC of serum lipoprotein. Cooper *et al.* (1975) normalized *in vitro* both the morphology and the C/PL ratio of erythrocytes by adding saturated PC to incubating serum. *In vivo* rodents' erythrocytes are depleted of cholesterol after phospholipid infusion (Robins and Miller, 1974).

RC deformability is diminished in some pathological states such as peripheral arterial disease (Reid *et al.*, 1976b); in patients with advanced cirrhosis of the liver,

Serono Symposium No. 37, "Vascular Occlusion: Epidemiological, Pathophysiological and Therapeutic Aspects", edited by M. Tesi and J. Dormany, 1981. Academic Press, London and New York.

the splenic and hepatic sequestration of erythrocytes is proportional to the reduction of their deformability (Teitel, 1967). For these reasons, we have studied both
the RC deformability with regard to the lipid composition of their membranes
and the possibility of improving it pharmacologically by means of polyunsaturated
phosphatidylcholine infusions, in patients with peripheral arterial disease and
advanced cirrhosis of the liver.

MATERIALS AND METHODS

Subjects

We studied 12 inpatients (8 males and 4 females) aged 45–63 years, with
advanced cirrhosis of the liver, and 12 inpatients (11 males and 1 female) aged
45–70 years with circulatory insufficiency of the legs; they were compared with
12 normal subjects matched for age and sex. Eight patients with cirrhosis of the
liver and eight with peripheral arterial disease were infused with polyunsaturated
phosphatidylcholine (EPL, Nattermann, Rome), containing 70% of linoleic acid,
2 g daily for 5 days; before and after the infusion osmotic fragility, deformability
and lipid composition of erythrocytes were studied.

Methods

RC deformability was measured in whole blood in duplicate according to
Reid *et al.* (1976a); fasting whole blood, collected with EDTANa$_2$, was filtered
through discs of polycarbonate (diameter 13 mm, pore size 5 μm) (Nucleopore,
Pleasanton, Ca., USA) under a negative pressure of 20 cm of water. The results
are expressed as the volume of packed cells filtered per minute. Erythrocyte
count, haematocrit and mean corpuscular volume (MCV) were determined with
a Coulter Counter. Plasma fibrinogen concentration was measured by the clot
weight method, and the osmotic fragility was estimated using a graded sequence
of concentration of NaCl. Washed RC were extracted with chloroform: methanol
(1:1 v/v); aliquots of the chloroformic phase were used for cholesterol and phospholipids determination and the value of the C/PL molar ratio was calculated.
The correlation between RC deformability and the C/PL molar ratio was calculated by linear regression analysis.

RESULTS

The volume of the erythrocytes filtered per minute is reported in Table I. Their
deformability was reduced in both groups of patients with respect to controls. The
mean corpuscular volume in the groups studied was similar (84.62 ± 3.96 in the
controls, 90.01 ± 7.09 in patients with cirrhosis of the liver and 91.95 ± 4.12 in
patients with peripheral arterial disease). The values of the C/PL molar ratio of RC
membranes were higher in both groups of patients with respect to controls (Table
I). The correlation between RC deformability and the C/PL molar ratio was signi-

Table I. Deformability and cholesterol/phospholipid molar ratio of erythrocytes in normal subjects and in patients with liver cirrhosis or peripheral arterial disease.

	No. of subjects studied	Deformability[b]	C/PL
Controls	12	0.36 ± 0.13 (0.23 − 0.66)	0.67 ± 0.11 (0.45 − 0.88)
Liver cirrhosis	12	0.08 ± 1.04[a] (0.02 − 0.29)	1.04 ± 0.17[a] (0.72 − 1.29)
Peripheral arterial disease	12	0.07 ± 0.04[a] (0.02 − 0.16)	0.93 ± 0.11[a] (0.68 − 1.08)

Mean ± s.d. and range of the values. Statistical analysis with Student's "t" test: [a]$P < 0.01$ with regard to normal subjects; [b]deformability of red blood cells is expressed as ml of packed cells filtered per minute.

Table II. Changes of deformability and cholesterol/phospholipid molar ratio of erythrocytes after polyunsaturated phosphatidylcholine infusions in patients with liver cirrhosis or peripheral arterial disease.

		Deformability	C/PL
Liver cirrhosis (8 patients)	Before	0.05 ± 0.02 (0.02 − 0.10)	1.09 ± 0.14 (0.91 − 1.29)
	After	0.20 ± 0.14[a] (0.08 − 0.47)	0.93 ± 0.12[a] (0.78 − 1.15)
Peripheral arterial disease (8 patients)	Before	0.06 ± 0.21 (0.02 − 0.12)	0.92 ± 0.11 (0.68 − 1.08)
	After	0.21 ± 0.10[a] (0.09 − 0.35)	0.80 ± 0.07[a] (0.72 − 0.91)

Mean ± s.d. and range of the value. Statistical analysis by means of paired Student's "t" test: [a]$P < 0.01$

ficant ($r = -0.62$): the volume of RC filtered per minute is higher when the ratio is low. There was no correlation between RC volume, fibrinogenaemia, haematocrit and RC deformability. The number of the reticulocytes was higher ($P < 0.01$) only in patients with liver cirrhosis (88 750 ± 13 840 mmc) with respect to the controls (66 750 ± 12 840). The values of both the C/PL molar ratio and the volume of packed cells filtered per minute before and after EPL infusions are reported in Table II. The treatment reduces the values of C/PL ratio and increases the RC filtered per minute in both the groups of patients. The osmotic fragility was little influenced by treatment and the mean corpuscular volume did not change in patients with peripheral arterial disease (from 92.52 ± 4.78 to 91.28 ± 6.24) or with liver cirrhosis (from 92.08 ± 7.63 to 90.83 ± 6.45), nor did haematocrit values. Reticulocytes did not change during EPL infusion.

DISCUSSION

The erythrocyte deformability is reduced in the patients with cirrhosis of the liver and with peripheral arterial disease. The volume of RC filtered per minute through the polycarbonate sieve is inversely correlated with the C/PL molar ratio of RC membranes. The ability of RC to pass through the channels of a polycarbonate sieve (like capillaries of small diameter) depends on a complex interaction between cell shape, intrinsic membrane deformability and the fluidity of RC content (Chien *et al.*, 1967). Our results demonstrate a reduced filterability of RC membrane when the C/PL molar ratio of erythrocyte membrane increases.

It is well recognized that red blood cell lipids are regulated by the exchange with plasma lipids (Shohet, 1971); cholesterol exchanges more rapidly than phospholipids (Reed *et al.*, 1968); the cholesterol content of RC membranes increases when plasma free cholesterol is high (D'Hollander and Chevallier, 1972). In patients with severe parenchymal liver disease, plasma-free cholesterol is high, causing the high cholesterol content in RC membranes. The reason for the high C/PL ratio in patients with peripheral arterial disease is not clear: hyperlipaemia is present in these patients and recently Hui and Harmony (1979) found that low density lipoproteins induce the dephosphorylation of spectrin, causing a crenated form of erythrocytes. Both the depletion of adenosine triphosphate and the accumulation of calcium make the red cell membranes more rigid; also the fatty acid-lecithin exchange, an energy dependent reaction, may be depressed in RC of patients with vascular disease (Shohet, 1971).

Phosphatidylcholine is incorporated as an intact molecule in the circulating membranes (Wagener, 1972), reducing C/PL molar ratio in the erythrocytes (Salvioli *et al.*, 1978) and in lipoproteins (Thompson *et al.*, 1976); in our previous study, the infusion of the same amount of lecithin changed the lipid composition of plasma lipoprotein and increased the initial low percentage of linoleic acid in RC lecithin of patients with liver cirrhosis (Salvioli *et al.*, 1978).

These may be the reasons for both the reduction of C/PL molar ratio and the improvement of RC deformability in EPL-treated patients. In fact, no changes of other factors reducing erythrocyte deformability such as osmotic fragility or plasma concentration of fibrinogen or mean corpuscular volume were observed after the treatment. Recently, Leblond and Coulombe (1979) found an inverse correlation between RC deformability and the percentage of reticulocytes, which have a greater volume. Only the patients with liver cirrhosis showed an increase in the number of reticulocytes but this, in comparison with the total number of red cells, seems too small to influence the filtration through micropore membranes.

REFERENCES

Bruckdorfer, K. R., Demel, R. A., De Gier, J. and Van Deenen, L. L. M. (1969). *Biochimica Biophysica Acta* **183**, 334.

Chien, S., Usami, S., Dellenback, L. J. and Gregersen, M. I. (1967). *Science* **157**, 827.

Cooper, R. A., Diloy-Puray, M., Lando, P. and Greenberg, M. S. (1972). *Journal of Clinical Investigation* **51**, 3182.

Cooper, R. A., Arner, E. C., Wiley, J. S. and Shattil, S. J. (1975). *Journal of Clinical Investigation* **55**, 115.
D'Hollander, F. and Chevallier, F. (1972). *Journal of Lipid Research* **13**, 733.
Evans, E. A. and LaCelle, P. L. (1975). *Blood* **45**, 29.
Gregersen, M. I., Bryant, C. A., Hammerle, W., Usami, S. and Chien, S. (1973). *Science* **157**, 825.
Hui, D. and Harmony, J. A. K. (1979). *Biochimica Biophysica Acta* **550**, 425.
Leblond, P. F. and Coulombe, L. (1979). *Journal of Laboratory and Clinical Medicine* **94**, 133.
Reed, C. F., Murphy, M. and Roberts, G. (1968). *Journal of Clinical Investigation* **47**, 749.
Reid, H. L., Barnes, A. J., Lock, P. J., Dormandy, J. A. and Dormandy, T. L. (1976a). *Journal of Clinical Pathology* **29**, 855.
Reid, H. L., Dormandy, J. A., Barnes, A. J., Lock, P. J. and Dormandy, T. L. (1976b). *Lancet* **1**, 666.
Robins, S. J. and Miller, A. (1974). *Journal of Laboratory and Clinical Medicine* **83**, 436.
Salvioli, G., Rioli, G., Lugli, R. and Salati, R. (1978). *Gut* **19**, 844.
Shohet, S. B. (1971). *Journal of Lipid Research* **12**, 139.
Teitel, P. (1967). *Nouvelle Revue Française d'Hématologie* **7**, 321.
Thompson, G. R., Jadhav, A., Nava, M. and Gotto, A. M. Jr. (1976). *European Journal of Clinical Investigation* **6**, 941.
Wagener, H. (1972). *In* "Phospholipide in Biochimie, Experiment and Klinik", (G. Schettler ed.), 59–71, Thieme, Stuttgart.

ON THE POSSIBLE ROLE OF A HEMOSTASIS ACTIVATING TISSUE FACTOR (HAF) IN HEMOSTASIS AND THROMBOGENESIS

K. Breddin, N. Bender, C. M. Kirchmaier and R. Wiedemann

Department of Internal Medicine, J. W. Goethe University,
Frankfurt am Main, W. Germany

PLATELETS AND HEMOSTASIS AFTER VASCULAR LESIONS

Platelets have a decisive role in primary hemostasis. During the first seconds after a vascular lesion, platelets are stimulated within the lumen, in the wall and outside the vessel. Usually, the first steps of primary hemostasis are explained in the following way: after a vascular lesion, platelets stick to the damaged vessel wall, probably especially to collagen of type III, aggregate and release their ingredients, which further activate platelets and coagulation. New results in our group have led us to assume a modified scheme for the first reactions in primary hemostasis which has been partially substantiated experimentally. Many of today's concepts on the mechanism of primary hemostasis or on the first steps of thrombus formation have been derived from results obtained with aggregometer studies. But *in vitro* induced or spontaneous aggregation occurs only if the platelets have already changed their shape to some extent.

These activated platelets are also more adhesive than the disc-like platelets circulating *in vivo*. The contact of platelets with foreign surfaces and the reduced temperature (25°C or less) induce this kind of platelet stimulation within 10–30 min. If hemostasis or thrombus formation are studied in an animal model, such as in rat mesenteric vessels, a rapid shape change of the adhering platelets can be observed outside and within the damaged vessel. What is responsible for this rapid platelet stimulation *in vivo*? In our laboratory, we define stimulated platelets as

Serono Symposium No. 37, "Vascular Occlusion: Epidemiological, Pathophysiological and Therapeutic Aspects", edited by M. Tesi and J. Dormany, 1981. Academic Press, London and New York.

Table I. Correlation between percentage of platelet shape change and blood sampling technique.

n = 10	
Exact venepuncture	Deliberate improper venepuncture
33%	64.5%

platelets which are sphered, show pseudopodia and adhere faster than non-stimulated platelets to different surfaces. Stimulated platelets may transform back to the original disc-like platelet form *in vitro* and *in vivo* within minutes. When we investigated morphological platelet changes directly after blood sampling, we observed that in some samples of citrated or whole blood, fixed directly after venepuncture, up to 80% of the platelets were morphologically changed, compared with the 20% we usually find in normal individuals. It seemed possible that this effect was due to the admixture of tissue fluid at blood sampling.

When we deliberately punctured the vessel wall in 10 healthy individuals and tried to aspirate some tissue fluid before drawing the blood in samples fixed in glutaraldehyde, a few seconds after blood drawing we found 64% of the platelets were morphologically changed (Table I).

Apparently, the addition of small amounts of tissue fluid introduced at blood sampling did induce a platelet shape change within seconds or even within parts of a second. We first concluded that this effect might be due to some yet unknown effect of thromboplastin. Therefore, we tried to prepare extracts of intra-operatively obtained, subcutaneous human tissue and later from different tissues of different animal species. We expected that thromboplastin might be responsible for the platelet changes observed and we also wanted to evaluate if the tissue extracts had other effects on platelet functions besides changing their shape.

METHODS

Platelet shape change was investigated as described by Bender *et al.* (1979). Tissue extracts were obtained as described by Kirchmaier *et al.* (1979) by tissue homogenization in 30% proponal, subsequent centrifugation and chromatography of the intermediate fraction on Sephadex LH 60. The effect of these extracts on platelet retention was investigated using a modified Hellem system with a short, glass bead column, which gave a basal retention in healthy individuals of 5–15%. The effect of the extracts on aggregation was investigated using PAT III method (Breddin *et al.*, 1976) or Born's method with the Braun Melsungen aggregometer.

RESULTS

Effects of the Tissue Extracts

The tissue extracts of subcutaneous human or porcine tissue contain some thromboplastic activity. Some phospholipids, especially lysolecithin in higher concentration induced platelet shape changes similar to those observed with

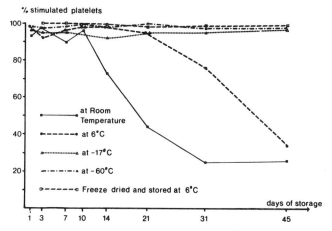

Fig. 1. Tissue extracts incubated at room temperature or at 6°C lose their platelet stimulating activity after 1–2 weeks. Deep frozen or lyophilized these extracts retain their platelet
stimulating activity for more than 45 days.

the tissue extracts (Bender *et al.*, 1979). Even in a dilution of 1:1000, the extract
stimulated 60% of the platelets within 2–3 s, while thromboplastin was practically
inactive in high and low concentrations.

After storage at room temperature, the tissue extracts lost their activity within
10 days. Deep frozen or lyophilized, they retained their platelet-stimulating activity for more than 45 days (Fig. 1).

Effect on Platelet Retention

The addition of 200 µl of tissue extract to 2 ml of citrated blood increased
platelet retention from 10–15% to a mean of 61% in normal individuals. In nine
patients with severe von Willebrand's disease with a very low factor VIII ass.
antigen and a missing ristocetin co-factor, the addition of 100 µl/ml of the tissue
extract directly to blood sampling did not enhance platelet retention in the
samples of these patients. But if a cryoprecipitate from normal platelet rich

Table II. The effect of tissue extracts (HaF) and cryoprecipitate (%) on platelet
retention in von Willebrand syndrome.

Citrated blood 1.8 ml		+0.2 ml NaCl	+0.1 ml cryo. +0.1 ml NaCl	+0.1 ml HaF +0.1 ml NaCl	+0.1 ml HaF +0.1 ml cryo.
Normal values	X̄	12.9	16.3	33.1	53
(n = 10)	s	4.4	5.2	10.5	13
V.W.S. (n = 8)	X̄	12.4	13.4	15.1	37.1
(Rist.Co-F.0%,	s	2.8	3.2	2.2	14.2
F.VIII-ass.Ag.0–10%)					
V.W.S. n = 6	X̄	12.3	15.1	27.8	44.6
(Rist.Co-F. 1–10%,	s	2.7	3.5	3.5	4.1
F.VIII-ass.Ag.X̄ 44.7%)					

K. Breddin et al.

Table III. Platelet stimulation and retention in Hermansky-Pudlak syndrome.

	normal values %	patient (M.P.) %
HAF-induced platelet shape		
Change	75–90	80
Platelet retention		
Without HAF	5–15	12
With HAF (100 μl/ml citr. blood)	33	17
With cryoprecipitate	16	14
With HAF + cryoprecipitate	53	18

plasma was added to the patient's blood together with the tissue extract at blood sampling, similar retention values were obtained as for normal individuals. In this test system, cryoprecipitate alone did not enhance platelet retention (Table II). In a young patient with Hermansky-Pudlak syndrome we also found a markedly reduced platelet retention, which could not be stimulated by the addition of tissue extract. But in this patient the tissue extract induced a rapid change of platelets comparable to that observed in normal individuals (Table III).

DISCUSSION

The results described so far show that the platelet-stimulating effect of the tissue extracts differs from thromboplastin activity. Both activities may act together and lead to effective hemostasis *in vivo*.

Even highly diluted, the tissue extracts stimulate the platelet shape change and enhance platelet retention or platelet adhesion. But the tissue extracts have no direct aggregating effect. We have named the lipoprotein responsible for these effects hemostasis activating factor (HAF). Certainly platelets can adhere, change their shape and aggregate without this stimulation, as shown in different *in vitro* tests, but *in vivo* HAF may be an important and effective accelerator of platelet stimulation. The stimulating effect of these tissue extracts is very short-lasting.

Even *in vitro* platelets retain their disc-like form within minutes, if incubated with the extract at 37°C. It seems likely that HAF is rapidly inactivated. Some results in different laboratory animals make it likely that inactivation occurs even faster in some animals than in man. The mechanism which inactivates HAF is of special interest and should be further elucidated.

Our results in patients with von Willebrand syndrome make it likely that the von Willebrand factor or factor VIII ass. antigen is essential for the rapid stimulating effect of HAF on platelet adhesion and, in a few of our patients, also for their rapid shape change. *In vitro* shape change and retention are normalized by cryoprecipitate. Cryoprecipitate did not influence the defective retention in the Hermansky-Pudlak syndrome.

We come to the following hypothesis of the first platelet reaction in primary hemostasis (Table IV): circulating disc-like platelets are rapidly stimulated after

Table IV.   Platelet reactions in hemostasis.

circulating disk-like platelets	*stimulation by*	
Hemostasis activating factor (HAF)	+	
von Willebrand factor	stimulated platelets	enhanced aggregability
shape change (sphering and pseudopode formation)	release	
increased adhesiveness		

contact with lipoproteins from damaged cells of the extravascular and vascular tissue. This stimulation is accelerated in the presence of the von Willebrand factor.

Stimulation enhances platelet adhesion and the platelets change their shape by sphering and pseudopodia formation. Shape change and increased adhesiveness apparently do not directly depend on each other, as our results in Hermansky-Pudlak syndrome and von Willebrand's disease indicate. Stimulated platelets stick to subendothelial structures such as collagen and basal membranes and especially to other platelets. Release, activation of coagulation and the formation of an effective platelet plug follow.

Acetylsalicyclic acid is a mild inhibitor of platelet stimulation. This effect of ASA lasts for only a few hours after a single dose. This inhibiting effect on platelet stimulation may be more important for antithrombotic effect than the longer lasting inhibition of thromboxane formation. We have therefore begun to test different antiplatelet drugs for their effect on HAF-induced platelet stimulation.

REFERENCES

Bender, N., Kirchmaier, C., Bartsch, B., Lindenborn, D. and Breddin, K. (1979). *Thrombosis Research* **14**, 341–351.

Breddin, K., Grun, H., Krzywanek, H. J. and Schremmer, W. P. (1976). *Thrombosis and Hemostasis (Stuttgart)* **35**, 669–691.

Kirchmaier, C., Bender, N., Wilhelm, B., Al-Sayegh, A. and Breddin, K. (1979). *Thrombosis Research* (In press.)

PROSTAGLANDIN FORMATION IN PLATELETS FOLLOWING ACUTE MYOCARDIAL INFARCTION

F. R. Matthias, W. Palinski and T. H. Schöndorf

Department of Internal Medicine, Justus Liebig University, Giessen, Germany

INTRODUCTION

In patients suffering from an acute myocardial infarction, and especially when undergoing episodes of circulatory shock, an activated coagulation system has often been found. This is documented best by the detection of soluble fibrin in the plasma of these patients (Matthias *et al.*, 1977; Matthias, 1978).

Thrombocytes are also involved in these states of hypercoagulability by production and liberation of pro-coagulant and pro-aggregatory substances. Prostaglandins (prostaglandin endoperoxides, thromboxane A_2) formed in platelets are assumed to play an important role in platelet thrombus formation, mainly in the arterial part of the vascular system. It seems a question, still undecided, whether fibrin and platelet thrombi or emboli are involved as a causal factor of an acute myocardial infarction, or whether they follow the acute onset as complicating events (Jørgensen, 1976; Roberts *et al.*, 1976). It is well known that endogenous catecholamines are elevated in a patient's plasma following myocardial infarction and in circulatory shock.

Catecholamines—dopamine, epinephrine and norepinephrine—are drugs often used to improve cardiac output and to sustain blood pressure in these clinical situations. Epinephrine and norepinephrine stimulate prostaglandin formation in platelets. The purpose of the investigations described below is to elucidate the relationship between the plasma coagulation system and the prostaglandin system in platelets of patients following myocardial infarction, as well as to study the effect of different catecholamines—especially dopamine—in respect to their prostaglandin forming potency in thrombocytes.

Serono Symposium No. 37, "Vascular Occlusion: Epidemiological, Pathophysiological and Therapeutic Aspects", edited by M. Tesi and J. Dormany, 1981. Academic Press, London and New York.

MATERIALS AND METHODS

Patients after myocardial infarction, from whom blood samples had been taken, were diagnosed and grouped as described earlier (Matthias, 1978). Soluble plasma fibrin was quantified by affinity chromatography (Heene and Matthias, 1973; Matthias et al., 1977). The ethanol gelation test and platelet aggregation were performed according to the original methods (Godal and Abildgaard, 1966; Matthias, 1978). Platelet suspensions in buffer or plasma were obtained from platelet rich plasma as previously described (Matthias, 1978). Prostaglandin endoperoxides—measured as nmol of malondialdehyde (MDA)—were determined in accordance to Smith et al. (1976). N-ethylmaleimide (NEM, final concentration in all platelet suspension: 1 mmol/l) was used to induce endoperoxide accumulation (Stuart et al., 1975). MDA recovery from buffer and plasma was estimated according to Smith et al. (1976).

In control persons (A) and patient groups (B and C), prostaglandin endoperoxide production of platelets in buffer was measured after 10 min of incubation with NEM at 37°C (Fig. 1 and Fig. 2). In the patient shown in Fig. 3, endoperoxides were measured after 60 min of platelet incubation in plasma together with NEM. In the in vitro experiments with dopamine (Giulini, Hannover, Germany), epinephrine and norepinephrine (Hoechst, Frankfurt am Main, Germany) the final concentration of the catecholamines was 600 μmol/l, or 91, 109 and 100 μg/ml, respectively. Platelet count was 7-10 x 10^8 platelets/ml in all experiments. After 30 min of incubation with catecholamines NEM was added, and after a further 30 min the endoperoxides were measured. In the rabbit experiments (2.0-2.5 kg; mean 2.3 kg body weight), after infusion of 0.60 μmol/l catecholamines in 10 ml 0.9% sodium chloride over 1 h, platelets were suspended in plasma (1.5-2.0 x 10^9 platelets/ml), incubated for 60 min at 37°C together with arachidonic acid (final concentration 10^{-5} mol/l) and NEM (final concentration 1 mmol/l). In each case endoperoxides were measured before incubation and/or infusion.

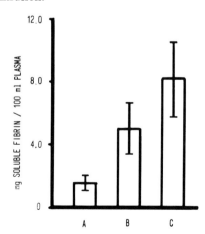

Fig. 1. Soluble fibrin in plasma. Mean values ± s.d. A = healthy donors (n = 11); B = patients after myocardial infarction (n = 7); C = patients after myocardial infarction suffering from circulatory insufficiency under norepinephrine and/or dopamine administration (n = 7).

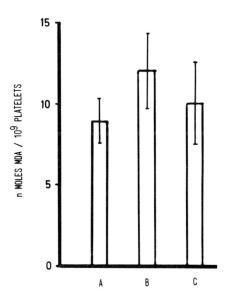

Fig. 2. Prostaglandin endoperoxides (measured as nmol/l MDA) per 10^9 platelets after 10 min of incubation in buffer together with NEM. Same donors as in Fig. 1. (See Fig. 1 for explanation of A, B and C). The difference between A and B is significant ($P < 0.01$).

RESULTS

The mean value of soluble fibrin in the plasma of normal donors (A) measured by affinity chromatography was 1.5 mg/100 ml plasma (Fig. 1). In patients after myocardial infarction but without circulatory insufficiency (B) the mean plasma fibrin content is 5.0 mg/100 ml (range 2.5–7.0 mg/100 ml), it rises in patients under norepinephrine and/or dopamine administration (C) up to 8.2 mg/100 ml (range 4.0–11.3 mg/100 ml). The differences are significant ($P < 0.01$ or $P < 0.05$). According to these results plasma thrombin action seems more pronounced in the latter group of patients.

The recovery of MDA from buffer was 98 ± 3.4% s.d. (n = 4) and from plasma 76 ± 3.1% s.d. (n = 4). This was taken into account. Before starting the incubation MDA was from 0% to 5% of the final amount in each experiment. In normal control persons (group A), prostaglandin endoperoxide formation of buffer-suspended platelets was 8.9 nmol/10^9 platelets (Fig. 2). In patients of group B, endoperoxide formation increased significantly to 11.9 nmol/10^9 platelets ($P < 0.01$). The platelets of group C produced more endoperoxides than the normal platelets did. The amounts, however, did not differ significantly from those of normals and of patients of group B. The mean value was 9.9 nmol/10^9 platelets.

As an example of the relationship between soluble plasma fibrin and prostaglandin endoperoxide formation over a longer period post-myocardial infarction, Fig. 3 shows the data obtained from a patient of group C. Comparable results were observed in other patients of this group. In one case, prostaglandin endoperoxides were measured after suspending platelets of a normal donor in his own plasma and in this patient's plasma. In the other case, the patient's platelets were suspended in normal plasma and in the patient's own plasma. When the data

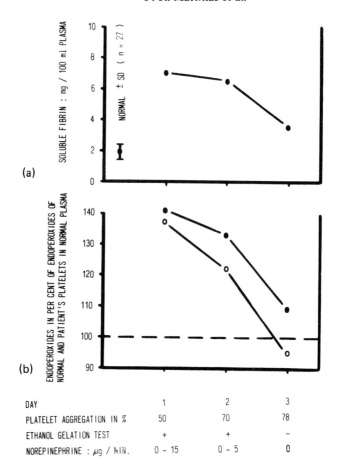

DAY	1	2	3
PLATELET AGGREGATION IN %	50	70	78
ETHANOL GELATION TEST	+	+	−
NOREPINEPHRINE : μg / MIN.	0 - 15	0 - 5	0

Fig. 3. (a) Soluble fibrin in plasma of a patient after myocardial infarction. (b) Prostaglandin endoperoxide formation in the patient's plasma after 60 min of incubation with NEM. o = Normal platelets in patient's plasma; ● = patient's platelets in patient's own plasma; 100% = normal or patient's platelets in normal plasma, respectively.

obtained from control and patient's platelets in normal plasma were calculated as 100%, the peak value of normal platelets in patient's plasma is 137% and of patient's platelets in his own plasma 141% (Fig. 3). After 3 days, patient's plasma showed no more differences in prostaglandin-producing potency when compared with the plasma of the normal donor. The plasma fibrin concentration, which had been measured simultaneously, was highest on the first day—7.0 mg/100 ml plasma—and declined to 3.5 mg/100 ml plasma on the third day. Concomitantly, the other parameters improved: platelet aggregation increased, the ethanol gelatio: test became negative. Norepinephrine administration could be discontinued.

To elucidate the platelet-activating prostaglandin-producing effect of the catecholamines—dopamine, epinephrine and norepinephrine—the experiments illustrated in Fig. 4 and Fig. 5 were performed. Adding the different catecholamir in a relatively high concentration to human platelets suspended in plasma, the

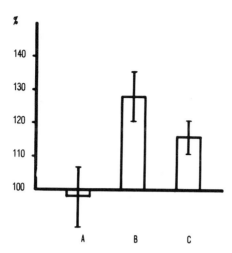

Fig. 4. Prostaglandin endoperoxide formation in human platelets suspended in plasma, after *in vitro* addition of dopamine (A), epinephrine (B) and norepinephrine (C); 100% = endoperoxide formation after addition of an equal volume of 0.9% NaCl (n = 5).

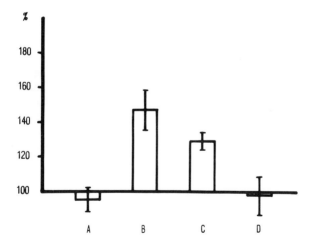

Fig. 5. Prostaglandin endoperoxide formation in rabbit platelets suspended in plasma after infusion of 10 ml 0.9% NaCl containing 0.60 μmol/l dopamine (A), epinephrine (B), norepinephrine (C) or NaCl only (D). Duration of infusion: 1 h. 100% = Endoperoxide formation before infusion (n = 5).

following results were obtained. The data are indicated as a percentage of the control experiments with 0.9% sodium chloride under the same conditions. The solution medium of the drugs did not influence the results. Dopamine has only a slight prostaglandin-producing effect on platelets when compared with the control experiments. In contrast, the prostaglandin endoperoxide-forming activity of epinephrine and norepinephrine was very marked; the difference to 0.9% sodium chloride and to dopamine are highly significant in all experiments.

When infusing the catecholamines into rabbits, similar results were obtained. Prostaglandin endoperoxides in platelets before infusion were defined as 100%. After infusion of 1 h, the values obtained by the experiments with 0.9% sodium chloride and with dopamine did not differ significantly from the values before starting the infusion in each group of animals. This means that the experimental procedure *per se* has no effect on platelets' prostaglandin system and that dopamine has no activating potency. Highly-significant augmented values, however, can again be observed after infusion of epinephrine and norepinephrine in respect to the pre-infusion prostaglandin production in each group as well as to dopamine and 0.9% sodium chloride.

DISCUSSION

Following myocardial infarction, a stimulated coagulation system has been found. In the experiments presented, activation of the plasmatic coagulation factors was confirmed by the detection of soluble fibrin in plasma via affinity chromatography and by the ethanol gelation test. In states of hypercoagulability, platelets are also involved. When compared with normal platelets, those of the patients under investigation showed an increased prostaglandin formation as an indicator of their pro-coagulant and pro-aggregatory activity (Fig. 1 and Fig. 2). This effect was less pronounced in patients suffering from circulatory insufficiency. This may be due to drugs depressing the prostaglandin system or to the concomitantly infused dopamine (see later). In accordance with our results, Abbate (personal communication) has also found an increased malondialdehyde production in platelets of patients after acute myocardial infarction.

In addition to this, patients' plasma exhibited a promoting effect on platelet prostaglandin endoperoxide formation (Fig. 3). The increase of prostaglandins formed by the platelets was paralleled by an elevation of plasma fibrin. This indicates a functional relationship between platelets and the plasma coagulation factors, probably partly linked by intravascular thrombin action. Endoperoxides were highest during norepinephrine administration. Heparin in the concentrations administered to the patients did not influence the prostaglandin endoperoxide formation. The reduced aggregability of platelets observed in these situations was discussed in a previous paper by Matthias (1978).

In the patient observed over a longer period of time, soluble fibrin was markedly lowered on the third day and endoperoxide formation in platelets did not differ from controls. This may be an indirect indication that plasma fibrin and the prostaglandin-dependent hyper-reactivity of the platelets increase as a consequence of the acute event, only after myocardial infarction and are not a pre-existing phenomenon. This may be supported by the fact that patients surviving for one or two days show a thrombotic occlusion of the coronary arteries in many cases. In patients who die immediately after the acute ischemic attack, this observation, however, is relatively rare (Chandler *et al.*, 1974). Antiplatelet drugs have not been used in the acute phase of infarction until now. A hyper-reactivity of patients' platelets and a stimulating effect of patients' plasma on the prostaglandin system of the platelets was found by Szczeklik *et al.* (1978) but for longer periods of time after myocardial infarction.

Dopamine, epinephrine and norepinephrine by themselves, or in combination, are drugs often used in circulatory shock. To elucidate the platelet activating, pro-aggregating effect of the different catecholamines as far as the prostaglandin system is involved, the experiments shown in Fig. 4 and Fig. 5 were performed. In equal doses—on a molar base—epinephrine and norepinephrine exhibit a highly-stimulating effect on platelets' prostaglandin endoperoxides. Dopamine has little or no activity in this respect. This is the case after *in vitro* as well as *in vivo* administration.

Dopamine induces platelet aggregation *in vitro*. Compared with the other cate-cholamines, the aggregation tracings of dopamine show a delayed course without a clear demonstration of the two phases. Moreover, dopamine inhibits the pro-aggregatory effect of epinephrine to some extent when added together to platelet rich plasma (Rossi *et al.*, 1978). This has been explained by the lack of one hydroxyl group in the dopamine molecule. The hydroxyl groups are supposed to be responsible for the interactions with the α-receptor of platelet membranes (Rossi *et al.*, 1978).

The amounts of the three catecholamines (18 μmol/h) infused into rabbits corresponded to 46–55 μg/min given to human beings of a body weight of 70 kg. Such doses of epinephrine and norepinephrine are reached in severe shock situations. In man, dopamine is given in larger amounts ranging between 200 μg/min and 1000 μg/min or even higher. When in our *in vitro* and *in vivo* experiments dopamine was administered in a four-fold amount, in respect to the other cate-cholamines, similar results were obtained as described above. In clinical situations, when shock patients necessarily need catecholamines, dopamine may induce only a weak prostaglandin stimulation in platelets if any. This could produce a desirably weak pro-aggregatory, pro-coagulant effect on platelets in states of hypercoagulability. When used in combination with other catecholamines dopamine might attenuate the production of procoagulant activities in platelets (Fig. 2, group C).

REFERENCES

Abbate, R. (1978). Personal communication.

Chandler, A. B., Chapman, I., Erhardt, L. R., Roberts, W. C., Schwartz, C. J., Sinapius, D., Spain, D. M., Sherry, S., Ness, P. M. and Simon, T. L. (1974). *Am. J. Card.* **34**, 823.

Godal, H. C. and Abildgaard, U. (1966). *Scand. J. Haematol.* **3**, 342.

Heene, D. L. and Matthias, F. R. (1973). *Thromb. Res.* **2**, 137.

Jørgensen, L. (1976). *In* "Thrombosis, platelets, anticoagulation and acetylsali-cyclic acid." (E. Donosi and J. I. Haft, eds). 131–142. Stratton Intercontinental Medical Book Corporation, New York.

Matthias, F. R. (1978). *Haemostasis* **7**, 273.

Matthias, F. R., Reinicke, R. and Heene, D. L. (1977). *Thromb. Res.* **10**, 365.

Roberts, W. C. and Ferrans, V. J. (1976). *Sem. Thrombos. Hemostas.* **2**, 123.

Rossi, E. C., Lous, G. and Zeller, E. A. (1978). *In* "Platelet function testing."

(H. J. Day, H. Holmsen and M. B. Zucker, eds). 99–103. US Dept. of Health, Education and Welfare Publication No. (NIH) 78-1087.
Smith, J. B., Ingerman, C. M. and Silver, M. J. (1976). *J. Lab. clin. Med.* **88**, 167.
Stuart, M. J., Murphy, S. and Oski, F. A. (1975). *New Engl. J. Med.* **292**, 1310.
Szczeklik, A., Gryglewski, R. J., Musial, J., Grodzińska, L., Serwonska, M. and Marcinkiewicz, E. (1978). *Thrombos. Haemostas.* **40**, 66.

BLOOD PLATELET FUNCTION, PLASMA PROSTAGLANDIN-LIKE ACTIVITY AND CYCLIC NUCLEOTIDE LEVEL IN PATIENTS WITH ATHEROSCLEROTIC ARTERIOPATHY*

A. Bodzenta, M. Bielawiec, B. Kiersnowska-Rogowska, M. Myśliwiec and F. Rogowski

Department of Haematology, Institute of Internal Medicine and Department of Toxicology, Institute of Pharmacology and Toxicology, Medical School, Białystok, Poland

INTRODUCTION

Interaction of the vascular wall and blood cells plays an important role in the homeostasis of circulation. Both the vascular wall and the blood cells contain prostaglandins as well as cyclic nucleotides which can influence the platelet function (Samuelsson *et al.*, 1975; Haslam *et al.*, 1978; Moncada and Vane, 1979). A relationship between cyclic AMP and vasodilatation was also found (Kukovetz and Poch, 1970; Vigdahl *et al.*, 1971).

In many pathological states and especially in atherosclerosis, disorders in the homeostasis of the circulation may play a very important role. Recently it has been suggested that a balance between thromboxane A_2, prostacyclin and cyclic AMP is very important in the pathogenesis of atherosclerosis (Moncada and Vane, 1978; Gryglewski, 1978).

The relationship between these factors is still not clear. Therefore, in this paper the blood platelet function, plasma-prostaglandin-like activity and cyclic nucleotide level were studied in patients with atherosclerotic arteriopathy and in healthy subjects. The influence of nicotinic acid derivatives on these parameters was also investigated in this group of patients.

*This work was supported by Project 10–RMZ–I.

Serono Symposium No. 37, "Vascular Occlusion: Epidemiological, Pathophysiological and Therapeutic Aspects", edited by M. Tesi and J. Dormany, 1981. Academic Press, London and New York.

MATERIAL AND METHODS

The investigations were carried out on 20 patients (2 females and 18 males), aged between 42 and 68 years, suffering from obliterative arteriosclerosis of the lower limbs. The control group consisted of ten healthy subjects (four females and six males), aged between 38 and 52 years, without symptoms of atherosclerosis. Ten patients suffering from obliterative arteriosclerosis of the lower limbs were treated with an intravenous injection of 300 mg nicotinic acid derivative (NAD-Sadamin "Polfa").

Blood for the investigations was drawn from the cubital vein, without stasis, into 3.8% sodium citrate solution in a proportion of 9:1. Blood samples for determining the platelet adhesiveness and cyclic nucleotide concentrations were mixed with EDTA. The following parameters were investigated in the plasma: platelet adhesiveness by the method of Sharp (1965); extraction and bioassay of the prostaglandin-like material using the method of Unger *et al.* (1971) and Vane (1957); cyclic AMP and GMP were radioimmunochemically assayed by the use of a cyclic AMP and cyclic GMP assay Kit (The Radiochemical Centre, Amersham, England). Student's t test was used for statistical analysis.

RESULTS

Figure 1 shows platelet adhesiveness in the patients suffering from obliterative arteriosclerosis of the lower limbs and in healthy subjects. The mean value of platelet adhesiveness in the investigated group of the patients was found to be $54 \pm 4.5\%$ and was statistically higher ($P < 0.001$) in comparison with the healthy subjects ($44 \pm 12\%$).

Figure 2 illustrates the mean level of prostaglandin-like activity in the patients with obliterative arteriosclerosis. The level of prostaglandin-like activity was

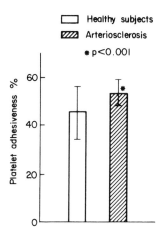

Fig. 1. Platelet adhesiveness in the patients suffering from obliterative arteriosclerosis of the lower limbs and in healthy persons.

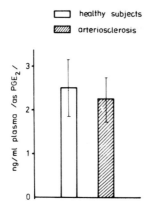

Fig. 2. The level of prostaglandin-like activity in the patients with obliterative arteriosclerosis and in healthy persons.

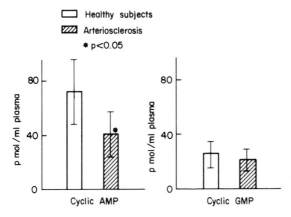

Fig. 3. The plasma concentrations of cyclic AMP and cyclic GMP in the patients with obliterative arteriosclerosis and in healthy persons.

found to be 2.27 ± 0.58 ng PGE_2/ml plasma. Similar values were found in the healthy subjects 2.5 ± 0.79 ng PGE_2/ml plasma. There was no statistically significant difference between these values in the two groups ($P < 0.25$).

Figure 3 presents the plasma concentrations of cyclic AMP and cyclic GMP in the blood of the investigated groups of patients and in the healthy subjects. The mean concentration of cyclic AMP in the investigated group of patients was found to be 40.4 ± 25.6 pmol/ml plasma. Statistical significance was observed ($P < 0.05$) in comparison with the healthy subjects (74.0 ± 24.0 pmol/ml plasma). No statistically significant changes were observed in the concentration of cyclic GMP in the blood of the investigated patients and healthy subjects (21.0 ± 12.8 pmol/ml plasma and 23.2 ± 15.4 pmol/ml plasma, respectively).

Figure 4 shows platelet adhesiveness, plasma prostaglandin-like activity and concentrations of cyclic AMP and cyclic GMP in the patients with obliterative

A. Bodzenta et al.

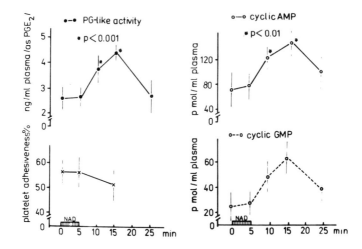

Fig. 4. Platelet adhesiveness, plasma prostaglandin-like activity and concentrations of cyclic AMP and cyclic GMP in the patients with obliterative arteriosclerosis after intravenous injec tion of 300 mg nicotinic acid derivative (NAD–Sadamin "Polfa").

arteriosclerosis after an intravenous injection of 300 mg NAD. No significant difference in the platelet adhesiveness was found after injection of NAD (from 56 ± 9% to 51 ± 10%). Five minutes after an injection of NAD, the level of prostaglandin-like activity was found to be 3.8 ± 0.71 ng PGE_2/ml plasma and it increased significantly and statistically to 4.4 ± 0.38 ng PGE_2/ml plasma during the next 5 min observation ($P < 0.01$). 20 min after injection of NAD, the level of prostaglandin-like activity approached the initial value before administration of NAD (2.7 ± 0.8 ng PGE_2/ml plasma and 2.27 ± 0.52 ng PGE_2/ml plasma, respectively). The concentration of cyclic AMP, 5 min after injection of NAD, was 124.0 ± 22 pmol/ml plasma and a gradual increase to 138.8 ± 25.6 pmol/ml plasma was observed during the next 5 min observation. Twenty minutes after administration of NAD, a fall in the concentrations of cyclic AMP occurred. There were statistically significant differences between these values as compared with the initial value before administration of NAD ($P < 0.01$).

Similar changes were observed in the concentrations of cyclic GMP after injection of NAD (48.0 ± 15 pmol/ml plasma and 62.6 ± 13.8 pmol/ml plasma, respectively).

DISCUSSION

Blood platelet-endothelial cell interactions play a role in several pathological processes including thrombosis and atherosclerosis. Endothelial cell injury leads to formation of platelet aggregates. The released platelet mitogenic factor promotes muscle cell growth in the vessel wall (Harker *et al.*, 1976). Migration of hypertrophied muscle cells into the intima is considered to be the first step to atherosclerosis (Bourgain, 1977). On the other hand, hyperfunction of platelets can lead to platelet aggregate formation even when the endothelium is intact. Subsequently, it leads to endothelial cell injury and the processes are similar.

We have found an increase in platelet adhesiveness in patients with atherosclerosis which may be one of the pathological factors in thromboembolic complications which often appear in this pathological state. The function of platelets is influenced by their environment. The role of platelet cyclic AMP and cyclic GMP in their aggregation has been reviewed quite extensively (Yamazaki *et al.*, 1978; Barber, 1976). It is well known that cyclic AMP prevents platelet aggregation. In general, agents which inhibit platelet aggregation increase cyclic AMP levels, whereas agents which induce platelet aggregation lower platelet cyclic AMP levels. It was suggested that cyclic AMP blocks the cyclo-oxygenase pathway of arachidonic acid (Nalbandian and Henry, 1978). We were interested in the plasma cyclic nucleotide level in patients with atherosclerosis. We noted a decrease in cyclic AMP levels in atherosclerotic subjects, cyclic GMP remained unchanged. Cyclic AMP level depends on adenylate cyclase and phosphodiesterase activities. One of the activators of the former enzyme is prostacyclin. The main sources of this prostaglandin are the lung and kidney, but large amounts of prostacyclin are produced in the vascular endothelium. The very marked increase in blood prostaglandin-like activity and in the cyclic nucleotide level following NAD infusion would seem to confirm this. Atherosclerotic plaques do not produce prostacyclin (D'Angelo *et al.*, 1978) and atherosclerotic arteries produce only small amounts of prostacyclin (Zinzinger and Silberbauer, 1978). Gryglewski *et al.* (1976) and Moncada and Vane (1979) suggested that the basic metabolic disturbance in atherosclerosis is related to impaired generation of vascular prostacyclin. This could be caused by lipid peroxides, the concentration of which increases in advanced atherosclerotic lesions. Lipid peroxides can inhibit prostacyclin formation by the vascular wall without impairing thromboxane A_2 generation by the platelets, thus increasing platelet function and lowering the defence mechanism giving protection against thrombosis. Cyclic GMP does not have any apparent effect on platelet aggregation (Apitz-Castro and De Murciano, 1978), but both cyclic AMP and cyclic GMP are now recognized as key intracellular regulators in several biological functions, including growth and morphogenesis (Greengard and Kebabian, 1974). At an early stage of induction of cell proliferation by several mitogens, the intracellular concentration of cyclic GMP was elevated up to 10-fold (Hadden *et al.*, 1972; Seifert and Rudland, 1974). Cyclic GMP inhibits the cyclic AMP–dependent protein kinase activity in isolated platelet plasma membranes. The membrane phosphoglycoprotein plays a central role in the triggering of platelet aggregation and it is also suggested that modulation of its degree of phosphorylation may be exerted through some cyclic AMP/cyclic GMP relationship, which in the basic state may be critical for platelet responsiveness (Apitz-Castro and De Murciano, 1978). Schultz *et al.* (1977) have found that in smooth muscle, many relaxant drugs such as sodium nitroprusside increase cyclic GMP levels, by as much as 50-fold. It is possible that NAD acts in a similar way, thus producing an increase in cyclic GMP levels in other cells including perhaps the vascular endothelium.

The metabolic processes in atherosclerosis are much more complex than those discussed on the basis of our results. Nevertheless, our investigations have shown that cyclic nucleotides may play an important role in atherosclerosis and in the response to vasoactive drugs.

170   *A. Bodzenta et al.*

REFERENCES

Apitz-Castro, R. and De Murciano, A. (1978). *Biochim. Biophys. Acta* **544**, 529.
Barber, A. J. (1976). *Biochim. Biophys. Acta* **444**, 579.
Bourgain, R. (1977). *Acta Clin. Belg.* **32**, 403.
D'Angelo, V., Villa, S. and Myśliwiec, M. (1978). *Thromb. Haemost.* **39**, 535.
Greengard, P. and Kebabian, J. W. (1974). *Fedn. Proc.* **33**, 1059.
Gryglewski, R. J. (1978). *Kardiol. Pol.* **21**, 489 (In Polish).
Gryglewski, R. J., Bunting, S., Moncada, S., Flower, R. J. and Vane, J. R. (1976). *Prostaglandins* **12**, 685.
Hadden, J. W., Hadden, E. M., Haddox, M. K. and Goldberg, N. D. (1972). *Proc. Natn. Acad. Sci. USA* **69**, 3024.
Harker, L. A., Ross, R. and Glomset, J. (1976). *Ann. N.Y. Acad. Sci.* **275**, 321.
Haslam, R. J., Davidson, M. M. L., Fox, J. E. B. and Lynham, J. A. (1978). *Thrombos. Haemostas. (Stuttgart)* **40**, 232.
Kukovetz, W. R. and Poch, G. (1970). *Naunyn-Schmiedebergs Arch. Pharmakol.* **267**, 189.
Moncada, S. and Vane, J. R. (1978). *Br. Med. Bull.* **34**, 129.
Moncada, S. and Vane, J. R. (1979). *New Engl. J. Med.* **300**, 1142.
Nalbandian, R. M. and Henry, R. L. (1978). *Seminars in Thrombos. Haemost.* **5**, 2, 87.
Samuelsson, B., Granström, E., Green, K., Hamberg, M. and Hammarström, S. (1975). *Prostaglandins* **44**, 669.
Seifert, W. E. and Rudland, P. S. (1974). *Nature* **248**, 138.
Sharp, A. A. (1965). *Lancet* **II**, 1296.
Schultz, K. D., Schultz, K. and Schultz, G. (1977). *Nature* **265**, 750.
Unger, W. G., Stamford, I. F. and Bennett, A. (1971). *Nature. Lond.* **233**, 336.
Vane, J. R. (1957). *Br. J. Pharmac. Chemother.* **12**, 344.
Vigdahl, R. L., Mongin, Jr., J. and Marquis, N. R. (1971). *Biochem. Biophys. Res. Commun.* **42**, 1088.
Yamazaki, H., Motomiya, T., Mashimoto, N., Asano, T. and Hidaka, H. (1978). *Thrombos. Haemost.* **39**, 158.
Zinzinger, H. and Silberbauer, K. (1978). *Atherogenese* **3**, 123.

ENHANCED *IN VIVO* PLATELET RELEASE REACTION IN DIABETIC PATIENTS WITH RETINOPATHY

J. Zahavi, D. J. Betteridge, N. A. G. Jones, J. Leyton, D. J. Galton
and V. V. Kakkar

*Thrombosis Research Unit, King's College Hospital Medical School,
London, UK and
Diabetes and Lipid Research Laboratory, St. Bartholomew's Hospital,
London, UK*

INTRODUCTION

Diabetes mellitus is one of the most common metabolic disorders. It is a proven risk factor for the development of atherosclerosis and its vaso-occlusive complications (Kannel *et al.*, 1971). These complications, as well as microangiopathy are frequent in diabetic patients. Platelets may play a central role in arterial thrombosis (White and Hespinstall, 1978) as well as in increased tendency to intravascular thrombosis in diabetes mellitus (Mansolf, 1975). However, no simple and reliable method as yet exists for measuring platelet function *in vivo*.

Recent developments have included measurement of plasma β-thromboglobulin and platelet factor 4 which are specific platelet proteins (Moore *et al.*, 1975; Niewiarowski *et al.*, (1968). β-Thromboglobulin is stored within the platelets in concentrations of $30-10^4$ times higher than in other tissues (Ludlam, 1979). It is extruded to the surrounding plasma during platelet aggregation (Holmsen, 1975), and is regarded as a useful indicator of *in vivo* platelet activation and release reaction. In previous studies, an increased sensitivity to various aggregating agents has been demonstrated *in vitro* in platelets from diabetic patients—the levels being highest in a small number of patients with neuropathy and retinopathy (Preston *et al.*, 1978; Burrows *et al.*, 1978). In one of these studies however, the patients were not compared with age and sex-matched controls (Burrows *et al.*,

Serono Symposium No. 37, "Vascular Occlusion: Epidemiological, Pathophysiological and Therapeutic Aspects", edited by M. Tesi and J. Dormany, 1981. Academic Press, London and New York.

J. Zahavi et al.

1978). Such a comparison is important since we and others have shown a significant increase in the plasma levels of β-thromboglobulin and platelet factor 4 with age (Zahavi *et al.*, 1979; Ludlam, 1979), and a sex difference in old healthy subjects (Zahavi *et al.*, 1979).

This study reports the levels of plasma β-thromboglobulin and platelet factor 4 in a large group of diabetic patients with and without retinopathy compared with age and sex-matched controls.

PATIENTS AND METHODS

One hundred and two patients (mean age 55.9 years) were studied (Table I). Forty-six patients were on insulin treatment, the remaining 56 on diet and/or oral hypoglycaemic drugs. Thirty patients suffered from retinopathy, 12 from peripheral vascular disease, two from ischaemic heart disease and in the remaining 58 there was no clinical evidence of vascular complications. The mean duration of

Table I. Clinical details of diabetic patients[a] and age and sex-matched controls.

	M	F	Age (years) Mean and range	Duration (months) Mean and range
30 Retinopathy	22	8	54.2 (28–73)	208.9 (33–480)
14 LVD[b]	9	5	63.9 (48–79)	209.8 (60–360)
58 NVD[c]	25	33	54.9 (20–76)	119.1 (14–295)
102 Controls	56	46	55.5 (19–83)	

[a]44 patients were on insulin, the remaining 56 on diet and/or oral hypoglycaemic drugs.
[b]Large vessel disease.
[c]No vascular disease.

the disease was beyond 10 years, it was lowest in patients without vascular disease. Patients were compared with age and sex-matched apparently healthy individuals. Plasma β-thromboglobulin level was determined in all the patients and platelet factor 4 in 67 of them. The 2 proteins were measured by radio-immunoassay as previously described (Zahavi *et al.*, 1979).

Statistical Analysis

Chi-squared analysis was used to test for non-normality distribution. In addition, the non-parametric Mann Whitney, Wilcoxon and Spearman tests (Siegel, 1956) were used in the analysis of data.

RESULTS

Plasma β-Thromboglobulin

The values for plasma β-thromboglobulin were not normally distributed and we have used therefore non-parametric statistical tests for the analysis of the data. The mean plasma level was 77.3 ng/ml in the 102 patients compared with only

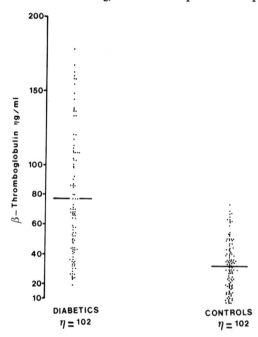

Fig. 1. Mean (horizontal lines) and distribution of plasma β-thromboglobulin levels in 102 patients with diabetes mellitus and age and sex-matched controls.

Table II. Plasma levels of β-thromboglobulin (β-TG) and platelet factor 4 (PF4) in diabetic patients and age and sex-matched controls.

	βTG ng/ml		PF4 ng/ml	
	No. studied	Mean and range	No. studied	Mean and range
Controls	102	33.2 (8–74)	67	14.9 (6.8–41.5)
Diabetic patients	102	77.3) (19–218)	67	51.5 (9–193)
P^a		≤ 0.0005		≤ 0.0005

P^a Wilcoxon pair differences test comparing patients to controls

33.2 ng/ml in the controls (Fig. 1, Table II). There was some overlap between patients and controls, however in 44 patients (43.1%), plasma β-thromboglobulin level was beyond the upper control range (Fig. 1). Statistically, the difference between patients and controls was highly significant (Table II).

Plasma Platelet Factor 4

The mean plasma platelet factor 4 level was 51.5 ng/ml in the 67 patients compared with 14.9 ng/ml in the controls (Fig. 2, Table II). Here again, there was some overlap between patients and controls. However, in 32 patients (48%), plasma platelet factor 4 level was beyond the upper control range (Fig. 2). Statistically, the difference between patients and controls was highly significant (Table II).

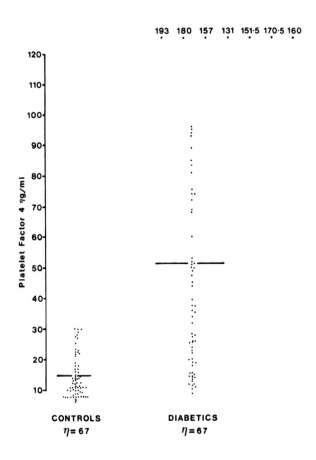

Fig. 2. Mean (horizontal lines) and distribution of plasma platelet factor 4 levels in 67 patients with diabetes mellitus and age and sex-matched controls.

Correlation of β-Thromboglobulin to Platelet Factor 4

Using the Spearman test, there was a significant positive correlation between plasma β-thromboglobulin and platelet factor 4 in the 67 patients studied and their age and sex matched controls (Table III). These results suggest that both proteins are released from the same platelet pool and presumably at the same rate.

Table III. Correlation between plasma β-thromboglobulin (βTG) and platelet factor 4 (PF4) in 67 diabetic patients and age and sex-matched controls.

	R^a	P
Controls	0.5012	$\leqslant 0.001$
Diabetic patients	0.7776	$\leqslant 0.001$

R^aCoefficient of correlation from the Spearman test.

COMPARISON OF β-THROMBOGLOBULIN AND PLATELET FACTOR 4 IN RETINOPATHY AND NON-RETINOPATHY PATIENTS

The mean plasma β-thromboglobulin and platelet factor 4 was higher in diabetic patients with retinopathy compared with those patients without (Table IV). There was an overlap between the two groups (Figs 3 and 4). However, in 15 (50%) of

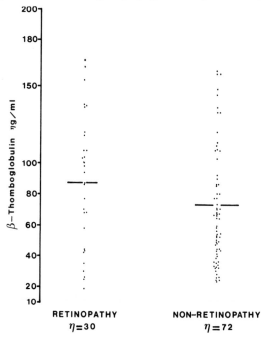

Fig. 3. Mean (horizontal lines) and distribution of plasma β-thromboglobulin levels in 30 retinopathy and 72 non-retinopathy patients.

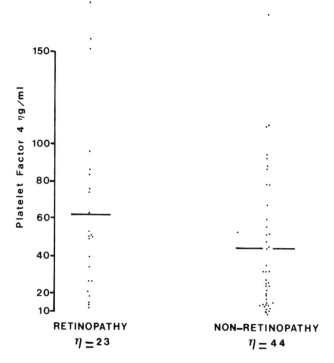

Fig. 4. Mean (horizontal lines) and distribution of plasma platelet factor 4 levels in 23 retinopathy and 44 non-retinopathy patients.

Table IV. Plasma levels of β-thromboglobulin (βTG) and platelet factor 4 (PF4) in patients with retinopathy.

	βTG ng/ml		PF4 ng/ml	
	No. studied	Mean and range	No. studied	Mean and range
Retinopathy	30	87.5 (19–167)	23	61.9 (11.5–181.5)
Non-retinopathy	72	73.1 (23–218)	44	46.1 (9–193)
P^a		≤ 0.046		≤ 0.031

P^aMann Whitney U-test comparing retinopathy to non-retinopathy patients.

the retinopathy compared with only 17 (23.6%) of the non-retinopathy patients, plasma β-thromboglobulin level was beyond 95 ng/ml (Fig. 3). Regarding platelet factor 4, in 13 (56.5%) retinopathy patients compared with only 15 (34%) non-retinopathy patients, the plasma level was beyond 49 ng/ml (Fig. 4). Statistically, the difference between the two groups was significant for both proteins (Table IV). There was no significant difference between diabetic patients with no vascular disease (mean level of β-thromboglobulin 73 ng/ml and of platelet factor 4 44.6 ng/ml) and patients with large vessel disease (peripheral vascular disease and ischaemic heart disease) (mean level of β-thromboglobulin 73.4 ng/ml and of platelet factor 4 55 ng/ml). Yet the last two groups of patients differed significantly from age and sex-matched controls (Wilcoxon test, $P \leqslant 0.0005$ for β-thromboglobulin and platelet factor 4).

Finally, there was no apparent difference in the plasma level of the 2 proteins between the 46 diabetic patients on insulin and the 56 on diet and/or oral hypoglycaemic drugs.

DISCUSSION

This study provides evidence that *in vivo* platelet activation and release reaction indicated by the increased plasma β-thromboglobulin and platelet factor 4 levels, is enhanced in diabetic patients and may lead to a pre-thrombotic state. The more pronounced increase in plasma β-thromboglobulin and platelet factor 4, in the diabetic patients with retinopathy than diabetics with no vascular complications or with large vessel disease, suggests that platelets may play an important role in the pathogenesis of diabetic microangiopathy. The duration of diabetes and its control by insulin or oral hypoglycaemic drugs, does not seem to influence the abnormal platelet function.

REFERENCES

Burrows, A. W., Chavin, S. I. and Hockaday, T. D. R. (1978). *Lancet* 1, 235.
Heath, H., Bridgden, W. D., Canever, J. V., Pollock, J., Hunter, P. R. and Kelsey, J. (1971). *Acta Diabetol.* 7, 308.
Holmsen, H. (1975). *In* "Biochemistry and Pharmacology of Platelets." Ciba Foundation Symposium 35. p. 175. Elsevier, North Holland.
Kannel, W. B., Castelli, W. P., Gordon, T. and McNamara, P. M. (1971). *Ann. Intern. Med.* 74, 1.
Ludlam, C. A. (1979). *Br. J. Haemat.* 41, 271.
Mansolf, F. A. (1975). *In* "The Eye in Systemic Disease." C. V. Mosby, St. Louis.
Moore, S., Pepper, D. S. and Cash, J. D. (1975). *Biochem. Biophys. Acta* 379, 360.
Niewiarowski, S., Poplawski, A., Lipinski, B. and Fabrizewski, R. (1968). *Exp. Biol. Med.* 3, 121.
O'Malley, B. C., Timperley, W. R., Ward, J. D., Porter, N. R. and Preston, F. E. (1975). *Lancet* 2, 1274.
Preston, F. E., Ward, J. D., Marcola, B. H., Porter, N. R., Timperley, W. R. and O'Malley, B. C. (1978). *Lancet* 1, 238.
Siegel, S. (1956). *In* "Non-parametric Statistics for Behavioural Sciences." McCraw Hill–Kogakuola Press, Tokyo.
White, A. M. and Hespinstall, S. (1978). *Br. Med. Bull.* 34, 123.
Zahavi, J., Jones, N. A. G., Leyton, J., Dubiel, M. and Kakkar, V. V. (1979). *Thromb. Res.* (In press.)

ALTERED PLATELET FUNCTION IN DIABETES MELLITUS. DECREASE OF VASCULAR PROSTACYCLIN, ANALYSIS OF PLASMA β-THROMBOGLOBULIN AND PLATELET FACTOR 4 ACCORDING TO STATE OF METABOLIC CONTROL AND DIABETIC MICROANGIOPATHY STAGES

G. Schernthaner, H. Sinzinger, K. Silberbauer and H. Freyler

Department of Medicine II and Department of Ophthalmology I, University of Vienna, Austria and Ludwig Boltzmann Institute for Clinical Endocrinology and Nuclear Medicine, Vienna, Austria

A number of factors are held responsible at present for the initiation or perpetuation of diabetic microangiopathy. Abnormal hemostasis for instance with increased activity of coagulation factors and reduced fibrinolytic activity, has long been considered a possible mechanism in the pathophysiology of diabetic angiopathy. In this connection, disturbed platelet function has received increased attention.

In diabetes mellitus, a variety of disturbed platelet functions has been found (Hassanein *et al.*, 1972; Heath *et al.*, 1978; Bensoussan *et al.*, 1975; Colwell *et al.*, 1976) and has been connected with the pathogenesis of late diabetic manifestations. Platelet-like aggregates were found in small vessels of patients with microangiopathy (Timperley *et al.*, 1974; Fagerberg *et al.*, 1959) and preliminary data have shown increased appearance of "circulating" reversible platelet aggregates in diabetes mellitus (Silberbauer *et al.*, 1978; Preston *et al.*, 1978).

Recently, it has been reported (Halushka *et al.*, 1976) that platelets from patients with diabetes mellitus produce more prostaglandin-E-like material than platelets from normal subjects when exposed to ADP, epinephrine or collagen. These data show that platelet hypersensitivity in diabetes may be related to an altered prostaglandin metabolism in the platelets, Preliminary data have shown

Serono Symposium No. 37, "Vascular Occlusion: Epidemiological, Pathophysiological and Therapeutic Aspects", edited by M. Tesi and J. Dormany, 1981. Academic Press, London and New York.

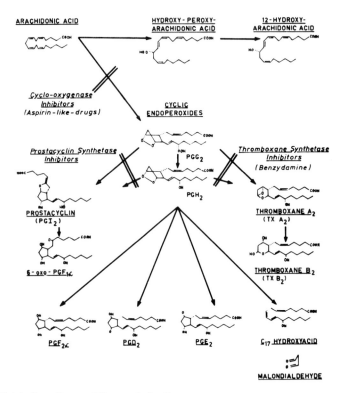

Fig. 1. Metabolic pathway of the prostaglandin system.

(Silberbauer *et al.*, 1979a, Johnson *et al.*, 1979) that the endogenous suppressor of platelet aggregation, also a member of the prostaglandin series (Fig. 1), is diminished in the vessel walls of diabetic patients.

In this review, the data of platelet functions currently available and their control mechanisms in diabetes mellitus are analysed in the context of the state of metabolic control and the stage of diabetic angiopathy.

PATIENTS, MATERIAL AND METHODS

Two hundred and fifty patients with juvenile onset diabetes mellitus (type I-diabetes) and 250 patients with "maturity onset" diabetes (type II) as well as 100 healthy individuals were studied. Plasma levels of β-thromboglobulin (β-TG) and platelet factor 4 (PF4)–platelet specific proteins which are released when platelets aggregate–were measured by radioimmunoassay accord to Bolton *et al.* (1976a) and Bolton *et al.* (1976b) respectively. Metabolic control of the patients was assessed by measurement of the actual blood glucose concentrations, the 24-h glucosuria and the concentrations of the glycosylated hemoglobin A_1.

Glucose concentrations were measured by the glucose-oxidase method and hemoglobin A_1 by ion-exchange chromatography. Prostacyclin (PGI$_2$-similar compounds) was determined immediately after removal of small venous segments which were removed by microsurgery from the lower arm under local anesthesia, in 15 juvenile diabetics and 15 healthy indivuduals using the bioassay described by Moncada *et al.* (1977). The ADP-induced platelet aggregation was used as an indicator in a turbidometric system. The generation of PGI_2 was calculated by standard curves of varying concentrations of a synthetic PGI_2 standard kindly provided by Dr Pike of the Upjohn Company, USA. Fluorescein angiography was the main parameter for the assessment of diabetic retinopathy: Stages: Stage 0 (normal ophthalmoscopic picture, normal angiogramm). Stage I: preretinopathy (normal ophthalmoscopic picture, fluorescein leakage and capillary occlusion in the angiogram); mainly exudative = Ia; predominantly occlusive = Ib. Stage II: non-proliferative diabetic retinopathy (stage I + microaneurysms, waxy exudates, cotton wool patches, retinal edema and hemorrhages; in the angiogram, these ophthalmoscopic lesions + dye leakage and capillary occlusion); mainly exudative = IIa, predominantly occlusive = IIb. Stage III: proliferative diabetic retinopathy (stage II + newly-formed vessels).

RESULTS

Plasma concentrations of β-TG and PF4 were significantly increased in the patients with type-I diabetes (n = 250) as well as in type-II diabetes (n = 250) in comparison to healthy individuals (n = 100; Fig. 2). A highly significant correlation was found between the plasma-levels of β-TG and PF4 in the type-I diabetics (Fig. 3; n = 75; r = 0.80, r = 0.80, $P < 0.005$) and in the type-II diabetics (n = 60, r = 0.88, $P < 0.005$). No correlation could be observed between the plasma-β-TG-levels and the actual blood glucose concentrations or the degree of 24-h glucosuria either in patients with type-I or in patients with type-II diabetes. In addition, no connection could be noted between the values of glycosylated hemoglobin (para-

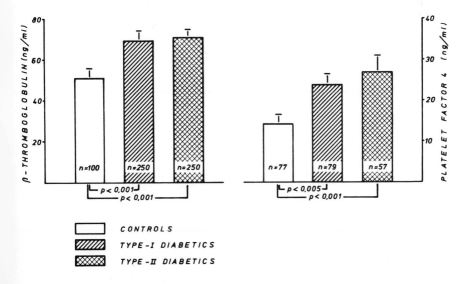

Fig. 2. Plasma concentrations of β-thromboglobulin and platelet factor 4 in patients with type I diabetes, type II diabetes and healthy controls.

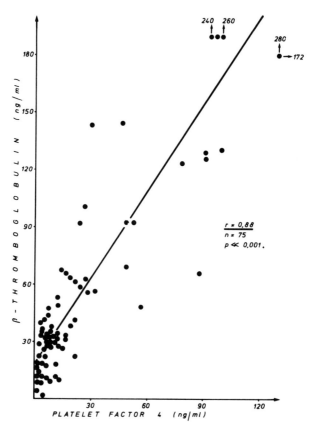

Fig. 3. Close correlation between plasma concentrations of β-thromboglobulin and platelet factor 4 in 75 type I diabetics.

meter of diabetic long-term control) and the plasma concentrations of the platelet "release products" either in patients with type-I or in patients with type-II diabetes (Fig. 4). The analysis of the plasma concentrations of β-TG in type-I diabetic patients with different stages of diabetic retinopathy is shown in Table I.

A tendency to a positive correlation between the severity of diabetic retinopathy and the increase of plasma β-TG was found, although the relation did not reach levels of significance. Plasma β-TG concentrations were higher in the patients with occlusive retinal lesions than in those with an exudative form of diabetic preretinopathy or non-proliferative retinopathy. Comparative examination of vessel segments of insulin-dependent diabetics (type I diabetics) with age- and sex-matched controls showed that vessel walls of insulin-dependent diabetics have diminished generation of PGI_2 in comparison to the vessel walls of healthy individuals (Fig. 5).

DISCUSSION

In the present study, significantly increased plasma-concentrations of β-TG or PF4 were found in a representative number of type-I and type-II diabetics, which

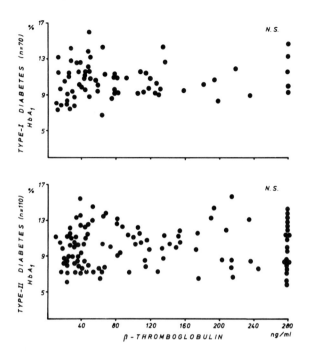

Fig. 4. Lack of correlation between plasma β-thromboglobulin and glycosylated haemoglobin (HbA₁) in patients with type I diabetes and type II diabetes.

Table I. Plasma β-thromboglobulin concentrations (mean ± s.e.) in type I diabetics with different stages of diabetic retinopathy.

Stages of diabetic retinopathy	β-Thromboglobulin (ng/ml)	
Stage 0	55.5 ± 7.2	(12)[a]
Stage 1	66.1 ± 8.6	(27)
1a	51.8 ± 8.3	(9)
1b	73.3 ± 12.2	(18)
Stage 2	77.6 ± 17.4	(9)
2a	67.0 ± 12.5	(4)
2b	86.2 ± 32.8	(5)
Stage 3	95.2 ± 26.9	(10)
All stages	70.7 ± 6.1	(58)

[a]Number of patients.

confirms data previously reported (Burrows *et al.*, 1978; Preston *et al.*, 1978; Schernthaner *et al.*, 1979a). The levels of β-TG and PF4 showed a strong positive correlation in the plasma, suggesting that both platelet proteins are released from the same platelet pool. Plasma-β-TH-levels are also reported to be increased in deep vein thrombosis (Ludlam *et al.*, 1975), acute myocardial infarction (Denham

G. Schernthaner et al.

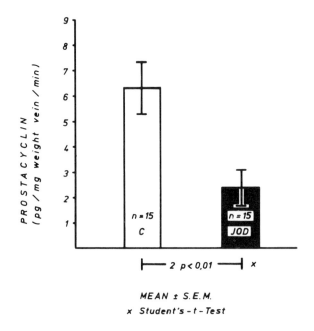

Fig. 5. Significantly decreased prostacyclin generation in vessel walls of type I diabetics (JOD) compared with healthy controls (C).

et al., 1977), pre-eclampsia (Redman et al., 1977), prosthetic heart valves (Ludlam et al., 1975), coronary artery disease (Mühlhauser et al., 1980), peripheral vascular disease (Cella et al., 1979), polycythemia vera and multiple myeloma (Schernthaner et al., 1979b) and are assumed to be reliable indicators for quantitating platelet function in vivo (Ludlam, 1979).

In this investigation, no connection could be observed between the stage of metabolic control and the plasma-levels of the platelet specific proteins either in 70 type-I diabetics or in 110 type-II diabetics. These data, however, do not exclude the existence of a correlation between platelet function and metabolic control in some diabetics, especially when extreme situations of diabetes control are taken into account. Preliminary data in favour of this hypothesis were reported in a very small number of patients by Peterson et al. (1977) and by Preston et al. (1978).

Interestingly, the data of Betteridge et al. (1979) confirmed the lack of correlation (Schernthaner et al., 1979c) between the concentrations of glycosylated hemoglobin and β-TG. To date, it is not known to what extent β-TG levels are correlated to the degree of diabetic microangiopathy. Preston et al. (1978) reported that the mean plasma β-TG level of diabetics with complications was higher than that of patients without late manifestations, although there was a wider overlap in β-TG between the two relatively small patient groups. In the present study, β-TG concentrations were analysed in 58 well-defined insulin-dependent, juvenile-onset diabetic patients, who were staged for diabetic retinopathy by repeated fluorescein angiography. Higher mean levels of β-TG were noted in patients with increasing severity of diabetic retinopathy. Type-I diabetics with predominantly occlusive retinal lesions showed higher β-TG levels than patients with mainly exudative retinal changes in the fluorescein angiogram. Interestingly, the occlusive form of diabetic pre-retinopathy or non-proliferative retinopathy has a particular tendency to progress (Freyler, 1975). Our preliminary data suggest that repeated measurements of plasma β-TG may be a useful marker for the recognition of patients with a higher risk of a progressive form of diabetic microangiopathy. In this context, it must be taken into consideration that the renal function may play a significant role, since the plasma β-TG-concentration is determined by the rate of its release from the platelets into, and the rate of its clearance from the circulation.

The significantly decreased generation of prostacyclin—the most important endogenous suppressor of platelet aggregation *in vivo*—in the vessel walls of 15 juvenile diabetics compared with age- and sex-matched controls indicates that an altered prostaglandin metabolism is an important factor for the hyperactive stage of platelets in diabetes mellitus. In the relatively small number of patients tested, no significant correlation could be observed between the prostacyclin activity and the duration of disease, the state of metabolic control and the presence of diabetic microangiopathy. The diminished PGI_2-generation in the vessel walls of diabetics could be caused by reduced ability of arachidonic acid to form membrane phospholipids or by a diminished activity of cyclo-oxygenase or PGI_2-synthetase (Fig. 1). However, a faster *in vivo* or *in vitro* PGI_2 degradation to 6-oxo-$PGF_{1\alpha}$—a stable metabolite of PGI_2—could not be excluded by the present available data. Recently, Johnson *et al.* (1979) also described a diminished vascular prostacyclin activity in three diabetic patients. The data obtained in humans (Silberbauer *et al.*, 1979a; Johnson *et al.*, 1979) were supported by experimental studies in streptocotocin Wistar-rats and in Göttingen-minipigs (Harrison *et al.*, 1978; Silberbauer *et al.*, 1979b). Further studies will be essential in order to clarify whether the decreased vascular prostacyclin generation in diabetes is a disease-associated phenomenon or a sequence of metabolic disturbance. Preliminary data (Schernthaner *et al.*, 1979d) have shown that significantly increased β-TG levels in diabetics with proliferative retinopathy can be lowered by treatment with dipyridamole, which is assumed to potentiate prostacyclin or directly stimulate the release of this thromboregulatory hormone. In the future, administration of prostacyclin or prostacyclin-analogs might be a new approach in the prevention or treatment of diabetic angiopathy.

REFERENCES

Bensoussan, D., Levy-Toledano, S., Passa, P., Caen, J. and Canivet, J. (1975). *Diabetologia* 11, 307.

Betteridge, D. J., Zahavi, J., Jones, N. A. G., Patel, H., Leyton, J. and Kakkar, V. V. (1979). *Excerpta Medica JCS* 481, 23.

Bolton, A. E., Ludlam, C. A., Pepper, D. S., Moore, S. and Cash, J. D. (1976a). *Thrombosis Research* 8, 51.

Bolton, A. E., Ludlam, C. A., Moore, S., Pepper, D. S. and Cash, J. D. (1976b). *British Journal of Haematology* 32, 73.

Burrows, A. W., Chavin, S. I. and Hockaday, T. D. R. (1978). *Lancet* 1, 235.

Cella, G., Zahavi, J., Haas de, H. A. and Kakkar, V. V. (1979). *British Journal of Haematology* 43, 127.

Colwell, J. A., Halushka, P. V., Sarji, K., Sagel, J. and Nair, R. M. G. (1976). *Diabetes* 25, 826.

Fagerberg, S. E. (1959). *Acta Medica Scandinavica* 3, 45.

Freyler, H. (1975). *Wiener Klinische Wochenschrift* 87, Suppl. 41.

Halushka, P. V., Lurie, D. and Colwell, J. A. (1977). *New England Journal of Medicine* 297, 1306.

Harrison, H. E., Reece, A. H. and Johnson, M. (1978). *Life Sciences, 23,* 351.

Hassanein, A. A., El-Graf, Th. and El-Baz, S. (1972). *Thrombosis Diathesis Haemorrhagica* 27, 114.

Heath, H., Bridgen, W. D., Canever, J. V., Pollock, J., Hunter, P. R., Kelsey, J. and Bloom, A. (1978). *Diabetologia* 7, 308.

Johnson, M., Harrison, H. E., Raftery, A. T. and Elder, J. P. (1979). *Lancet* 1, 325.

Ludlam, C. A. (1979). *British Journal of Haematology* 41, 271.

Ludlam, C. A., Bolton, A. E., Moore, S. and Cash, J. D. (1975). *Lancet* 2, 259.

Moncada, S., Higgs, E. A. and Lane, J. R. (1977). *Lancet* 1, 18.

Mühlhauser, I., Schernthaner, G., Silberbauer, K. and Kaindl, F. (1980). (In press)

Peterson, C. M., Jones, R. L., Koenig, R. J., Melvin, E. T. and Lehrman, M. L. (1977). *Annals of Internal Medicine* 86, 425.

Preston, F. E., Ward, J. D., Marcola, B. H., Porter, N. R., Timperley, W. R. and O'Malley, B. C. (1978). *Lancet* 1, 238.

Redman, C. W. G., Allington, M. J., Bolton, F. G. and Sirrat, G. M. (1977). *Lancet* 2, 248.

Schernthaner, G., Silberbauer, K., Sinzinger, H., Piza-Katzer, H. and Winter, M. (1979a). *European Journal of Clinical Investigation* 9, II, 31.

Schernthaner, G., Ludwig, H. and Silberbauer, K. (1979b). *Acta Haematologia* (In press.)

Schernthaner, G., Silberbauer, K., Sinzinger, H. and Müller, M. (1979c). *Thrombosis Haemostasis* 42, 334.

Schernthaner, G., Mühlhauser, I. and Silberbauer, K. (1979d). *Lancet* 2, 748.

Silberbauer, K. F., Schernthaner, G., Ludwig, H., Sinzinger, H. and Freyler, H. (1978). (In press.)

Silberbauer, K., Schernthaner, G., Sinzinger, H., Piza-Katzer, H. and Winter, M. (1979a). *New England Journal of Medicine* 300, 366.

Silberbauer, K., Schernthaner, G., Sinzinger, H., Clopath, P., Piza-Katzer, H. and Winter, M. (1979b). *Thrombosis and Haemostasis* 42, 303.

FACTOR VIII COMPONENTS IN OCCLUSIVE ARTERIAL DISEASE AND THEIR RESPONSE TO VENOUS OCCLUSION

O. Ponari, C. Manotti, A. Megha, M. Pini, R. Poti and A. G. Dettori

Centro per le Malattie Emostatiche, Ospedali Riuniti di Parma, Parma, Italy

The aim of this investigation was to examine Factor VIII (F VIII) complex (coagulant activity: F VIII:C; protein related antigen: F VIII R:Ag and von Willebrand activity: F VIII R:vW) in the plasma of a group of patients with peripheral vascular disease, and evaluate its changes in response to venostasis.

MATERIAL AND METHODS

The investigation was carried out on 30 male subjects, mean age 61.2 years (range 39–73 year), with atherosclerosis obliterans of the legs, Fontaine class II and III. Diagnosis was made on clinical and instrumental grounds (oscillometry, Doppler sonography and arteriography whenever possible). The control group comprised 21 male subjects, mean age 60.1 years (range 30–73 year), free of clinical manifestations of atherosclerosis.

Blood was taken without stasis from an antecubital vein of resting subjects in the morning, then venous stasis was induced in one arm by means of a sphygmomanometer cuff, inflated at a level intermediate between systolic and diastolic pressure for 10 min. Immediately before deflating the cuff, a second sample of blood was drawn from the compressed arm. F VIII:C was determined with a one-stage method (Reagents and method from General Diagnostic, Morris Plains, NY, USA). F VIII R:Ag was determined by electroimmunodiffusion (Laurell, 1966). F VIII R:vW was measured by the method of Weiss *et al.* (1973).

As a reference plasma for the determination of coagulant activity, the "Reference Plasma 100% F VIII" of Immuno Diagnostika, Vienna, Austria, was

Serono Symposium No. 37, "Vascular Occlusion: Epidemiological, Pathophysiological and Therapeutic Aspects", edited by M. Tesi and J. Dormany, 1981. Academic Press, London and New York.

employed. A pool of plasma from 20 normal male and female subjects, aged between 18 and 70 years, was used as a reference plasma for antigen and von Willebrand activity.

RESULTS AND COMMENT

Comparisons

Comparisons between patient and control group are reported in Fig. 1. Mean values of the single component of F VIII complex and ratios between them, both before and after venostasis, are considered. There are no statistically significant variations between the two groups for any parameter considered. In other words,

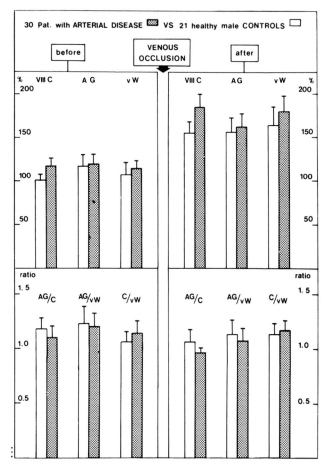

Fig. 1. Comparison between patients and controls for components of factor VIII complex and ratios between them, under basal conditions (left) and after venous occlusion (right). Differences between means were analysed by Student's "t" test for unpaired data.

the mean plasma levels of F VIII complex in patients with advanced atherosclerosis obliterans of the legs are similar to those of a healthy control group, either under basal conditions or after venostasis. The same is true of the ratios between the single components of F VIII complex. In both groups, plasma levels of the three components are, on average, higher than the levels of the reference plasma. The rather old age of the subjects may account for this finding, since plasma levels of F VIII are reported to increase with age (Cooperberg and Teitelbaum, 1960; Meade and North, 1977).

Effects

The effect of venostasis on the single F VIII components is reported in Table I. Stasis induces a marked increase of the activities examined, with a significant difference in the mean values for each component, either in patient or control groups.

Table II reports changes induced by venostasis on the ratios between the single F VIII components. In the control group, the ratios do not change; in the patient group, there are significant variations in the ratio Ag/C.

These findings demonstrate that a standardized venostasis induces an increase in plasma levels not only of F VIII C, as previously known (Egeberg, 1963; Ponari *et al.*, 1973) but of all the F VIII components. In the same way as other stimuli (adrenaline: Ingram, 1961; Gader *et al.*, 1973; physical exercise: Rizza, 1961; Prentice *et al.*, 1972; Denson, 1973), venostasis causes a release of F VIII

Table I. Changes induced by venous occlusion on components of factor VIII complex.

	Basal m̄ (se)	Ven. Occl. m̄ (se)	Differences[a] t	P
CONTROL (n = 21)				
F VIII: C	100.62 (8.13)	155.57 (12.46)	7.57	< 0.001
F VIII R: AG	116.67 (12.82)	155.71 (16.26)	6.25	< 0.001
F VIII R: VW	108.00 (12.39)	161.28 (21.20)	3.74	< 0.01
PATIENTS (n = 30)				
F VIII: C	117.27 (8.50)	185.60 (15.17)	7.29	< 0.001
F VIII R: AG	120.43 (11.31)	162.00 (14.74)	7.57	< 0.001
F VIII R: VW	114.73 (9.00)	180.20 (18.11)	4.11	< 0.001

[a]Differences between means before and after stasis analysed by Student's "t" test for paired data.

Table II. Changes induced by venous occlusion on ratios between factor VIII components.

		Basal $\bar{m}$ (se)	Ven. Occl. $\bar{m}$ (se)	Differences[a] t	P
CONTROLS (n = 21)					
AG/C	Ratio	1.18 (0.12)	1.06 (0.11)	1.79	NS
AG/VW	Ratio	1.23 (0.15)	1.13 (0.10)	1.37	NS
C/VW	Ratio	1.06 (0.09)	1.13 (0.10)	1.08	NS
PATIENTS (n = 30)					
AG/C	Ratio	1.10 (0.10)	0.96 (0.08)	3.25	< .01
AG/VW	Ratio	1.19 (0.12)	1.07 (0.11)	1.13	NS
C/VW	Ratio	1.14 (0.11)	1.17 (0.09)	0.27	NS

[a]Differences between means before and after stasis analysed by Student's "t" test for paired data (NS = $P > 0.05$).

from vascular endothelium, the site of its synthesis and storage can be hypothesized. The increase of the single components, which maintain the same ratios before and after venostasis, is consistent with the release of a preformed F VIII molecule(s). The differences shown by atherosclerotic patients only in the ratio Ag/C indicate, on the other hand, a more variable response of these patients. The increase of F VIII : C in local blood after venostasis is, however, difficult to explain in terms of release. In fact vascular endothelium has been shown to contain only F VIIIR:Ag and F VIII R:vW (cf. Bloom, 1978). It has to be assumed that the released F VIII complex may rapidly acquire coagulant activity in the peripheral blood.

REFERENCES

Bloom, A. L. (1978). *Haematologica* **63**, 101.
Cooperberg, A. A. and Teitelbaum, J. (1960). *British Journal of Haematology* **6**, 281.
Denson, K. W. E. (1973). *British Journal of Haematology* **24**, 491.
Egeberg, O. (1963). *Scandinavian Journal of Clinical and Laboratory Investigation* **15**, 20.
Gader, A. M. A., Clarkson, A. R. and Cash, J. D. (1973). *Thrombosis Research* **2**, 9.
Ingram, G. I. C. (1961). *Journal of Physiology* **156**, 217.
Laurell, C. B. (1966). *Analytical Biochemistry* **15**, 45.

Meade, T. W. and North, W. R. S. (1977). *British Medical Bulletin* **33**, 283.
Ponari, O., Civardi, E., Megha, A., Pini, M., Poti, R. and Dettori, A. G. (1973). *British Journal of Haematology* **24**, 463.
Prentice, C. R. M., Forbes, C. D. and Smith, S. M. (1972). *Thrombosis Research* **1**, 493.
Rizza, C. R. (1961). *Journal of Physiology* **156**, 128.
Weiss, H. J., Hover, L. W., Rickles, F. R., Varma, A. and Rogers, J. (1973). *Journal of Clinical Investigation* **52**, 2708.

ANTITHROMBIN III IN PATIENTS WITH ATHEROSCLEROTIC VASCULAR DISEASE

G. Avellone, V. Mandala, F. P. Riola and A. Pinto

Institute of Clinical Medicine and Medical Therapy of University of Palermo, Palermo, Italy

Antithrombin III (AT III) by operating both on factor X and on thrombin, has clinical interest because it has been shown to be decreased by Mackie *et al.* (1978) and Sas *et al.* (1974) in patients with familial thrombophilia, in the post-operative period (Stathakis *et al.*, 1973), in thrombophlebitis of limbs (von Kaulla and von Kaulla, 1967; Hedner and Nilsson, 1973), in young women submitted to estrogen-progestogen oral contraceptive therapy (Fagerhol *et al.*, 1970; von Kaulla and von Kaulla, 1970) and in atherosclerotic vascular disease.

In patients with myocardial infarction, Hedner and Nilsson (1973) have shown low levels of AT III by both biological and immunological methods; these results are confirmed by O'Brien (1974). In a study on atherosclerotic patients with myocardial infarction, angina pectoris, essential hypertension and stroke, Banerjee *et al.* (1974) shown a decrease of AT III activity; this decrement was also found in a group of diabetic patients. Hardin *et al.* (1975), studying patients with stroke, noticed that those with serious illness had a progressive increase of high weight molecular complexes of fibrinogen degradation (HWMFD) in the days following the acute cerebrovascular accident. In a group of patients with coronary heart disease subjected to coronary angiography, Yue (1976) has shown that a decrease of AT III activity is a high-risk factor in acute coronary thrombosis, and assumes that coronary heart disease is a gradual process linked to progressive decrease of the inhibitor mechanism and suggests a possible therapeutic approach with heparin.

Serono Symposium No. 37, "Vascular Occlusion: Epidemiological, Pathophysiological and Therapeutic Aspects", edited by M. Tesi and J. Dormany, 1981. Academic Press, London and New York.

Innerfield et al. (1976) has shown by coronary angiography that an excellent correlation exists between low AT III activity and one, two or three coronary vessel occlusions. In a group of male patients submitted to coronary angiography, Stormorken and Herkssen (1977) showed patients with stenosis or blockage of a coronary vessel had a significant decrease of AT III activity.

MATERIALS AND METHODS

We examined 211 patients, 75 of which were the control group, (M. 39–F. 36, age mean 41.5), who on the grounds of clinical and ECG patterns were divided into three groups.

(a)   Forty patients with coronary heart disease (CHD), 30 with ECG findings of ischemia at rest and ten with a myocardial infarction history at least 36 months before.

(b)   Thirty patients with cerebral vascular disease (CVD): 20 of which had clinical symptoms of progressive mental change (unreliable memory, vertigo, tinnitus, decreased power of concentration, emotional instability or sleep disorder); ten with a stroke history from at least 8 months before.

(c)   Sixty-eight patients with peripheral vascular disease (PVD): graded on clinical symptoms (according to Fontaine) and pathological rheography were divided into: 29 patients at stage I; 28 patients at stage II; 11 patients at stage III.

After an observation period of at least 4 days, during which time the administration of drugs was reduced to the essential minimum, all had venous blood drawn from an antecubital vein without venostasis. Patients with pathology that might influence the biological determination of AT III activity were excluded. The determination of AT III was executed by a modified von Kaulla method. The values, expressed as a percentage of activity and read off a datum-line, were obtained from the pooled serum of 10 healthy donors and verified periodically in our laboratory.

RESULTS

The results have shown that in patients with atherosclerotic vascular disease, AT III activity is decreased compared with a control group (Fig. 1). In patients with CHD, the mean value of AT III activity is 81.77% s.d. 33.88), a low value compared with the control group which had a mean of 113.17% (s.d. 18.63). A value slightly higher is shown in patients with CVD who have a mean value of 73.59% (s.d. 29.05). The highest value was shown by patients with PVD at 79.14% (s.d. 32.39). It was possible to define two sub-groups of CHD ischemia (value 88.77%-s.d. 35.01) and myocardial infarction history (mean value 73.57%-s.d. 29.88), AT III activity was lowest in patients with a myocardial infarction history (Fig. 2).

Patients with cerebral atherosclerosis had a lower value with a stroke history (70.77%–s.d. 29.04) than patients with progressive mental changes (74.99%–s.d.

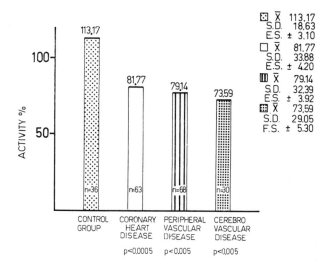

Fig. 1.

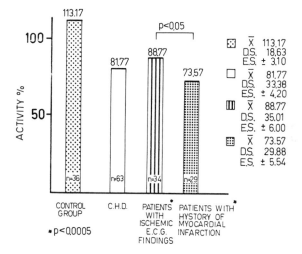

Fig. 2.

29.70) (Fig. 3). Lastly, in the group with atherosclerosis of the lower limbs, the lowest value was shown by patients in stage III (58.73%–s.d. 39.12). The value at stage I was 83.18% (s.d. 29.66) (Fig. 4).

CONCLUSION

The decreased AT III activity shown in patients with atherosclerotic vascular disease confirms an increase of fibrinogen forming processes, influenced by

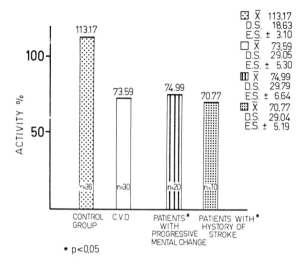

Fig. 3.

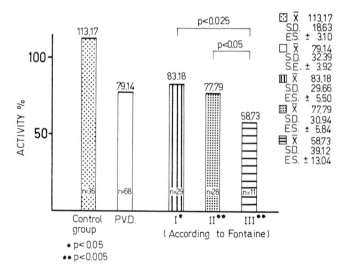

Fig. 4.

inhibitor activity. The action of thrombin on fibrinogen giving high molecular weight complexes of fibrinogen is certainly one factor altering flow and the formation of an occluding thrombus.

Therefore the finding of a decreased AT III activity suggests the use of therapy aimed at increasing the inhibitor activity.

REFERENCES

Banerjee, R. N., Sahni, A. L., Kumar, V. and Arya, M. (1974). *Thromb. Diath. Haemorrh.* **32**, 116–123.

Fagerhol, M. K., Abildgaard, U., Bergsjo, P. and Jacobsen, J. K. (1970). *Lancet* May 30, 1175.

Hardin, W. *et al.* (1975). *Stroke*.

Hedner, U. and Nilsson, I. M. (1973). *Thromb. Res.* **3**, 631–641.

Innerfield, I. *et al.*(1976). *Am. J. Clin. Pathol.* **65**, 64–68.

von Kaulla, E. and von Kaulla, K. N. (1967). *Am. J. Clin. Path.* **48**, 69–80.

von Kaulla, E. and von Kaulla, K. N. (1970). *Lancet* Jan. 3, 36.

Mackie, M., Bennet, B., Ogston, D. and Douglas, A. S. (1978). *Br. J. Haemat.* **22**, 341–351.

O'Brien, J. R. (1974). *Thromb. Diathes. Haemorr.* **32**, 116–123.

Sas, G. *et al.* (1974). *Thromb. Diathes. Haemorr.* **32**, 105–115.

Stathakis, N. *et al.* (1973). *Lancet* Feb. 24.

Stormorken, H. and Herkssen, J. (1977). *Thromb. Haemost.* **38**, 874–880.

FACILITATION OF ACTIVATOR INDUCED FIBRINOLYSIS WITH LOW DOSES OF PLASMIN AND SUBSEQUENT DECREASE IN α2-ANTIPLASMIN LEVEL

J. Choay, J. C. Lormeau, F. Toulemonde and G. Antoine

Institut Choay, Paris, France

INTRODUCTION

In the plasma, the fibrinolytic process initiated by plasminogen activators is slowed by two categories of inhibitors: firstly activation inhibitors, which oppose the enzyme action of the activators and thereby prevent the conversion of plasminogen to plasmin; secondly, plasmin inhibitors, which block the enzyme as it is formed and thereby interfere with the breakdown of fibrin.

Recent studies (Collen, (1976); Moroi and Aoki (1976); Mullertz and Clemmensen (1976); Wiman and Collen (1977)) have shown that the resistance of plasma to the induction of fibrinolysis comes essentially from the second category of inhibitors, and in particular an antagonist called α2-antiplasmin (α2-PI), a fast-acting plasmin inhibitor or primary inhibitor of plasmin. This glycoprotein, with a molecular weight of 65 000, present in the plasma at a concentration of 1 μmol/l, instantaneously and irreversibly forms an enzymatically inactive complex with plasmin. Moroi and Aoki (1976) have shown that this plasmin inhibitor has a certain affinity for lysyl-plasminogen and thereby interferes with fibrin lysyl-plasminogen interactions by obstructing the binding sites of the latter. The importance of the role of α2-PI led us to raise the possibility of lowering its inhibitory power using human plasmin and to study the consequences of this lowering both on the fibrinolysis induced by a plasminogen activator, urokinase, and on fibrin lysyl-plasminogen interactions. This study was carried out *in vitro*, by adding increasing amounts of human plasmin to human plasma;

Serono Symposium No. 37, "Vascular Occlusion: Epidemiological, Pathophysiological and Therapeutic Aspects", edited by M. Tesi and J. Dormany, 1981. Academic Press, London and New York.

in this plasma, residual α2-PI levels have been determined by an immunological technique, and clot lysis time measured as well as the binding level of lysyl-plasminogen.

MATERIAL AND METHODS

Human plasma, platelet poor plasma, citrated and stored frozen at $-35°C$; urokinase (Choay, Paris), human urinary origin, 54 000 mol/wt, specific activity 100 000 IU/mg of protein; lysyl-plasminogen (Choay, Paris), human placental extract (method: Lormeau, 1976), specific activity 2.5 μkat/mg of protein; plasmin, prepared by activation of lysyl-plasminogen by urokinase bound to agar gel, specific activity 2 μkat/mg, active sites: 80% according to the estimation of Chase and Shaw (1967); thrombin (Roche) bovin origin 50 NIH μ/mg; rabbit α2-PI serum, kindly supplied by Dr D. Collen, to whom our thanks are due. The measurement of α2-PI levels was made by the immunoelectrophoretic technique of Laurell (1966).

The measurement of plasma clot lysis time was made by the following being successively added to a series of haemolysis tubes placed in a water bath at $37°C$: 1 ml of plasma, plasmin in increasing amounts from 0 to 1 μmol/l of plasma; 3 μl of the mixture taken for estimation of α2-PI at each dilution; 60 Iu of uro-kinase then added to each tube, followed by 2 NIH units of thrombin. The lysis time of the clot formed varies according to the quantity of plasmin added. Clot lysis time is measured. A parallel series of tubes without addition of urokinase was set up in order to assess the degree of lysis caused by plasmin alone.

Measurement of the binding level of lysyl-plasminogen to fibrin is established by using the technique adapted from that developed by Vairel (1970) for deter-mining low plasmin activity. A clot is formed by recalcification of 0.5 ml of human plasma at the end of a glass tube. This clot is washed with saline until there is no further lysis observed in the presence of urokinase, which requires 1 to 2 h of washing. The clot is then left in contact for 1 h with a 0.1 mg/ml solution of lysyl-plasminogen in plasma containing varying doses of plasmin (from 0 to 1 μmol/l). The clot is then again washed for 1 h. It is finally left to incubate with a 20 IU/ml solution of urokinase at $37°C$ and clot lysis time measured. The greater or lesser binding level of lysyl-plasminogen to the clot is reflected by faster or slower fibrin clot lysis time after addition of urokinase.

RESULTS

Influence on Fibrinolysis of Decreased α2-PI Levels

Table I shows the level of residual α2-PI in relation to the amount of added plasmin and the clot lysis time with or without urokinase. While at the beginning of the addition of plasmin, the level of inhibitor decreases regularly by approxi-mately 10% with each addition of 0.1 μmol of plasmin, beyond 0.6 μmol the decrease is no longer proportional, and finally approximately 25% of inhibitor remains which does not appear to react with plasmin.

Table I. Clot lysis time under the influence of urokinase in plasma to which increasing amounts of plasmin have been added.

Added plasmin (μmol/l of plasma)	0	0.1	0.2	0.3	0.4	0.5	0.6	0.7	0.8	0.9	1
α 2-antiplasmin (residual) estimation according to Laurell, mean of 4 measurements (% of initial content)	100	91	82	69	58	45	39	34	31	27	25
Clot lysis time without addition of urokinase (min)	absence of lysis	absence of lysis	absence of lysis	absence of lysis	absence of lysis	140	70	30	17	5	3
Clot lysis time in the presence of 60 U of urokinase	60	36	19	11	6	4	2	1	<1	<1	<1

Table II. Fixation of lysyl-plasminogen on fibrin, in plasma to which increasing amounts of plasmin have been added.

Added plasmin (μmol/l of plasma)	0	0.1	0.2	0.3	0.4	0.5	0.6	0.7	0.8	0.9	1
α 2-antiplasmin (residual) estimation according to Laurell: mean of 4 measures (% of initial content)	100	91	82	69	58	45	39	34	31	27	25
Washed clot lysis time (min)	160	120	80	35	20	8	3	spontaneous lysis	spontaneous lysis	spontaneous lysis	spontaneous lysis

In the absence of urokinase, clot lysis time allows the detection of the presence or absence of plasmin activity in the plasma and the measurement of at what plasmin level the inhibitory power of α2-PI is completely suppressed: up to 0.4 μmol of plasmin, there is no clot lysis, at 0.5 μmol a very weak lysis is observed which subsequently becomes much faster. Plasma thus has the capacity of completely inhibiting approximately 0.5 μmol of plasmin per litre.

In the presence of urokinase clot lysis time allows assessment of the accelerating effect on fibrinolysis of the decrease in α2-PI level. With a normal level of inhibitor, fibrinolysis occurs in 60 min, while it occurs in 6 min for 0.4 μmol of plasmin per litre; this dose corresponds to a complete suppression of the inhibitory power of α2-PI. Between these two values, each fall in the inhibitor level was associated with an increase in the rate of fibrinolysis.

Influence on the binding of lysyl-plasminogen to fibrin by the decrease in *α2-PI level.* Using the technique described we have previously demonstrated variations in the fixation of different plasminogens. Thus, a washed clot—resistant to urokinase—after incubation became, in the presence of lysyl-plasminogen, much more sensitive to lysis by urokinase, while this was not the case after incubation in the presence of glutamyl-plasminogen. Thus lysis is directly related to the level of bound lysyl-plasminogen. Table II shows that in normal plasma the added lysyl-plasminogen binds to the fibrin of the washed clot inducing its lysis by urokinase in 160 min. Previous addition of plasmin to plasma shortens the lysis time which falls to 20 min for 0.4 μmol of plasmin per litre of plasma. This demonstrates an increase of the binding level. Up to 0.5 μmol/l, this increase is related to the amount of plasmin added, beyond this value the presence of free plasmin in the plasma causes spontaneous lysis of the clot.

DISCUSSION

The results of these *in vitro* studies brings us to the following statements: small doses of human plasmin added to plasma, not exceeding 0.5 μmol/l, are entirely taken up by α2-PI and the fibrinolytic activity of the enzyme does not appear. Beyond this threshold, a free plasmin activity appears in the plasma, even though there is immunological evidence of the presence of α2-PI. The effect is as if 20 to 30% of the inhibitor present in the plasma did not possess the property of complexing plasmin. This finding was already reported by Collen in 1977.

The neutralization of α2-PI by non-fibrinolytic doses of plasmin induces a marked decrease or even a suppression of its inhibitory power in the plasma; we show that this phenomenon has two essential consequences. First, when plasminogen activator is added to the plasma, the plasmin formed no longer meets any fast-acting inhibitor and its action on fibrin is thus greatly accelerated; secondly, when the fibrin clot is enriched in lysyl-plasminogen, there is an enhancement of the binding of pro-enzyme to fibrin. It can be concluded that a decreased plasma level of the fast-acting inhibitor produces a decreased interaction of the latter with lysyl-plasminogen, thereby liberating the binding sites of this pro-enzyme to fibrin. Furthermore, the extreme speed of the plasmin/α2-PI reaction, resulting in an inactive complex, makes one think that *in vivo* plasmin slowly injected in non-fibrinolytic dosage, will never be able to reach the liver where it is destroyed.

These findings indicate the possibility of new sequential thrombolytic therapy. Thus a slow injection of plasmin in an amount not exceeding 0.5 μmol (i.e. 50 mg/l) of plasma, prior to thrombolytic treatment with urokinase, could improve its results, widen the field of its application and possibly allow a reduction in dose.

Sequential thrombolytic therapy has already been introduced by Kakkar in 1975 in the treatment of deep venous thrombosis and by Brochier and Griguer in 1977 in the treatment of pulmonary emboli. The value of the administration of plasmin prior to this type of treatment can be envisaged.

REFERENCES

Brochier, M. and Griguer, P. (1979). *La Vie Médicale* 15, 1205–1216.
Chase, T. and Shaw, E. (1967). *Biochem. Biophys. Res. Commun.* 29, 508–514.
Collen, N. (1976). *Eur. J. Biochem.* 69, 209–216.
Collen, D. and Witman, B. (1979). *Blood* 53, 2, 313–324.
Laurell, C. B. (1966). *Anal. Biochem.* 15, 45–52.
Lormeau, J. C., Choay, J., Goulay, J., Sache, E. and Vairel, E. G. (1976). *Ann. Pharm. Franc.* 34, No. 7–8, 287–296.
Moroi, N. and Aoki, N. (1976). *J. Biol. Chem.* 251, 5956–5965.
Moroi, N. and Aoki, N. (1977). *Thrombos. Res.* 10, 851–856.
Mullertz, S. and Clemmensen, I. (1976). *Biochem. J.* 159, 545–553.
Vairel, E. G. (1970). *Prod. Pharm.* 25, 347–353.
Wiman, B. and Collen, D. (1977). *Eur. J. Biochem.* 78, 19–26.

FIBRINOLYTIC AND ESTERASE ACTIVITY IN
ARTERIOSCLEROSIS OBLITERANS

M. Kotschy, J. Kaniak, M. Kurzawska-Mielecka and M. Czarnacki

*Department of Angiology, Institute of Internal Medicine, Medical School
Wrocklaw, Poland*

The decreased fibrinolytic activity of the blood in patients with arteriosclerosis obliterans (AO) of the lower extremities, as observed by some authors (Nestel, 1959; Czarnecki, 1960; Gibiński and Nowak, 1961; Craven and Cotton, 1968; Bugar *et al.*, 1969; Perlick, 1969) is mostly based on determinations of the fibrinolysis time, obtained by dissolving an area of fibrin, and the fibrinogen level. These methods reflect only the level of the plasminogen activator in blood. To get a better insight into the fibrinolytic potential of blood as well as fibrinolysis time of euglobulin clot and fibrinogen content with Folin-Ciocalteau reagent we also determined plasminogen and antitrypsin by the caseinolytic method, fibrinogen/fibrin degradation products (FDP) according to Merskey *et al.* (1969) and antithrombin activity using TAME as a substrate. To recognize the activation of factor XII and kallikreinogen better, TAM-esterase activity of plasma, spontaneous and kaolin-induced after 1 and 5 min activation, was also determined by the method of Colman *et al.* (1969).

Our investigations were carried out on 170 patients with AO of lower extremities, 146 men and 24 women of the age 54 ± 10.3 with different types of arterial occlusion and at different stages of peripheral arterial insufficiency. They were compared with a control group of 72 persons. The fibrinolytic potential of these patients with different types of occlusion and different stages of arterial insufficiency are illustrated in Table I.

In the group of patients examined with AO, a prolongation of fibrinolysis time, higher fibrinogen, FDP and antitrypsin levels and simultaneous decrease of plasminogen and antithrombin activity, were observed. Higher fibrinogen content

Serono Symposium No. 37, "Vascular Occlusion: Epidemiological, Pathophysiological and Therapeutic Aspects", edited by M. Tesi and J. Dormany, 1981. Academic Press, London and New York.

Table I. Fibrinolytic activity in patients with AO.

	Control No. = 72	AO No. = 170	P
Fibrinogen μmol/l	9.12 ± 1.17	14.12 ± 4.11	0.001
Plasminogen Cas. U/l	1720 ± 60	1550 ± 210	0.001
Euglobulin lysis time (min)	127 ± 28	195 ± 66	0.001
Fibrin split products mg/l	8.6 ± 3.9	18.6 ± 7.0	0.001
Antitrypsin g tryps./l/h	0.80 ± 0.08	0.98 ± 0.24	0.01
Antithrombin mmol/l/h	254 ± 21	164 ± 52	0.001

Table II. Fibrinolytic activity in different phases of A.O.

	Uncomplicated	With gangrene	Exacerbation of ischemia
Fibrinogen μmol/l	13.23 ± 3.53	16.76 ± 3.82	10.0 ± 1.76 $P - 0.001$
Plasminogen Cas. U/l	1540 ± 223	1650 ± 220	1470 ± 150 $P - 0.01$
Euglobulin lysis time (min)	186 ± 60	225 ± 61	150 ± 48 $P - 0.001$
Fibrin split products mg/l	18 ± 5	15 ± 6	21 ± 6 $P - 0.001$
Antitrypsin g tryp/l/h	0.93 ± 0.14	0.84 ± 0.05 $P - 0.01$	0.86 ± 0.13 $P - 0.01$
Antithrombin mmol/l/h	217 ± 43	263 ± 24 $P - 0.001$	128 ± 29 $P - 0.001$

with lower antithrombin activity reflects increased coagulability in AO seen also by the use of other clotting methods (Czarnecki, 1960; Murphy and Mustard, 1962; Kaniak *et al.*, 1976). Significant decrease of plasminogen level with increased FDP values can be an indicator of the more potent activation of fibrinolysis occurring in AO. The longer fibrinolysis time observed in these patients in comparison

Table III. Fibrinolytic activity in ischemic limb in AO
(18 patients).

	Normal	Ischemic
Fibrinogen	13.83 ± 5.0	13.53 ± 4.41
Plasminogen Cas. U/l	1520 ± 180	1560 ± 320
Euglobulin lysis time (min)	196 ± 10	190 ± 67
Fibrin degradation product mg/l	15 ± 7	25 ± 9 *P* −0.001
Antitrypsin g tryps./l/h	0.97 ± 0.18	1.1 ± 0.20
Antithrombin mmol/l/h	217 ± 53	200 ± 48

Table IV. Plasma TAM esterase activity in patients with AO.

Investigated group	Plasma esterase activity on TAM mm/l/h		
	Spontaneous	Kaolin induced	
		1 min	5 min
Control No. = 21	4.6 ± 3.0 (1.62–7.58)	75.1 ± 14.0 (60.9–89.3)	34 ± 11.6 (22.4–45.6)
AO No. = 30	2.2 ± 1.78 (0–6.6)	64.9 ± 16.5 (38.1–75.4)	35.8 ± 9.9 (10.2–54.1)
P	0.001	0.05	−

to the control group indicates only a lower plasminogen activator content in the circulating blood. The fibrinolytic potential in different phases of AO, i.e. in AO uncomplicated, complicated by gangrene of the lower extremities and during an exacerbation of the ischemia, is shown in Table II.

In uncomplicated chronic ischemia, the determinants of the fibrinolytic potential behaved similarly to the group of patients with AO (Table I). A prolongation of fibrinolysis time, with higher fibrinogen, FDP and antitrypsin levels were observed together with a decrease in plasminogen and antithrombin activity. In AO with gangrene the levels of fibrinogen, plasminogen and antitrypsin were significantly higher, fibrinolysis time longer but FDP lower than in uncomplicated cases. During exacerbation of ischemia, lower values of fibrinogen, plasminogen, antitrypsin, antithrombin with higher FDP and shorter fibrinolysis times were observed. This indicates a consumption of these factors by a higher plasminogen-activator content of the blood, probably liberated from the tissues (Donner *et al.*,

1977). During exacerbation of ischemia thrombi were probably formed in the vessels of the ischemic legs with a tendency to lysis.

For a better understanding of the processes in ischemia, blood was also drawn from ischemic legs. The fibrinolytic potential in this blood was compared with one obtained from a healthy superior extremity of the same patient. The results are shown in Table III. The ischemic blood differs from the normal only in the significantly higher FDP values. The other parameters remain the same.

Table IV illustrates TAM esterase activity of plasma in 30 patients with AO in Stage IV peripheral arterial insufficiency according to Leriche-Fontaine. The spontaneous esterase activity in AO is significantly lower than in the control group. Probably the proteolytic enzymes such as activated factor XII, thrombin, plasmin and kallikrein are consumed or inhibited. The kaolin-induced esterase activity is, after 1 min activation, only a little lower in AO than in the control group. This activity belongs almost entirely to factor XII and kallikreinogen. Practically no differences were observed in the behavior of esterase activity induced with kaolin after 5 min activation. This expresses the action of antiproteolytic inhibitors.

In our investigated group of patients with AO, a tendency to increased clotting and fibrinolysis with a lower plasminogen activator content in the circulating blood was observed. In gangrene of the lower limbs, there exists a greater tendency to hypercoagulability and inhibition of fibrinolysis. Higher values of FDP in the venous blood of an ischemic leg in comparison to a healthy one confirms the occurrence of a more intensive clotting and fibrinolytic process in the ischemic extremity.

The formation of intravascular thrombus, its liquefaction and activation of kallikreinogen and kinins decides the clinical consequences of chronic peripheral ischemia in AO.

REFERENCES

Bugar, K. and Meszaros Cserveny, H. (1969). *Magyar belorv. Archiv.* 22, 318.
Colman, R. W., Mason, J. W. and Sherry, S. (1969). *Ann. Intern. Med.* 71, 763.
Constantin, R., Hilbe, G., Spöttel, T. and Holzknecht, F. (1972). *Thrombos. Diath. Haemorrh.* 27, 649.
Craven, J. L. and Cotton, R. C. (1968). *Angiology* 19, 307.
Czarniecki, W. (1960). *Pol. Arch. Med. Wewn.* 30, 487.
Donner, L., Klener, P. and Roth, Z. (1977). *Thrombos. Diath. Haemorrh.* 37, 436.
Gibiński, K. and Nowak, A. (1971). *Pol. Arch. Med. Wewn.* 31, 308.
Kaniak, J., Kurzawska, M., Kotschy, M., Włodarczyk, J. and Prastowski, W. (1976). *Pol. Tyg. Lek.* 31, 1757.
Murphy, E. A. and Mustard, J. P. (1962). *Circulation* 25, 114.
Nestel, J. P. (1959). *Lancet* 2, 373.
Perlick, E. (1969). *Antikoagulantien (Leipzig)* p. 166.

IMPAIRED BLOOD AND TISSUE FIBRINOLYSIS BUT NORMAL PROSTACYCLIN-LIKE ACTIVITY IN PATIENTS WITH RECURRENT VENOUS THROMBOSIS

N. Ciavarella, M. Schiavoni, V. De Mitrio, G. Lucarelli, T. Frontera and
A. Ciccolella

Hemophilia and Thrombosis Centre Policlinico, Bari, Italy

Impaired fibrinolytic activity has been shown in the blood and in the vessel walls of patients with recurrent venous thrombosis (RVT) (Nilsson and Isacson, 1973; Browse *et al.*, 1977). Shortened platelet and fibrinogen survival time have been noted in these subjects (Steele *et al.*, 1978). Recently, great attention has been given to prostacyclin, which is produced in the vessel walls and may prevent intravascular platelet aggregation. The aim of our studies was to establish the role of blood and tissue fibrinolytic activity in the pathogenesis of RVT. Moreover, we looked at the prostacyclin-like activity of the vein walls in some of these patients.

MATERIALS AND METHODS

Studies were undertaken in 74 patients (p) with RVT: 25 were men and 49 were women with an average age of 58 years (range 18 to 69 years). The majority of patients had a history of RVT well documented clinically and phlebographically. Studies were performed 3 months after the acute phase of thrombosis. Almost all of the patients were on an anticoagulant treatment with warfarin. To estimate the indices of blood fibrinolytic activity, 44 healthy volunteers (14 men and 30 women with an average age of 30 years, between 18 and 45 years), were considered as controls (c). Venous biopsy was performed in 40 patients and in 10 controls (5 men and 5 women with an average age of 28 years, between 18 and 45 years) to

Serono Symposium No. 37, "Vascular Occlusion: Epidemiological, Pathophysiological and Therapeutic Aspects", edited by M. Tesi and J. Dormany, 1981. Academic Press, London and New York.

investigate tissue fibrinolytic activity and prostacyclin-like activity. Inhibitors of coagulation and fibrinolysis in some subjects were also checked.

Blood fibrinolytic activity was estimated by acetate-buffered dilute clot lysis time (DCLT) according to Gallimore's modified method of Fearnley. Citrated plasma was used to determine euglobulin lysis time (ELT) and lysis area of resuspended euglobulin precipitate on unheated fibrin plates (FP) according to Olow and Nilsson (Nilsson, 1973). The same tests were performed after 10 min venous occlusion (fibrinolytic capacity). Plasma plasminogen (PLG) was determined by immunological assay on an immunoplate (Behring).

Plasmatic antithrombin III, as an inhibitor of coagulation, (AT III) was measured by immunological assay on an immunoplate (Behring). Serum α2-macroglobulin (α2-M) and plasma α1-antitrypsin (α1-AT), as inhibitors of the fibrinolytic system, were also studied by immunological assays on an immunoplate (Behring), plasmatic antiplasmin (AP) was detected by chromogenic assay (Kabi S-2251). Tissue fibrinolytic activity was studied according to a modified histochemical technique by Todd-Pandolfi. The fibrinolytic activity was expressed in arbitrary units, the medium value found at our laboratory in 10 healthy volunteers was 6.5 (range 5 to 9). Prostacyclin-like activity (PLA) was evaluated in 20 vein biopsy specimens by the modified technique described by Moncada *et al.* (1976).

RESULTS

The spontaneous fibrinolytic activity was found significantly lower in patients than controls, as detected by: DCLT (patient average: 344 ± 93 min; control average: 202 ± 95 min, $P < 0.001$) (Fig. 1). ELT (patient average: 348 ± 98 min; control average: 228 ± 142 min, $P < 0.001$) (Fig. 2). FP (patient average: 57 ± 44 m^2; control average: 116 ± 26 mm^2, $P < 0.001$) (Fig. 3). Plasma PLG, checked in 48 out of 74 patients compared with 18 controls was significantly higher in patients than in controls: (patient average 12 ± 2 mg/100 ml; control average 10 ± 0.6, $P < 0.005$) (Fig. 4).

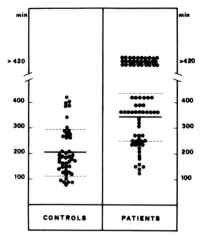

Fig. 1. Fibrinolytic "activity" in 44 controls and 74 patients with recurrent venous thrombosis by acetate-buffered dilute clot lysis time (DCLT) $P < 0.001$.

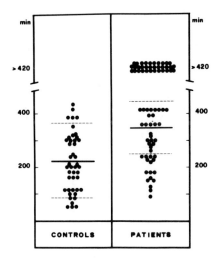

Fig. 2. Fibrinolytic "activity" in 44 controls and 74 patients with recurrent venous thrombosis by euglobulin lysis time (ELT) $P < 0.001$.

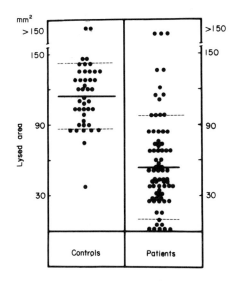

Fig. 3. Fibrinolytic "activity" in 44 controls and 74 patients with recurrent venous thrombosis by fibrin plates assay (FP) $P < 0.001$.

Fibrinolytic capacity tested by venous occlusion gave reduced results in the patients compared with the controls: DCLT (patient average: 166 ± 129 min; control average 73 ± 43 min, $P < 0.001$) (Fig. 5). ELT (patient average: 184 ± 144 min; control average 79 ± 44 min, $P < 0.001$) (Fig. 6). FP (patient average: 193 ± 127 mm^2; control average 328 ± 46 mm^2, $P < 0.001$) (Fig. 7).

The tissue plasminogen activator content in the venous specimens was pathologically low in about 60% of patients (patient average: 4.5 ± 1.5).

Plasma AT III checked in 38 out of 74 patients compared with 30 controls was

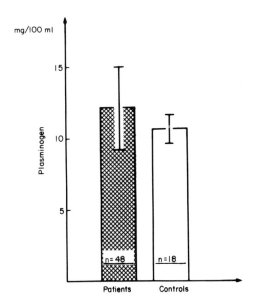

Fig. 4. Behaviour of PLG in patients with recurrent venous thrombosis.

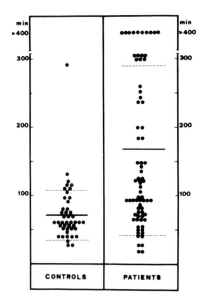

Fig. 5. Fibrinolytic "capacity" in 44 controls and 74 patients with recurrent venous thrombosis by acetate-buffered dilute clot lysis time (DCLT) $P < 0.001$.

significantly lower in patients than the controls: (patient average: 24 ± 5 mg/100 ml; control average 27 ± 3 mg/100 ml, $P < 0.01$).

Serum $\alpha2$-M, checked in 38 out of 74 patients compared with 10 controls was

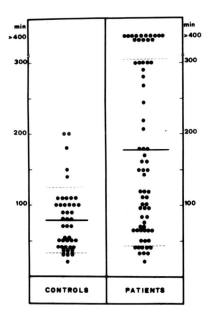

Fig. 6. Fibrinolytic "capacity" in 44 controls and 74 patients with recurrent venous thrombosis by euglobulin lysis time (ELT) $P < 0.001$.

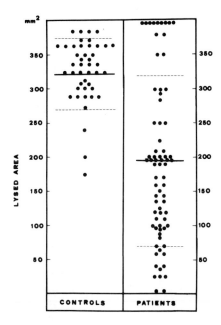

Fig. 7. Fibrinolytic "capacity" in 44 controls and 74 patients with recurrent venous thrombosis by fibrin plates assay (FP) $P < 0.001$.

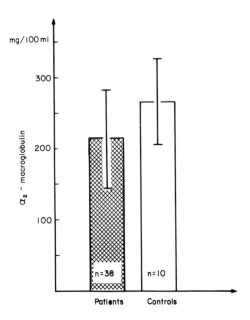

Fig. 8. Behaviour of α2-M in patients with recurrent venous thrombosis.

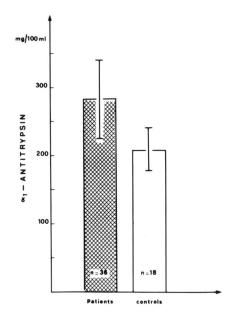

Fig. 9. Behaviour of α1-AT in patients with recurrent venous thrombosis.

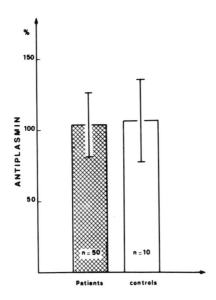

Fig. 10. Behaviour of plasma antiplasmin in patients with recurrent venous thrombosis.

slightly lower in patients than the controls: (patient average 216 ± 67 mg/100 ml; control average 263 ± 59 mg/100 ml, $P < 0.05$) (Fig. 8).

Plasmatic $\alpha 1$-AT, checked in 36 out of 74 patients and compared with 18 controls was significantly higher in patients than controls: patient average 281 ± 5 mg/100 ml; control average 204 ± 29 mg/100 ml, $P < 0.001$) (Fig. 9).

Plasma antiplasmin, checked in 50 out of 74 patients and compared with ten controls showed no differences between patients and controls: (patient average 103 ± 23 mg/100 ml; control average 105 ± 28 mg/100 ml, P: NS) (Fig. 10). The PLA was measured in only 20 patients out of 74. Normal content or release of this activity was found in all but four venous specimens. In three samples, it was apparently increased, while in the last one, a patient with uterine carcinoma, it was completely absent.

DISCUSSION

It is generally accepted that the indices we have used (DCLT, ELT, FP, PLG and tissue activator activity) give reliable information about the fibrinolytic system. Utilizing these tests, we found a reduction of fibrinolytic activity in the majority of patients if measured by DCLT, ELT and FP, while on the other hand, an increase of plasma PLG was observed. Thus we can confirm the observation of other investigators (Nilsson and Isacson, 1973; Browse *et al.*, 1977) that the patients with RVT have a low spontaneous fibrinolytic activity in the blood. The increase of PLG could be caused by a defect in the utilization of the protein by its activator or of excessive synthesis. It has also been suggested that the local increase of fibrinolytic activity after venous occlusion can indicate the ability of vascular endothelium to release activators in the bloodstream. Although a 10 min venous occlusion test is not sufficient to release all the activator from the vessel stores, it can at least reveal a major deficiency of fibrinolytic activity in the vein walls. The local increase of plasminogen activator during venous occlusion was found deficient in our patients with RVT. Tissue plasminogen activator content was also found to be abnormally low in about 60% of patients with RVT. We observed that the majority of subjects with a poor content of plasminogen activator in the vessel walls also have a low increase of fibrinolytic activity. This agreement suggests a defect of synthesis associated with a deficiency of release of activators. From these results it may therefore be concluded that patients with RVT frequently have a defect of the fibrinolytic system.

The decrease of AT III has been associated with thrombotic episodes (Egeberg, 1965). We found a statistically significant decrease of this protein as measured by immunological assay.

Normal or increased content of inhibitors of the fibrinolytic system has been reported in the literature in patients with thrombotic diseases (Nilsson, 1973). Our study shows a statistically significant decrease of one such protein, α2-M, and conversely an increase of α1-AT. We have also registered normal amounts of plasma antiplasmin activity in our patients. At the moment we are not able to explain these conflicting results.

Circulating prostacyclin prevents platelets from clumping by increasing platelet cAMP. It is possible that a deficiency of prostacyclin could not prevent circulating platelet aggregates. As our determination of PLA is not a quantitative method, we cannot argue about the differences between patients with RVT and controls.

CONCLUSIONS

Defective spontaneous fibrinolytic activity, reduced local fibrinolytic activity after venous occlusion and a pathologically low content of plasminogen activator in the vessel walls with an increase of plasmatic plasminogen, were demonstrated in the majority of patients with RVT. Moreover, a reduced plasma AT III, a decrease of α2-M and increase of α1-AT with normal plasma antiplasmin activity was observed. The PLA measured in vein biopsy specimens was found to be normal in the majority of patients examined.

REFERENCES

Browse, N. L. et al. (1977). British Medical Journal 1, 478.
Egeberg, O. (1965). Thrombosis and Diathesis Haemorrhagica 13, 516.
Moncada, S. et al. (1976). Nature 263, 663.
Nilsson, I. M. and Isacson, S. (1973). Progress in Surgery 11, 46.
Steele, P. et al. (1978). American Journal of Medicine 64, 441.

HAEMOSTATIC BALANCE AND CENTRAL RETINAL
VEIN THROMBOSIS

G. Lippi,[1] A. La Torre,[2] A. Resina,[1] P. Santoro,[2] G. Venturi[2] and A. Doni[1]

[1] Cattedra di Chimica e Microscopia Clinica, Firenze, Italy
[2] Istituto di Clinica Oculistica I, Firenze, Italy

Venous retinal thrombosis may be connected, as everybody knows, with coagulative-fibrinolytic system variations in the general circulation. For this reason there is much documentation about changes of one or more factors in either system. It is not easy to draw general conclusions from the great quantity of available data which are anyway difficult to compare because of the different procedures which have been followed.

We thought it right to have a retrospective look at the data we obtained from the study of patients suffering from retinal central vein (and/or its branches) thrombosis from September 1978 to June 1979. The method we followed in this field consisted of recording data expressing the state of the coagulation system in order to highlight the existence, amount and character of the haemostatic imbalance.

MATERIALS AND METHODS

Sixty-one subjects of both sexes, aged between 35 and 82 years (mean 62 years) suffering from retinal central vein thrombosis have been studied. Blood samples were taken just after the clinical instrumental diagnosis performed in every subject by a fluoroangioscopic survey, before any pharmacological treatment.

The haemostatic balance has been examined by studying the following parameters:

Serono Symposium No. 37, "Vascular Occlusion: Epidemiological, Pathophysiological and Therapeutic Aspects", edited by M. Tesi and J. Dormany, 1981. Academic Press, London and New York.

(A) Coagulation system:
  1. Cellular component:
    (a) Platelet count on PRP;
    (b) Platelet aggregation quota (PAQ) according to Born (1962) and
    Yamazaki *et al.* (1974).
  2. Plasma component:
    (a) aPTT, fibrinogenaemia, Quick's time, Normo-test, TEG; we have
    elaborated the index of thrombodynamic potential (ITP)
(B) Anticoagulation system:
  (1) Fibrinolysis time on whole blood.
(C) Evaluation of soluble complexes of fibrin monomers by the paracoagulation
tests:
  (1) Ethanol gelation test
  (2) Serial dilution protamine sulphate test (SDPS-test) according to Gurewich
  and Hutchinson (1971) modified by Doni *et al.* (1974).

ITP's values (usually between 5 and 12.5) have been utilized to quantify the
coagulation activation and the fibrinolysis time (normal values between 210 min
and 300 min) for the fibrinolytic potential. ITP and fibrinolysis time, in addition
to the data of the above mentioned tests, have been particularly useful in classi-
fying the cases; all the other data considered were normal except for the PAQ
which rose in 50.31% of the cases.

RESULTS

The examined cases (Fig. 1) can be divided as follows (Table I):
Four cases (6.56%) have normal haemostasis;

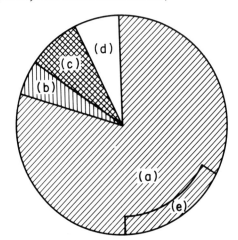

Fig. 1. (a) subjects with hyperhaemostatic imbalance, (b) subjects with hyperhaemostatic
compensated imbalance, (c) subjects with hypohaemostatic imbalance, (d) subjects with
normal haemostasis, (e) subjects with positivity of paracoagulation tests.

Table I. Occurrence of venous retinal thrombosis and coagulative-fibrinolytic system variations.

	No. of cases	
Normal Haemostasis		4 (6.56%)
Haemostatic Imbalances: —activation of the coagulation system + depressed fibrinolysis	26 (42.62%)	
—isolated activation of the coagulation system	17 (27.86%)	49 (80.32%)
—isolated activation of the fibrinolytic system	6 (9.84%)	
Hyperhaemostatic imbalance with activation of the coagulative and fibrinolytic system		3 (4.92%)
Hypohaemostatic imbalance caused by isolated activation of the fibrinolytic system		5 (8.2%)
		total 61 cases

Forty-nine cases (80.32%) have presented with imbalance of difference types.

Twenty-six cases (42.62%) had activation of the coagulation system and depressed fibrinolysis. (The paracoagulation tests, index of accelerated proteolytic activity (APA) are positive in nine of these cases);

Seventeen cases (27.86%) had isolated activation of the coagulation system (two cases had positive paracoagulation tests);

Six cases (9.84%) had isolated depression of the fibrinolytic system (only one case had a positive paracoagulation test);

Three cases (4.92%) had a hyperhaemostatic imbalance which was compensated by the activation of the coagulative and fibrinolytic systems.

Five cases (8.20%) had hypohaemostatic imbalance caused by the isolated activation of the fibrinolytic system.

CONCLUSIONS

The evaluation of the balance between the coagulation and the anticoagulation systems, on the grounds of our tests, has allowed us to demonstrate the existence of a hyperhaemostatic imbalance in most of the subjects suffering from retinal central vein (and/or its branches) thrombosis.

Certainly these changes in the general circulation cannot explain the pathogenesis of the retinal venous thrombosis alone, but surely are an important factor modulating the significance and the evolution of this pathology. We should be able to predict the most suitable pharmacological treatment in every case on the grounds of the type of imbalance.

BIBLIOGRAPHY

Born, G. V. R. (1962). *Nature* **194**, 927.

Doni, A., Resina, A., Moggi, A. and Bono, F. (1974). *La Ricerca* **4**, 83.

Fearnley, G. R., Balmforth, G. and Fearnley, E. (1957). *Clin. Sci.* **16**, 645.

Godal, H. and Abilgaard, U. (1966). *Scand. J. Haemat.* **3**, 342.

Gurewich, V. and Hutchinson, E. (1971). *Ann. Intern. Med.* **75**, 895.

Isacson, S. and Nilsson, J. M. (1972). *Acta Chir. Scand.* **138**, 179.

Nilsson, J. M. and Isacson, S. (1973). *Progr. Surg.* **11**, 46.

Pandolfi, M. (1974). *International Symposium on Ocular Angiology* **69**.

Pandolfi, M., Hedner, U. and Nilsson, J. M. (1970). *Am. J. Ophthal.* **1**, 482.

Raby, C. (1974). Masson et Cie.

Raitta, C. (1965). *Acta Ophthal, Kbh.* Suppl. **83**.

Valsecchi, A., Brunetti, A., Pullini, S., de Zio, A., Botti, C. and Gerhardinger, R. (1978). *Boll. Ocul.* **3**, 227.

Yamazaki, H., Sano, T., Shimamoto, T., Mashimo, N. and Takahashi, T. (1974). *Thromb. Diath. Haemorrh.* Suppl. **60**, 213.

DEEP VEIN THROMBOSIS AND TOURNIQUET ISCHAEMIA

N. A. G. Jones, P. S. F. Chan, P. J. Webb, F. Mistry and V. V. Kakkar

Thrombosis Research Unit, King's College Hospital Medical School, London, UK

INTRODUCTION

A number of different factors have been implicated in the pathogenesis of venous thrombosis. One of these factors is a reduction in the fibrinolytic activity of blood. The activators of plasminogen, which are responsible for the fibrinolytic activity of blood, are stored in vessel walls and released into the blood in response to various stimuli. Venous congestion leads to an increase in the fibrinolytic activity of blood in an occluded limb. This fact could be turned to advantage in the prevention of deep vein thrombosis (DVT). A trial of intermittent compression of the arms, during surgery, with inflatable sleeves reduced the incidence of leg DVT by more than half (Knight and Dawson, 1976). Several authors have therefore suggested that a completely occlusive tourniquet could be a simple form of prophylaxis against DVT (Kroese and Stiris, 1976; Klenerman et al., 1977).

The aims of this study have been to determine the effect of a pneumatic tourniquet on the following.

(1) The incidence of DVT in patients undergoing orthopaedic operations on the lower limb.

(2) Whether increased fibrinolytic activity is associated with the use of the tourniquet.

PATIENTS AND METHODS

In this study, 73 patients undergoing a variety of orthopaedic procedures on the lower limb have been studied. After exsanguination of the leg with an Esmarch

Serono Symposium No. 37, "Vascular Occlusion: Epidemiological, Pathophysiological and Therapeutic Aspects", edited by M. Tesi and J. Dormany, 1981. Academic Press, London and New York.

bandage, the tourniquet was routinely inflated to 400 mmHg. No patient was included whose tourniquet time was less than 30 min. Because of the inaccuracy of the ^{125}I-fibrinogen uptake test in the presence of surgical wounds, ascending venography was used between the seventh and fourteenth days post-operatively to diagnose DVT. Fifty four men and 19 women were studied, their mean age being 42.8 years (range 18–87). Sixteen patients underwent an Attenborough total knee replacement; 46 underwent menisectomy and 11 others had various other procedures.

In 13 consecutive patients, blood tests were performed to monitor changes in fibrinolytic activity during the operations and post-operative period. Four samples were withdrawn at the following intervals.

(1) Before induction of anaesthesia and application of the tourniquet (PRE).
(2) After 30 min of tourniquet ischaemia (MID-OP).
(3) Five minutes after release of the tourniquet (5 min POST-OP).
(4) Forty-eight hours after operation (48 h).

The following tests were performed: plasminogen; antiplasmin and α_2-macro-globulin; fibrinogen and fibrinogen/fibrin degradation products; euglobulin lysis time.

RESULTS

Incidence of DVT

Twenty-seven of the patients developed a DVT, an incidence of 37%. The tibial veins were involved in all these with the majority being significant thrombi greater than 5 cm. Five patients, in addition, had popliteal or femoral thrombi (Table I).

The effect of *age* and *tourniquet duration* is shown in Table II. There is a significant higher incidence in the older age group. Perhaps surprisingly, tourniquet duration made no difference to the incidence of DVT.

The type of operation might be expected to influence the incidence of DVT (Table III). Those undergoing total knee replacement might be expected to have the higher incidence of 62.5% DVT because of the operation's greater magnitude, longer immobility and possible local trauma during surgery. The incidence of 34.8% DVT in the menisectomy group is above the 25% incidence for major abdominal surgery.

Table I. Incidence of deep vein thrombosis.

Patients studied	73
DVT	27 (37%)
Tibial < 5 cm	3
Tibial > 5 cm	24
Popliteal	3
Femoral	2

Table II.   The effect of age and tourniquet duration on deep vein thrombosis.

Age			
< 40 years	8/34	(23.5%)	P 0.02[a]
> 40 years	19/39	(48.7%)	
Tourniquet duration			
< 60 min	18/49	(36.7%)	P NS
> 60 min	9/24	(37.5%)	

[a]Student *t* test

Table III.   Type of operation and deep vein thrombosis.

Total knee replacement (Attenborough)	10/16	(62.5%)
Menisectomy	16/46	(34.8%)
Others	1/11	(9.1%)

One major non-fatal pulmonary embolism occured in a 35-year-old man after a medial menisectomy. Twenty-three patients had venography of the non-operated leg and no DVT were detected; there were five DVT in this group on the operated leg.

Fibrinolytic Activity

The euglobulin lysis time (Fig. 1) showed a mean time of 2.5 h before induction. There was a small insignificant fall during surgery. Five minutes after release of the

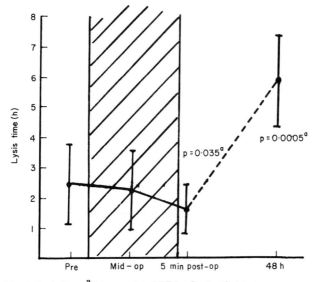

Fig. 1.   Euglobulin lysis time. [a]Compared to PRE by Student's *t* test.

Table IV. Fibrinolytic activity associated with tourniquet ischaemia[a]

	Pre-op	Mid-op	P	5 min post-op	P	48 h	P
Plasminogen (%)	99 ± 13.6	109 ± 12.2	NS[b]	103 ± 14.7	NS	103 ± 28.8	NS
Antiplasmin (%)	112 ± 18.0	106 ± 13.6	NS	112 ± 17.1	NS	119 ± 11.3	NS
α_2-macroglobulin (%)	92 ± 12.2	93 ± 12.0	NS	94 ± 15.2	NS	96 ± 11.8	NS
Fibrinogen ng/ml	2.14 ± 0.7	2.31 ± 0.85	NS	2.75 ± 1.24	NS	3.2 ± 1.31	0.044[c]
FDP μg/ml	4.55 ± 1.6	4.41 ± 2.26	NS	4.95 ± 2.3	NS	3.85 ± 1.3	NS

[a]Results are expressed as mean ± s.d. [b]Not significant. [c]Compared to pre-levels by Student's *t* test.

tourniquet there was a significant fall to 1.7 h ($P = 0.035$) indicating increased fibrinolytic activity. However, after 48 h, the lysis time of 5.8 h (mean) is significantly prolonged ($P = 0.0005$) Student's t test.

All the other parameters examined showed only a significant rise in fibrinogen level at 48 h as one expects after surgery (Table IV).

DISCUSSION

This study has shown an incidence of 37% DVT in a group of 73 patients undergoing orthopaedic operations on the leg requiring a pneumatic tourniquet. Over the age of 40 years, the incidence is 48.7%. Changes which have been found in fibrinolytic activity are similar to those reported by several workers after major surgery (Mansfield, 1972; Gordon-Smith *et al.*, 1974; Borwse *et al.*, 1977; Aberg and Nilsson, 1978). Fibrinolytic activity is enhanced during surgery and immediately post-surgery but by 48 h "fibrinolytic-shutdown" takes place when the euglobulin lysis time is long.

These findings do not support the hypothesis that the tourniquet enhances fibrinolytic activity, thus reducing deep vein thrombosis. Our study has not answered the question of what happens in the deep veins of the leg below the tourniquet. It may be that reperfusion of ischaemic veins leads to endothelial stripping of cells and the initiation of a thrombosis (Cherry *et al.*, 1974). Our findings are consistent with those of Larsson and Risberg (1977) and as further discussed by Risberg (1977).

Since these patients have significant thrombi, which may be associated with pulmonary embolism, they should be protected against DVT. The value of a combination of heparin and dihydroergotamine (which increases flow in the deep veins) in such patients requires further investigation.

REFERENCES

Aberg, M. and Nilsson, I. M. (1978). *British Journal of Surgery* **65**, 259.

Browse, N. L., Gray, L. and Morland, M. (1977). *British Journal of Surgery* **64**, 23.

Cherry, G. W., Ryan, T. J. and Ellis, J. E. (1974). *Thrombosis et Diathesis Haemorrhagica* **32**, 659.

Gordon-Smith, I. C., Hickman, J. A. and Le Quesne, L. P. (1974). *British Journal of Surgery* **61**, 213.

Klenerman, L., Mackie, I., Chakrabarti, R., Brozovic, M. and Stirling, Y. (1977). *Lancet* **1**, 970.

Knight, M. T. N. and Dawson, R. (1976). *Lancet* **2**, 1265.

Kroese, A. T. and Stiris, G. (1976). *Injury* **7**, 271.

Larsson, J. and Risberg, B. (1977). *Thrombosis Research* **11**, 817.

Mansfield, A. O. (1972). *British Journal of Surgery* **59**, 754.

Risberg, B. (1977). *Lancet* **2**, 360.

EVALUATION OF ACTH, CORTISOL AND THYROID HORMONES IN SUBJECTS WITH PERIPHERAL ATHEROSCLEROTIC ARTERIOPATHY

S. Abeatici and A. M. Raso

*Second School of General Clinical Surgery and Surgical Therapy,
University of Turin, Italy*

In an examination of hormone parameters in subjects with atherosclerotic arteriopathy, attention was directed to the relationship between stress, its relation to various hormones and their possible consequences on the underlying disease. It was therefore decided to examine a sample series of subjects with ulcers and a second control series of patients with diseases not related to stress. A search was made for changes in ACTH, cortisol and T_3 and T_4 levels. In this respect, the study was the counterpart of investigations carried out in the search for atherosclerosis in subjects with hypophyseal, adrenal and thyroid alterations (Bastenie *et al.*, 1971; Goodman, 1959; Kalbak, 1972; Tullock *et al.*, 1973).

MATERIAL AND METHOD

ACTH, plasma cortisol and thyroid hormone values were determined in 30 males affected by peripheral atherosclerotic arteriopathy (Leriche 2 or 3), admitted to the second Surgical Clinic, University of Turin or to the Holy Cross Hospital, Cuneo, in 1977 and 1978. Atherosclerosis has been diagnosed and recorded angiographically and most subjects had already undergone direct or indirect vascular surgery. ACTH and cortisol were also evaluated in 30 males hospitalized in the same institutions over the same period with inguinal hernia or varices on the lower extremities. Their clinical pictures ruled out the possibility of atherosclerosis or

Serono Symposium No. 37, "Vascular Occlusion: Epidemiological, Pathophysiological and Therapeutic Aspects", edited by M. Tesi and J. Dormany, 1981. Academic Press, London and New York.

other diseases related to the hormones in question. The second control series consisted of 30 males with gastroduodenal peptic ulcer, drawn once again from the same hospitals during the same period. They were chosen because there is impressive evidence suggesting that peptic ulcer offers an almost textbook illustration of a stress mechanism.

Three age groups—under 45, 45–60 and over 60 years—were distinguished within each series. Each group consisted of ten subjects. Withdrawals for ACTH and cortisol determinations were always taken at 10 a.m. without a tourniquet, followed by immediate storage at $-20°C$ in a freezer, though the fact that a single daily withdrawal places a limit on the amount of information that can be obtained was not lost sight of.

The following parameters were evaluated: age, place of residence, occupation, ACTH and cortisol and ACTH and cortisol in relation to age. Thyroid hormones were determined radioimmunologically (T_3 in ng/100 ml and T_4 in μg/100 ml) in the 30 arteriopathy patients and 30 similar controls. The age of the subjects examined varied, with a predominance of persons over 50. The control group was thus selected to obtain a similar age pattern. The following parameters were considered: age, place of residence, occupation, T_3 and T_4, and T_4 in relation to age.

RESULTS

ACTH and Cortisol

The three series covered virtually the same age range: 37–76 years (average 54.96) in the atherosclerotics; 21–71 years (average 50.63) in the first control series; 28–76 years (average 51.3) in the gastroduodenal ulcer subjects. There were no substantial differences between the three series with regard to residence or occupation.

ACTH values (in pg/ml) varied noticeably, apparently a function of age, in the atherosclerotics: minimum 11 pg/ml in a 76-year-old subject; maximum 100 pg/ml in a 39-year-old subject. A similar pattern was observed in the two control series: mean = 29.7 pg/ml in the atherosclerotics, 28.1 in the first control series and 25.7 in the second. ACTH values decreases with age in the atherosclerotic patients. There was no statistically significant difference between the means in this series and the first control series, whereas there was such a difference between the three age groups; coupled with a non-significant interaction. The ulcer patients, on the other hand, displayed no appreciable difference in terms of age, as can be seen from Tables I–V.

In Table I, factorial analysis of variance revealed a significant difference between the age groups, while the absence of significant differences between the

Table I. Statistical comparison of ACTH values: atherosclerotics *vs* controls.

	F
Series	0.0059 (*NS*)
Age	3.55 (*P* < 0.05)
Interaction	0.502 (*NS*)

Table II.   Statistical comparison of ACTH values: ulcer patients *vs* controls.

	F
Series	0.17 (*NS*)
Age	0.92 (*NS*)
Interaction	2.99 (*NS*)

Table III.   Statistical comparison of cortisol values: atherosclerotics *vs* controls.

	F
Series	0.51 (*NS*)
Age	0.29 (*NS*)
Interaction	0.41 (*NS*)

Table IV.   Statistical comparison of cortisol values: ulcer patients *vs* controls.

	F
Series	10.45 ($P < 0.01$)
Age	0.24 (*NS*)
Interaction	0.35 (*NS*)

ulcer patients and the controls is apparent in Table II. Plasma cortisol covered a rather wide range in the atherosclerotics: 16 ng/ml in a 44-year-old patient to 530 ng/ml in one patient aged 67. The mean was 115.56. The first control series displayed a similar variability (mean 97.1), while the ulcer patients presented very high values, with a mean (217.9 ng/ml) that was very significantly higher ($P < 0.01$) than the means in the other two series. With regard to the relationship between cortisol and age, factorial analysis showed the absence of significant differences between the atherosclerotics and the first control series (age and interaction). By contrast, there was a very significant difference between the high cortisol levels in the ulcer patients and the controls; they were independent of age and the interaction was not significant.

The regression curves for ACTH and cortisol were calculated for each series: r = 0.091 in the atherosclerotic patients, r = 0.063 in the ulcer patients; r = 0.0627 and $P < 0.05$, i.e. similar to a physiological distribution, in the controls.

T_3 and T_4

Residence and occupation had much the same frequencies in the two series. The mean age of the atherosclerotics was 61.56 years. If 55 years is taken as a discrimimant, the series falls into two equal groups (up to 55 and over 55 years). The same is true of the control series, where the mean age was 57.83 years. There was little spread of T_4 values in the atherosclerotic series (mean 7.65 μg/ml). A similar uniformity was also apparent in the controls (mean 9.23 μg/ml). Crude analysis of the means shows that T_4 was much lower in the atherosclerotic patients

Table V. Statistical comparison between
T_4 and T_3.

	F
Between series	4.32 $(P < 0.05)$
Between ages	0.05 (NS)
Interaction	0.15 (NS)
Between series	0.09 (NS)

than in the controls. Analysis of variance, too, made it clear that the means were significantly different, i.e. values were really lower in the first series. Since both series (atherosclerotics and controls) were divided into two age groups, factorial analysis of variance was performed to see whether age had any influence on the difference between the means. The significance of that difference was confirmed (F = 4.32; $P < 0.05$), while the difference between the age groups was virtually nil.

A similar study was run on the T_3 values. The mean for the atherosclerotics was 97.97 ng/100 ml, as against 91.62 in the controls. This difference was not significant. Since age was of no significance in the case of T_4, the question was not pursued in the case of T_3, no difference, in fact, was noted between the two series.

CONCLUSIONS

The first point to note is that ACTH values were much the same (including the means) in the atherosclerotics and the controls. The mean in the ulcer patient series was also virtually the same as that of the control series. Plasma cortisol, on the other hand, was significantly higher in the ulcer patients than in either of their other series, and its behaviour seemed to fit that observed in "stress" ulcer showing that the influence of corticoids on the gastric mucosa forms part of the concept of stress (Abeatici *et al.*, 1975). In the arteriopathic patients, however, cortisol was within normal limits, in spite of the fact that the clinical and experimental evidence suggests that corticoids by no means play a negligible part in the induction of atherosclerosis through their alteration of fat metabolism, permissiveness with regard to catecholamines and action on the clotting process.

It will be noted that ACTH decreased with age in the atherosclerotics, whereas this was not the case in patients with ulcers. This finding was to some extent foreseeable on physiopathological grounds. It was not sufficiently constant, however, to enable it to be used as proof of involvement of the hypothalamus-hypophysis-adrenal axis in the pathogenesis of atherosclerosis.

This means that the findings, with regard to both ACTH and cortisol, lend no support to the view that the progress of atherosclerosis can certainly be attributed to a series of hormone changes which take the form of increased production of corticoids, i.e. the physiopathological substrate of stress, as in the case of ulcer.

Primarily on account of their action on the regulation of peripheral resistance and chronic arterial hypertonia, the thyroid hormones can definitely be regarded as responsible for changes in vessel wall metabolism and intramural flow, though their sole responsibility for atherosclerosis is universally denied.

It is usually taken for granted that, in hypothyroidism, blood cholesterol is enhanced. Its depression in hyperthyroid patients is also assumed. Slight hypocholesterolaemia, however, has been noted in hyperthyroidism, though the ratio between free and total cholesterol is within normal limits. This helps to explain why we have attributed little importance to cholesterol in thyroid patients in relation to arteriopathy, and also why T_3 and T_4 have not been related to cholesterol levels in this study. Furthermore, there is evidence that stress does not necessarily induce an increase in T_4 by means of a direct or mediated action on the thyroid, while various workers agree on the absence of changes due to T_3.

These data support our findings. In the first place, it should be noted that wide subject age differences in the atherosclerotics and in controls were in no way associated with changes in the two hormones. The idea that hypercholesterolaemia can be related to parenchymal and vascular involution of the thyroid would thus seem unacceptable. Equally unacceptable is the view that arteriopaths presumed to have hypercholesterolaemia are low on thyroid hormones. The data are statistically significant ($P < 0.05$) with regard to the higher circulating T_4 levels in the arteriopaths as opposed to the controls, with no difference between the age groups. This greater significance may perhaps be related to a mechanism that was first established when stress appeared, and then became a separate, independent entity, due to the need for an accelerated anabolic-catabolic mechanism in the arterial wall, subject to the action of catecholamines. Since catecholamines and CTH enhancement takes place at the expense of TSH, a feedback may lead to an increase in peripheral T_4 without the gland becoming constantly hyperactive (T_3 unchanged). Therefore, if stress, anxiety, hyperglycaemia and other risk-factors are held to be responsible for atherosclerosis, the conclusion that atherosclerosis, prior to its clinical manifestation, leads to hyperfunction of the thyroid, and hence the endocrine, anticatecholaminic defence of the blood vessel walls, becomes inescapable.

REFERENCES

Abeatici, S. *et al.* (1975). Valori della gastrinemia e della cortisolemia nei traumatizzati cranici.

Bastenie, P. A., Vanhaelst, L., Bonnyns, M., Neve, P., Staquet, M. (1971). *Lancet* 1.

Cannon, W. B. (1929). Bodily changes in pain, hunger, fear and rage.

Goodman, H. M. (1959). Mobilization of fatty acid by epinephrine in normal and hypophysectomized rhesus monkeys.

Kalbak, K. (1972). Ann. Rheum. Dis.

Tullock, B. R., Lewis, B., Fraser, T. R. (1973) *Lancet.*

STUDIES ON THE "HUNTING REACTION" IN SUBJECTS WITH RAYNAUD'S PHENOMENON: EFFECTS OF SYMPATHETIC BLOCK

G. Nuzzaci, M. Zoppi, L. Iacopetti, M. Maresca, G. P. Chiriatti and P. Procacci

Cardiovascular Unit and Pain Clinic, Institute of Medical Clinic, University of Florence, Italy

The purpose of this research was to examine the behaviour of the digital arterial flow in a group of healthy subjects (8) and in a group of patients with Raynaud's phenomenon (12) during immersion of the hand in cold water.

A block with local anaesthetic (lidocaine 1%) of the stellate ganglion was also induced in these patients to observe the effects of the block of the sympathetic activity on the examined function. The digital flow was measured by plethysmography, using strain gauges built for the purpose (Nuzzaci *et al*, 1976) and placed around the fingers completely insulated so that they could transduce the changes of digital flow during immersion in water.

The study group consisted of eight healthy subjects and 12 subjects with Raynaud's phenomenon. They were observed for 15 min in basal conditions, during 60 min of immersion in water at 10°C, and for 30 min after immersion. The arterial flow was measured every minute.

Subjects with Raynaud's phenomenon were observed before the sympathetic block, 15 min after the block and 24 h after the block. Figure 1 shows the behaviour of the digital flow in a normal subject. It confirms the classic finding described by Lewis (1930) of the "hunting reaction", consisting of periodic vasoconstrictions and vasodilatations induced by cold. According to Lewis (1930) and Keatinge (1970), the "hunting reaction" is independent of sympathetic control because it takes place after complete denervation.

Serono Symposium No. 37, "Vascular Occlusion: Epidemiological, Pathophysiological and Therapeutic Aspects", edited by M. Tesi and J. Dormany, 1981. Academic Press, London and New York.

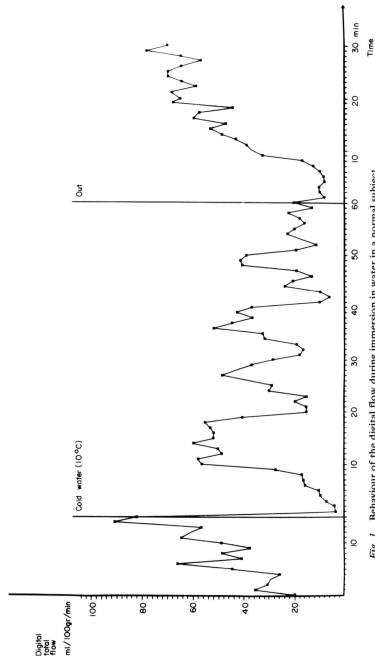

Normal subject

Digital
total
flow

ml/100gr/min

Cold water (10°C)

Out

Time

30 min

Fig. 1. Behaviour of the digital flow during immersion in water in a normal subject.

Subject with Raynaud phenomenon

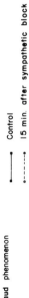

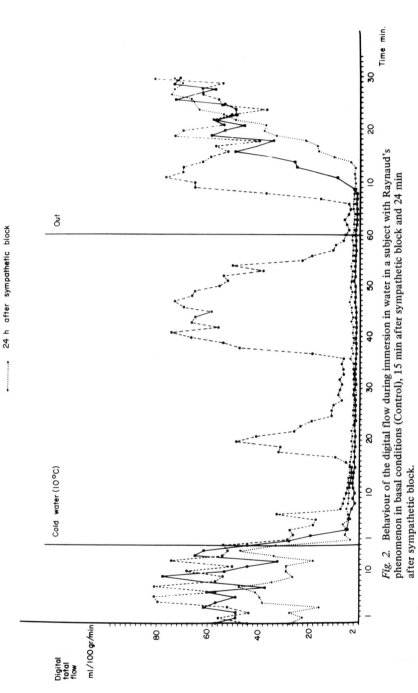

Control
15 min. after sympathetic block
24 h after sympathetic block

Out

Cold water (10°C)

Digital total flow
ml/100gr/min

Time min.

Fig. 2. Behaviour of the digital flow during immersion in water in a subject with Raynaud's phenomenon in basal conditions (Control), 15 min after sympathetic block and 24 min after sympathetic block.

In Figure 2 the behaviour of the flow in a subject with Raynaud's phenomenon is shown. In these subjects during immersion of the hands in cold water the vaso-constriction was steady and the "hunting reaction" never appeared.

A block of the stellate ganglion, induced in these patients, was confirmed by the presence of the Horner's syndrome and by the disappearance of the galvanic skin reflex. In those patients examined 15 min after the block, the reaction was present; when the sympathetic activity was completely restored 24 h after the block, the behaviour of the flow was the same as before the block. We are now carrying out the analysis of the periodic functions but the examples shown are quite typical of what happens in all subjects.

On the basis of our results, we may conclude that while in healthy subjects, the sympathetic efferents probably did not control the "hunting reaction", in the pathological subjects the interaction between sympathetic efferent discharge and responsiveness of the arterial wall was altered in the sense of an abnormal vasoconstriction. The "hunting reaction" appeared during the sympathetic block because one of the two factors was eliminated.

REFERENCES

Keatinge, W. R. (1970). *In* "Physiological and Behavioural Temperature Regula-tion" (J. D. Hardy, A. P. Gagge and J. A. A. Stolwijk, eds) 231–236, Charles C. Thomas, Springfield, Illinois.

Lewis, T. (1930). *Heart* **15**, 177.

Nuzzaci, G., Procacci, P., Francini, F., Zoppi, M. and Maresca, M. (1976). *In* "Proceedings of the Tenth International Congress of Angiology of the Union Internationale d'Angeiologie", (K. Seki and Y. Mishima, eds) 351. Tokio.

VENOUS EFFECTS OF ORAL CONTRACEPTIVES. STRAIN GAUGE PLETHYSMOGRAPHIC STUDY OF VENOUS CAPACITANCE, TONE AND DISTENSIBILITY IN THE LOWER LEGS OF YOUNG FEMALES

M. Guerrini, S. Pecchi, R. Cappelli, F. Bruni and S. Forconi

Istituto di Patologia Speciale Medica, Università di Siena, Italy

The possible association between circulatory diseases and the use of oral contraceptives has aroused much interest and conflict of opinion. Oral contraceptives have been reported to increase the risk of thromboembolic events by acting on blood clotting, fibrinolysis and platelet adhesiveness (Alkjaersig *et al.*, 1975; Burrow and Luce, 1977; Carvalho *et al.*, 1977; Kannel, 1979) or on the vascular wall or endothelium (Almén *et al.*, 1975; Gammal, 1976). The risk of thromboembolism occurs not only in venous but also in arterial circulation as reported by Barrillon *et al.* (1977) and Jick *et al.* (1978) for myocardial infarction, and by Kay (1975) for hypertension. Also serum lipids concentration may be affected by oral contraceptives and the consequent changes have been correlated to their possible atherogenic effect (Anrell *et al.*, 1966; Basdevant *et al.*, 1977).

Epidemiological studies (Grant, 1969; Boston Collaborative Drug Surveillance Programme, 1973) confirmed that the most important side-effects of oral contraceptive were to be found in the venous system. Therefore, in order to evaluate the role of these compounds on venous function, we studied with the pletysmographic method, a group of young females who were taking oral contraceptives with or without symptoms of venous disorders. The results were compared with those of a group of normal women who were not taking the "pill".

Serono Symposium No. 37, "Vascular Occlusion: Epidemiological, Pathophysiological and Therapeutic Aspects", edited by M. Tesi and J. Dormany, 1981. Academic Press, London and New York.

MATERIAL AND METHODS

The study was carried out on three groups of women: Group 1 included 14
women, age varying from 19 to 35, taking oral contraceptives for over 6 months
with symptoms of venous disorders in the lower legs (tiredness, heaviness, cramps,
swelling, restless legs). Women with varicose veins or phlebitis were excluded.
Group 2 included 12 women, age varying from 19 to 32, taking oral contraceptives
for more than 6 months, but without symptoms in their legs. Group 3 was comprised of 14 control women, age varying from 16 to 25, not taking oral contraceptives and with no symptoms or sign of venous disorders.

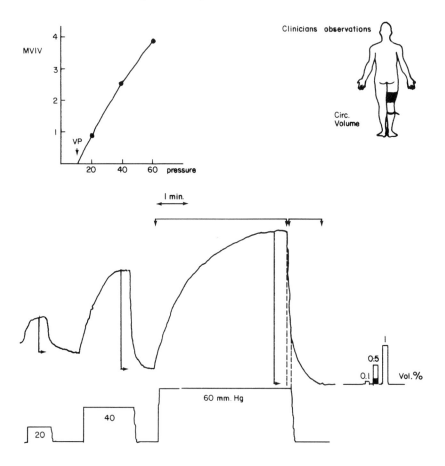

Fig. 1. Tracing obtained with the Periflow in a study of the venous circulation. Upper
tracing: volume changes during periods of venous occlusion at various pressure levels of the
cuff. Lower tracing: continuously controlled occluding pressure. On the right side is the
calibration and on the left side, the method for calculating venous pressure, plotting MVIV
against cuff pressure. The tracings involved a young female with a moderate prevaricosis,
in supine position, foot 15 cm above the heart level. Strain gauge at the calf, cuff at the thigh.
MVIV (20 mmHg) = 0.88 ml/100 ml; MVIV (40 mmHg) = 2.52 ml/100 ml; MVIV (60 mmHg)
= 3.88 ml/100 ml; MVIV = 212 s; MVO = 76 ml/100 ml/min; tTE = 57 s; VD = (3.88–2.52):
(60–40) = 0.06 VT = 14.70.

The venous function was studied by means of a strain-gauge plethysmograph (Periflow), as described elsewhere (Forconi *et al.*, 1979) with the women in the supine position and with both legs posed with the feet 15 cm above the heart level, using venous occlusion at 20, 40 and 60 mmHg, in order to calculate (Fig. 1):

(a) maximal venous incremental volume (MVIV) at various pressure levels in ml/min; (b) maximal venous incremental volume time (tMVIV); (c) maximal venous outflow (MVO) in ml/100 ml/min, from the tangent of the initial slope of the curve after release of the cuff inflation; (d) time of the total emptying (tTE); (e) dV/dP, by dividing the difference between two MVIV by the difference of the respective pressures, as an index of venous distensibility (VD); (f) the inverse of VD (dP/dV) as an index of the venous tone (VT); (g) venous pressure (VP).

The means and the standard deviations, calculated for every parameter, were compared in the three groups using the analysis of variance.

RESULTS

The results are reported in Table I. In the women of the first group ("pill", with symptoms) it can be seen that there is a decisive and significant increase in MVIV, tMVIV, MVO, tTE and VD, while VT is significantly lower than in the control group. In group 2 ("pill", no symptoms), while MVIV appears at the same level as in the control group and MVO and tTE are unchanged, we can see that VT is significantly lower and that VD is significantly higher than in the control group. VP appears to be the same in the three groups.

DISCUSSION

The most important fact emerging from these results is that the venous function is impaired in women taking the "pill" and having symptoms in their legs. In fact, in comparison with the control group, the increase in MVIV indicates a higher capacitance of the venous system, due to an increase of the venous distensibility and to a decrease of the venous tone (as suggested by the behaviour of the VD and the VT). This finding seems self-evident for it is not surprising that subjects who have symptoms of venous disorders show signs of an impaired venous function. What is most striking is that in group 2 (women taking the "pill" but without symptoms), while the venous capacitance (MVIV) does not differ from the control group, there are higher values of VD and lower values of VT. This suggests that the oestroprogestinic compounds may worsen venous function not only in symptomatic, but also in asymptomatic women.

This study confirms that of Keates *et al.* (1975) who, measuring the volume of the calf, reported a significant loss of venous tone in women using oral contraceptives, and that of Meszaros (1977) who plethysmographically demonstrated a decrease of the venous tone which could be pharmacologically corrected.

The impairment of the venous function can be attributed to the decreased capacity of the venous wall to resist the increase of pressure. This atony might be due to the influence of the female sex hormones on cardiovascular and smooth

Table I. Behaviour of the parameters of venous function in the three groups of women. Means ± s.d. ANOVA (for legends see text).

| | GROUP III | | GROUP II (no symptoms) | | GROUP I | | |
	Control n = 28	Pill n = 24	F	P	Pill n = 28	(symptoms) F	P
MVIV (40 mmHg)	1.3 ± 0.45	1.2 ± 0.33	0.4170	0.5270	2.1 ± 0.65	27.1571	0.00003
MVIV (60 mmHg)	2.3 ± 0.51	2.4 ± 0.44	1.5798	0.2121	3.5 ± 0.72	50.9947	0.000001
tMVIV	176 ± 40	202 ± 39	5.4996	0.0217	249 ± 46	40.1834	0.000004
MVO	54.9 ± 13.5	56.3 ± 14.2	0.1372	0.6747	75.4 ± 15.0	28.5590	0.00002
tTE	60 ± 13	66 ± 16	1.7513	0.1887	70 ± 10	9.3032	0.0038
VP	13.6 ± 2.8	14.4 ± 3.1	0.7893	0.3822	14.3 ± 3.0	0.6701	0.4218
dV/dP	0.045 ± 0.013	0.056 ± 0.009	7.3380	0.009	0.060 ± 0.013	36.7280	0.000007
dP/dV	23.0 ± 9.6	17.0 ± 2.9	4.1730	0.0450	15.0 ± 2.6	17.9139	0.0002

muscle physiology. Reynolds (1940) reported that oestrogens cause an increased production or release of acetylcholine which may account for the immediate increase of the distensibility; while Danforth *et al.* (1964) suggested the chronic effect of changing the supporting structures of the vessel wall. These effects observed during oral contraceptive therapy, are the same as those shown during the pregnancy; not only in the vascular smooth muscle but also in that of the ureter, gallbladder and uterus itself (Goodrich, 1966).

Our findings, along with many others already recorded in the literature, once more recommend prudence in the use of the "pill".

REFERENCES

Alkjaersig, N., Fletcher, A. and Burstein, R. (1975). *American Journal of Obstetrics and Gynecology* **122**, 199.

Almén, T., Hartel, M., Nylander, G. and Olivecrona, H. (1975). *Surgery Gynecology and Obstetrics* **140**, 938.

Anrell, M., Cramer, K. and Rybo, G. (1966). *Lancet* **1**, 291.

Barillon, A., Delachaye, J. P., Grand, A., Vorhauer, W., Allard, J., Quarente, J. J., Massey, J., Rucks, J., Rodriguez-Palmeira, M. and Gerbaux, A. (1977). *Archives Maladie Coeur* **9**, 921.

Basdevant, A., de Lignieres, B. and Mauvais-Jarvis, P. (1977). *Nouvelle Presse Médicale* **17**, 1469.

Boston Collaborative Drug Surveillance Programme (1973). *Lancet* **7817**, 1317.

Burrow, J. P. and Luce, J. K. (1977). *Post-graduate Medicine* **82**, 52.

Carvalho, A., Vaillancourt, R. A., Cabral, R. B., Lees, R. S. and Coleman, R. W. (1977). *Journal of the American Medical Association* **237**, 875.

Danforth, D. N., Manalo Estrella, P. and Buckingham, J. C. (1964). *American Journal of Obstetrics and Gynecology* **88**, 952.

Forconi, S., Jageneau, A., Guerrini, M., Pecchi, S. and Cappelli, R. (1979). *Angiology* **30**, 487.

Gammal, E. B. (1976). *British Journal of Experimental Pathology* **57**, 248.

Grant, G. C. (1969). *British Medical Journal* **11**, 73.

Goodrich, S. M. and Wood, J. E. (1966). *American Journal of Obstetrics and Gynecology* **96**, 407.

Kannel, B. W. (1979). *Circulation* **60**, 490.

Keates, J. and FitzGerald, E. D. (1975). *Bibliotheca Anatomica* **13**, 354.

Jick, H., Dinan, B. and Rothman, K. J. (1978). *Journal of the American Medical Association* **239**, 1403.

Meszaros, T. (1977). *Praxis* **66**, 209.

Reynolds, S. R. M. (1940). *Journal Pharmacology and Experimental Therapeutics* **68**, 173.

THE EFFECTS OF BETA-BLOCKING AGENTS ON ARTERIAL FLOW OF THE LOWER LIMBS USING STRAIN-GAUGE PLETHYSMOGRAPHY

A. Strano, S. Novo, A. Pinto and G. Davi

Institute of Clinical Medicine and Medical Therapy of University of Palermo, Italy

Beta-adrenoceptor-blocking drugs are widely recognized as being useful anti-hypertensive and anti-anginal agents. Nevertheless, in patients that also exhibit peripheral atherosclerotic vascular disease, these agents could increase peripheral vascular resistance and make the symptomatology worse. In fact, in animals and man, acutely administered intravenous propranolol increases the peripheral vascular resistance and inhibits the beta$_2$-adrenoceptor-mediated vasodilator response to infused isoprenaline (Ablad *et al.*, 1973; Ablad *et al.*, 1974; Johnsson, 1975a,b; Vaughan Williams, 1973; van Hervaarden, 1977, 79). The beta-blocking effects of oxprenolol on vascular resistance resemble those of propranolol (Vaughan Williams, 1973). The selective antagonists at beta-adrenoceptors seem to have different actions on peripheral vascular resistance and on increase of peripheral flow induced by isoprenaline; acutely administered metoprolol does not change significantly peripheral vascular resistance and does not inhibit the effects of the infusion of isoprenaline on peripheral blood flow (Ablad *et al.*, 1973; Ablad *et al.*, 1974; Johnsson, 1975a,b; van Hervaarden, 1977).

Unlike conventional beta-adrenoceptor-blocking drugs, acute administration of labetalol, a competitive antagonist at both alpha and beta-adrenoceptor sites, reduces peripheral vascular resistance like an alpha-adrenoceptor-blocking drug such as phenoxybenzamine (Brogden *et al.*, 1978).

The different action of non-selective, selective and alpha-beta-blocking agents on peripheral vascular resistance could give variations of the peripheral arterial flow, especially in patients with peripheral atherosclerotic vascular disease (Pratesi

Serono Symposium No. 37, "Vascular Occlusion: Epidemiological, Pathophysiological and Therapeutic Aspects", edited by M. Tesi and J. Dormany, 1981. Academic Press, London and New York.

et al., 1967). Many authors have observed that beta-adrenergic-blocking drugs such as propranolol may induce cold hands and feet, intermittent claudication or the Raynaud phenomenon (Leading Article of *Br. Med. J.* 1977; O'Brien, 1978).

Marshall *et al.* (1976) have recommended that beta-adrenergic-blocking drugs should be avoided in patients with peripheral ischemia, and this opinion is in agreement with Vale *et al.* (1977) and Ahlquist (1979), who include vascular peripheral disease among the contraindications in non-selective beta-adrenergic blocking drugs' use.

The aim of this study was to evaluate the effects of metoprolol, a cardio-selective beta-blocking agent and labetalol, an alpha-beta-blocking adrenergic agent compared with oxprenolol, a non-selective beta-blocking agent, on peripheral arterial flow.

MATERIALS AND METHODS

The study included 20 patients with obliterative atherosclerosis in the lower limbs, at second and third stage, aged between 40 and 55 years; 12 men and 8 females. Sixteen of these had a monolateral atherosclerotic lesion, eight had a bilateral one.

The arterial blood flow was measured, using a strain-gauge plethysmograph, under basal conditions and after the administration of placebo, oxprenolol, metoprolol and labetalol on different days. As well as the rest flow, in every session, we also determined the post-ischemic flow 3 min after arterial occlusion at 270 mmHg. We used NaCl 0.9% (10 ml in 5 min i.v.) as a placebo. The oxprenolol (0.1 mg/kg), metoprolol (0.1 mg/kg) and labetalol (1 mg/kg) were administered i.v. in 5 min. The rest flow (RF) was detected 5 min after the injection of the drugs and the post-ischemic flow (PF) 10 min after.

At the same time, the systolic and diastolic humeral blood pressure and the heart rate were measured. The basal vascular resistance was calculated by dividing the rest flow with the sum of diastolic blood pressure plus a third of the differential blood pressure. The lower vascular resistance was calculated dividing the peak flow with the same parameters. The results obtained from the lower limbs without atherosclerotic lesions (16) was correlated with those obtained from the lower limbs with atherosclerotic lesions (24).

RESULTS

Only labetalol significantly reduced the systolic and diastolic blood pressure, while the heart rate was lower after oxprenolol (Fig. 1).

In the legs with atherosclerotic lesions, the rest flow generally is reduced by oxprenolol ($P < 0.025$), while a significant increase is caused by labetalol ($P < 0.0025$); no variations were caused by metoprolol. The peak flow was increased appreciably only by labetalol ($P < 0.0025$–Fig. 2).

In the legs without atherosclerotic lesions, significant variation was obtained

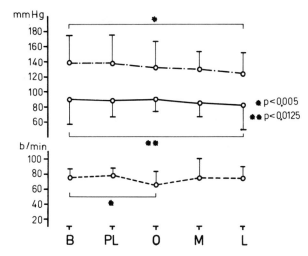

Fig. 1. Effect on systolic and diastolic blood pressure and blood flow after administration of drugs B, basal conditions; P1, placebo; 0, oxyprenolol; M, metoprolol; L, labetalol.

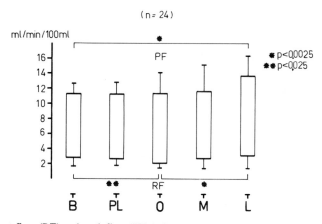

Fig. 2. Rest flow (RF) and peak flow (PF) in legs with artherosclerotic lesions.

between oxprenolol and metoprolol (P 0.05) for the rest flow, while only labetalol lowered the peak flow significantly ($P < 0.005$–Fig. 3). In the legs with atherosclerotic lesions, the basal vascular resistances (BVR) were lowered, with a significant difference by labetalol ($P < 0.0005$), while an increase was obtained with oxprenolol ($P < 0.005$–Fig. 4). The lower vascular resistances (LVR) were reduced by metoprolol ($P < 0.05$) and labetalol ($P < 0.0005$–Fig. 4).

In the legs without atherosclerotic lesions (Fig. 5), similar differences in the effects of oxprenolol, metoprolol and labetalol on BVR and LVR were observed.

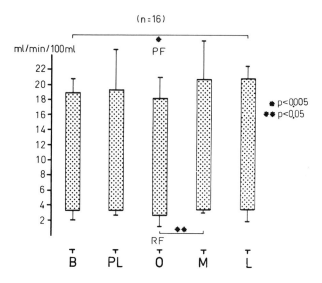

Fig. 3. Rest flow and peak flow in legs without atherosclerotic lesions.

LEGS WITH ATHEROSCLEROTIC LESIONS

	B.V.R.	p<	L.V.R.	p<
BASE	37,21± 5,31		9,26 ± 1,42	
PLACEBO	37,23± 5,08	N.S.	9,30 ± 1,27	N.S.
OXPRENOLOL	49,05± 5,05	0,0005	9,12 ± 0,93	N.S.
METOPROLOL	36,02 ± 3,95	N.S.	8,57 ± 1,21	0,05
LABETALOL	30,27 ± 5,47	0,0005	7,53 ± 1,86	0,0005

Fig. 4. Comparison of BVR and LVR in legs with atherosclerotic lesions on administration of drugs.

LEGS WITHOUT ATHEROSCLEROTIC LESIONS

	B.V.R.	p<	L.V.R.	p<
BASE	32,54± 5,14		5,54 ± 0,84	
PLACEBO	32,56± 4,32	N.S.	5,43±0,72	N.S.
OXPRENOLOL	39,15± 4,03	0,0005	5,60± 0,57	N.S.
METOPROLOL	29,58 ± 4,50	0,05	4,81 ± 0,80	0,01
LABETALOL	28,92± 4,72	0,025	4,68 ± 0,86	0,005

Fig. 5. Comparison of BVR and LVR in legs without atherosclerotic lesions on administration of drugs.

DISCUSSION

Our results confirm that the three beta-adrenergic blocking agents used at the dosage employed and under our experimental conditions, have different actions on the total peripheral arterial flow of the calf, without distinguishing between the skin blood flow and the muscle blood flow measured by strain-gauge plethysmography.

In the limbs without atherosclerotic lesions, the post-ischemic flow is increased significantly after labetalol, while in the rest flow it shows no variations. In the limbs with atherosclerotic lesions, the peak flow is increased by latetalol, while oxprenolol significantly lowers the rest flow. Metoprolol does not produce significant variations of the arterial flow.

Bracchetti *et al* (1971) obtained similar results with propranolol and McSorley and Warren (1978) observed a decrease of the skin temperature, rest flow and post-ischemic flow after propanolol and no significant variations after metoprolol. It is known that labetalol given intravenously lowers peripheral vascular resistance (Brodgen *et al*, 1978), increasing the peripheral arterial flow.

In fact, in our study, the fall in basal vascular resistance reached a statistically significant level after the injection of labetalol; a little decrease was obtained with metoprolol, while oxprenolol increased the basal vascular resistance. Similar differences were obtained in the limbs without atherosclerotic lesions.

These results must be confirmed after long-term oral treatment. Our findings suggest that in patients with peripheral vascular disease, labetalol or metoprolol have important advantages over oxprenolol in its effects on the peripheral circulation.

REFERENCES

Ablad, B., Carlsson, E. and Ek, L. (1973). *Life Science* 12, 107.
Ablad, B., Carlsson, E., Dahlof, C., Ek, L. and Hultberg, E. (1974). *Advances in Cardiology* 12, 290.
Ahlquist, R. P. (1979). *American Heart Journal* 97, 137.
Bracchetti, D., Maresta, A. and Russo, F. (1971). *Bollettino S.I.C.* XVII 3, 149.
Brogden, R. N., Heel, R. C., Speight, T. M. and Avery, G. S. (1978). *Drugs* 15, 251.
Johnsson, G. (1975a). *Acta Pharmacologica Toxicologica* 36, Suppl. 5, 59.
Johnsson, G. (1975b). Selectivity studies with adrenergic beta-receptor blockers in man. *In* "Pathophysiology and Management of Arterial Hypertension." Proceedings of a Conference in Copenhagen, Denmark, April 10–11.
Leading Article (1977). *British Medical Journal* 1, 529.
Marshall, A. J., Roberts, C. J. and Barritt, D. W. (1976). *British Medical Journal* 1, 1498.
McSorley, P. D. and Warren, D. J. (1978). *British Medical Journal* 2, 1598.
O'Brien, E. T. (1978). *Angiology* 29, 4, 332.
Pratesi, F., Corsi, C. and Spinelli, P. (1967). Differenze fra il distretto circolatorio muscolare e quello cutaneo in funzione dei recettori alfa e beta adrenergici nell'uomo. *Atti XXVIII Congresso Nazionale S.I.C.* 47.
Vale, J. A., Van de Pette, S. J. and Price, T. M. L. (1977). *Lancet* 2, 412.

van Hervaarden, C. L. A., Fennis, J. F. M., Binkhorst, R. A. and van't Laar, A. (1977). *European Journal of Clinical Pharmacology* **12**, 397.
van Hervaarden, C. L. A., Binkhorst, R. A., Fennis, J. F. M. and van't Laar, A. (1979). *British Heart Journal* **41**, 1, 99.
Vaughan Williams, E. M., Bagwell, E. E. and Singh, B. N. (1973). *Cardiovascular Research* **7**, 226.

PARTICIPATION OF LYMPHATIC SYSTEM IN
POST-PHLEBITIC SYNDROME

A. K. Cordeiro, F. F. Baracat, O. Tijerina and C. Sanchez y Fabela

Instituto Arnaldo Vieira de Carvalho, Sao Paulo, Brasil
University of Monterrey, Faculty of Medicine, Mexico Hospital General
Centro Medico Nacional IMSS, Mexico City

Mayall (1960) making lymphangiographic studies in the post-phlebitic syndrome showed disturbances of the lymphatic system. However, for many decades numerous clinical investigators had examined edema formation in post-phlebitic syndromes and thrombophlebitis (Zimmerman and Takats, 1931) and the general belief was that edema constituted simply an acute inflammatory process. Homans and Zollinger (1929) paid more attention to lymphatic blockage than venous obstruction. Reichert (1926) in his work on soft tissue sections in dogs concluded that in this type of edema a venous component and a lymphatic component coexisted, but these works were not confirmed by others (Zimmerman, 1931). Haller and Mays (1963) studied simple venous obstruction in dogs and they did not show edema. Only after venous ligature, followed by the filling of these veins with thrombotic material with consequent inflammatory reaction, could they produce a typical clinical picture of edema and concluded that lymphatic obstruction secondary to the inflammatory reaction that follows thrombophlebitis was the initial factor in edema formation.

MATERIALS AND METHOD

Our material constituted 50 patients of both sexes with determination of tissue pH, blood proteins, electrophoretic lipidogram, protein electrophoresis, proline and hydroxyproline studies in blood and urine, sexual chromatin, kariogram,

Serono Symposium No. 37, "Vascular Occlusion: Epidemiological, Pathophysiological and Therapeutic Aspects", edited by M. Tesi and J. Dormany, 1981. Academic Press, London and New York.

lymphangiography (Kinnmonth *et al.*, 1955) and radioisotopic lymphangiography (with [198]Au, coloidal sulphur marked by technetium), with pre- and post-operative controls.

RESULTS

Results obtained by us in the study of the role of the lymphatic system in the post-phlebitic syndrome in these 50 cases were as follows.

Edema of the post-phlebitic syndrome improves if not associated with a lesion of the superficial lymphatic system.

Association of lymphatic system lesions and the clinical picture in the post-phlebitic syndrome as a consequence aggravates the edema and dictates particular rules in its treatment.

One observes lymphangiographic disturbances of the superficial lymphatic system in the post-phlebitic syndrome that are characterized by: modifications of superficial lymph pathways that became transverse and meandering with varicose dilatations; blockages and modification of the lymphatic wall permeability with lymph trunk neoformation and dermal backflow (Figs 1, 2).

One observes traumatic lesions of the lymphatic superficial system after surgery for varices and in the post-phlebitic syndrome, such as: surgical lesions of the afferent superficial lymphatic trunks at the inguinal incision for surgery of varices, causing almost total section of the afferent superficial lymphatic trunks; distor-

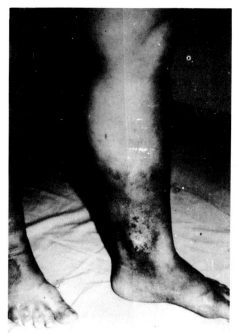

Fig. 1. Patient D.T.B.—Post-phlebitic syndrome of left lower limb. Ulcer on inferior third of left leg.

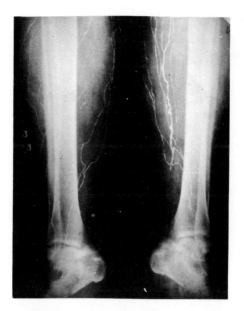

Fig. 2. Patient D.T.B.—Lymphangiography: Right—hypoplasia of superficial lymph system. Left—blockage of the superficial lymph system at the level of the ulcer. Superficial lymph trunks showing dilatation and varicosities.

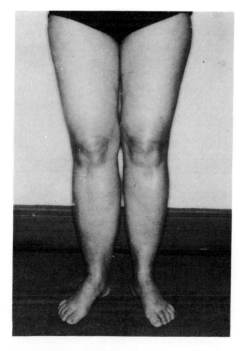

Fig. 3. Patient A.L.W.—Post-phlebitic syndrome.

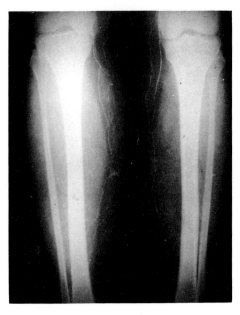

Fig. 4. Patient A.L.W.–Lymphangiography showing traumatic lesion of superficial lymph trunks in medial third of right leg produced during saphenectomy.

tion of the superficial lymphatic trunks at different levels making the formation of a collateral web necessary (Figs 3, 4, 5), or even interrupting nearly all of the superficial lymphatic trunks so that the patient shows a clinical picture of lymphatic hypoplasia, following surgery for varices or post-phlebitic syndrome (Fig. 6).

One also sees a disturbance of subcutaneous pH and collagen metabolism by disturbance of fibroblast metabolism, due to long-standing lymph stasis and hence subcutaneous fibrosclerotic changes.

DISCUSSION AND CONCLUSIONS

By Starling's law extracellular fluid is derived from blood by filtration through the capillary cellular membranes and it is the result of a balance that exists between blood pressure, which tends to force fluid out of the capillaries, and the osmotic pressure of plasma proteins that tries to retain it.

It is quite possible that small electrolyte molecules and water pass freely in both directions through the capillary membrane by free diffusion via small pores in the vascular wall, which impede the passage of high molecular weight proteins.

Peripheral edema can result from disturbances of any of these control factors. Increases of capillary permeability produced by a lesion causes an excessive accumulation of proteins that enrich the extracellular fluid. By osmosis more fluid leaves the vascular compartment. Venous obstruction increases capillary and venous pressure, resulting in an increase of fluid entering the tissues. If maintained, it produces a cessation of metabolite filtration and diffusion of oxygen precipitating stasis and chronic venous ulcers.

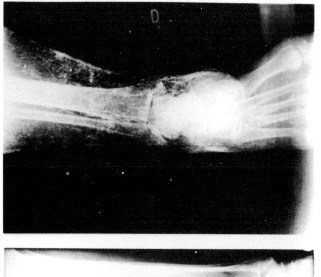
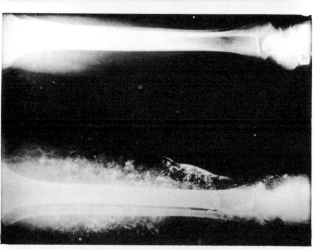
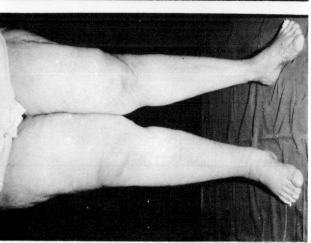

Fig. 5. Patient C.M.—Post-phlebitic syndrome plus post-phlebitic lymphedema of right lower limb after saphenectomy. In lymphangiography: intense colateral lymph circulation with intense dermal back-flow in the right leg and ankle.

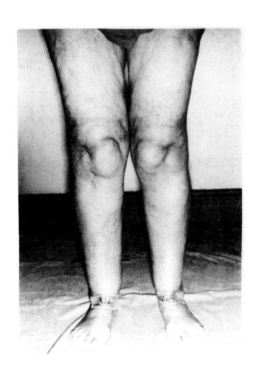

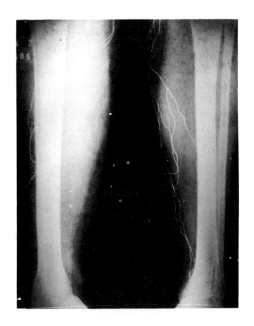

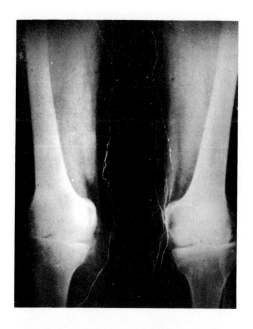

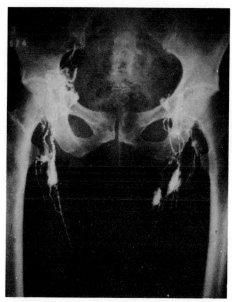

Fig. 6. Patient M.C.M.—Post-phlebitic lymphedema of the right lower limb. Lymphangio-graphy—traumatic avulsion of the superficial lymph system of right lower limb during saphenec-tomy. As a consequence we have an iatrogenic hypoplasic picture.

However, lymph system disturbance results in the difficulty of removal of high molecular weight proteins from the tissues. Osmotic pressure then increases bringing as a consequence an increase of intravascular fluid filtration through the capillary membrane to the tissues.

Under these conditions of lymph circulation disturbances, stasis in superficial lymphatic trunks, dilatation with valvular incompetence and dermal backflow through collateral lymphatic trunks to the dermal plexus results. Increase of high molecular weight proteins modifying skin pH excites fibroblast proliferation, causing increased oedema, diminished resistance to streptococcal and staphylococcal infections, decreased lymph capacity and increase of interstitial fibrosis.

High molecular weight proteins must be removed from the interstitial space by the lymph system and in order that the lymph system can perform its function there are certain conditions.

One of the main conditions is pH. If pH is disturbed there will be disturbances in subcutaneous tissue and subsequently the lymph system. In general, this pH is beween 5–7, but one can observe pH disturbances varying from 4 to 8 and we have found a range of 8 to 10. The pH disturbance of the interstitial space causes disturbances of high molecular weight protein absorption. These accumulate in the interstitial space and increase edema.

This increase of proteins in the interstitial space excites fibroblastic proliferation. The fibroblast reacts to the different metabolic conditions of modified pH, protein excess in the interstitial space, chemical and enzymatic disturbances altering the RNA metabolism of the fibroblast nucleus causing disturbances of hyaluronic acid conversion to condriotin sulphuric acid and neuraminic acid, by collagen deposition in the interstitial space (Cordeiro and Baracat, 1974).

This irregular collagen deposition plus metabolic disturbances, due to lymph system dysfunction, results in the appearance of a hard edema, pitting at the beginning when deposition is loose and not later when fibrosclerotic deposition occurs.

As a consequence of perilymphatic and interstitial fibrosclerotic disturbances, we observe superficial lymphatic trunk dilatation giving valvular incompetence and subsequent lymph reflux to the dermal plexus (dermal backflow). In lower limbs with the venous insufficiency of the post-phlebitic syndrome and long-standing chronic ulcers with subcutaneous fibrosis, increase of intralymphatic pressure occurs. Lymphography shows insufficient filling of the lymphatics by radiopaque contrast, owing to recurrent lymphangitis producing progressive blockage of the lymphatic trunks and sometimes distal dilatation with valvular incompetence (Figs 1, 2).

To this lymphangiographic picture are added the trauma of different techniques for surgical treatment of post-phlebitic syndrome or varices. Surgical treatment of varices can cause lymph system lesions by stripping or by the surgical incision in the inguinal region. We have observed, by lymphography, radiopaque contrast extravasation at the level of the incision and sometimes almost complete section of the afferent superficial lymphatic trunks. On the other hand, stripping produces localized lesions (Figs 3, 4) by pulling off the Y branches that surround the veins or tributaries (Fig. 6). In thrombophlebitis, lesions of superficial lymphatic system are shown by lymphography. In the lower leg, we find lymphatic trunks with transverse paths sometimes in small numbers, dilated and irregular. In the thighs they are generally not disturbed because few skin trophic lesions occur. We can find varicose dilatation of lymphatic trunks in patients with recanalized deep veins with strong distal venous stasis provoking a great lymphatic overload. Reduction of the number of lymphatic trunks is observed in patients that have suffered frequent erysipelatous crises. The radiological picture results from inflammatory obliteration of the superficial lymphatic trunks by a proliferant endolymphangitis, thrombolymphangitis or fibrotic lymphangitis.

As for neoformation of lymphatic trunks and dermal backflow, these are also observed in patients with subcutaneous fibrosclerotic lesions (Fig. 5). Modifications of the lymphatic wall permeability at the level of trophic disturbances is shown by extravasation of radiopaque contrast a little above the lesions.

Similarly, deep lymph system disturbances are observed in the legs and present as extravasation of contrast in this region. Post-phlebitic syndrome surgery also aggravates the superficial lymphatic system lesions by dividing superficial lymphatic trunks which soon become more irregular, dilated and varicose.

In conclusion, the post-phlebitic syndrome edema improves with rest if not associated with lymph system disturbances, since lymphatic capacity for removal of high molecular weight proteins is not impaired. Edema becomes permanent when disturbances of the superficial lymph system appear. Lymphangiographically these superficial lymph system disturbances present as irregular paths, varicose dilatations, obstructions, modifications of vascular lymphatic wall permeability, vessels neoformation and dermal backflow.

To these disturbances of superficial lymph system function are added associated chemical and enzymatic disturbances caused by long-standing stasis with subcutaneous pH disturbances, collagen metabolism disturbances and by fibroblast metabolism disturbances.

The lymph system is not a cause of post-phlebitic syndrome, but is implicated in lesions of this syndrome by alterations of subcutaneous tissue by nutrition disturbances, oxygenation disturbances and subsequent disturbances of high molecular weight protein absorption, secondary infections and fibrosis, so aggravating the edema.

REFERENCES

Collete, J. M., Vigoni, M. and Godart, S. (1966). *Phlebologie* **19**, 2, 125.
Cordeiro, A. K. and Baracat, F. F. (1974). *Rev. Bras. Cardiovasc.* **10**, 3, Jul-Sept, 155.
Haller, Jr, J. A. and Mays, I. (1963). *Am. Surg.* **29**, 567.
Haller, Jr, J. A. (1969). *Cientifico-Medica, Barcelona.*
Homans, J. and Zollinger, R. (1929). *Arch. Surg.* **19**, 992.
Jacques, H., Barbosa, C. G., Brum, F. A., Tavares, J. C., Vieira de Melo, A. and Mayall, R. C. (1965). *Rev. Bras. Cardiovasc.* **1**, 130.
Kinmonth, J. B., Taylor, G. W. and Harper, R. A. (1955). *Br. Med. J.* **1**, 940.
Mayall, R. C. (1960). *J. Cardiovasc. Surg., Torino* **1**(2), 176.
Mayall, R. C. and Barbosa, C. (1968). La grosse jambe; L'Expansion Scientifique (Ed), 88.
Reichert, F. L. (1926). *Arch. Surg.* **13**, 871.
Schobinger, R. A. and Ruzicka, F. F. (1964). "Vascular Roentgenology." 698. Macmillan, New York.
Zimmermann, L. M. and Takats, G. de (1931). *Arch. Surg.* **21**, 937.

SECTION III
DIAGNOSTIC TECHNIQUES

A NEW PULSE WAVE ANALYSIS IN OBLITERATING ARTERIOSCLEROSIS

I. Oliva and K. Roztočil

Cardiovascular Research, The Institute for Clinical and Experimental Medicine, Prague, Czechoslovakia

At present, the diagnosis of the initial stages of obliterating arteriosclerosis is difficult owing to the lack of suitable non-invasive techniques. One of them is the recording of the pulse wave and analysis of its morphology.

The object of this communcation is to propose a new simple pulse wave analysis based on the measurement of the distance between ascending and descending limbs of the pulse wave.

MATERIAL

Fifty-one men and three women aged 46–56 years were grouped, according to the *arteriographic* findings in lower limb arteries, into two groups. The first group involved 26 limbs with definite arteriosclerotic changes *without* occlusion; the second group involved 35 limbs *with* occlusion of the femoral arteries or one or two calf arteries.

Control measurements were performed in two groups of healthy individuals—in one, young individuals (mean age 22 years) where we examined 46 limbs and the second, older individuals (mean age 50 years) where we examined 26 limbs. For obvious ethical reasons we did not perform angiography of the lower limb arteries in healthy subjects. Both control groups were evaluated on the basis of case histories and objective clinical examination which showed palpable pulsation in lower limbs, normal values with the positional test and negative findings on auscultation of the pelvic and lower limb arteries after short physical exercise. In

Serono Symposium No. 37, "Vascular Occlusion: Epidemiological, Pathophysiological and Therapeutic Aspects", edited by M. Tesi and J. Dormandy, 1981. Academic Press, London and New York.

I. Oliva and K. Roztočil

both pathological groups we performed percutaneous femoral arteriography with a Seldinger technique (Seldinger, 1953), modified by Linhart *et al.* (1976). Using this technique, the distal descending aorta, the pelvic, femoral, popliteal, both tibial, fibular and both pedal arteries were visualized bilaterally.

METHODS

The pulse wave registration was performed by a transparent photoplethysmograph applied to the distal phalanx of the second toe. The individuals were examined in the recumbent position at a room temperature of 22-24°C. Using warm air, the instep and toes were warmed up to bring their skin temperature up to 31°C.

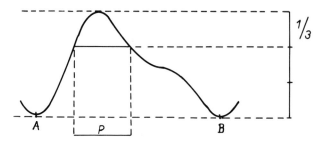

Fig. 1. Scheme of the proposed pulse wave analysis. P, distance between the ascending and descending limbs (at the border of the first and second third of the amplitude measured from the crest of the curve). AB, length of the pulse wave.

The pulse wave analysis was performed as follows (Fig. 1). A line was drawn between the ascending and descending limbs of the pulse wave parallel to the baseline at the junction of the first and second thirds of the amplitude measured from the crest of the curve. The length of this parallel line was in a constant proportion to the duration of the pulse wave, depending on the heart rate. To compare the curves of different lengths (of different heart rates), *the length of the parallel line was divided by the length of the pulse wave.*

RESULTS

The individual values obtained in each group of subjects are given in Fig. 2. The two healthy groups did not differ significantly from each other. The difference between the two pathological groups was significant ($P < 0.01$). The pathological groups differed significantly from both control groups ($P < 0.01$).

The mean values and standard deviations in the examined groups are given in Table I.

In addition to group evaluation, we attempted to predict the occurrence of obliterating arteriosclerosis in individual patients. We found no significant differences between the group of healthy young individuals and healthy

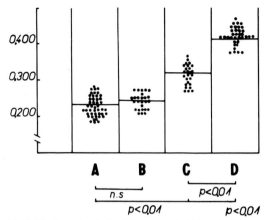

Fig. 2. Calculated individual results. A, healthy young individuals; B, healthy individuals; C, patients with arteriosclerosis of lower limbs without occlusion; D, ditto with occlusion. A.B − n.s.; C:D − $P < 0.01$; A:C − $P < 0.01$; A:D − $P < 0.01$.

Table I. The mean values and standard deviations in examined groups.

Mean value	s.d.	Groups
0.229	± 0.028	healthy young
0.243	± 0.026	healthy
0.316	± 0.028	without occlusion
0.411	± 0.033	with occlusion

individuals with the mean age 50 years. Therefore, two standard deviations from the mean in the group of healthy young individuals (where, in the absence of angiographical examination, the possibility of arteriosclerotic changes is deemed lower in the younger group than in the group of healthy individuals with the mean age of 50 years) were taken as an acceptable range of normal values (0.229 ± 0.056). This criterion would have made it possible to detect 100% of lower limbs with occlusion and 80.8% of lower limbs with definite arteriosclerotic changes but without occlusion.

This method is quick, simple and inexpensive. It makes it possible to screen subjects with arteriosclerotic changes within a few minutes and to distinguish between those with occlusion and with less advanced arteriosclerotic changes.

REFERENCES

Seldinger, S. J. (1953). *Acta Radiol.* **39**, 368.
Linhart, J., Dejdar, R., Spáčil, J., Pavlovič, J., and Broulíková, A. (1976). *In* "Proceedings of the X International Congress of Angiology, " Tokyo.

PLETHYSMOGRAPHY REVISITED AS A TOOL FOR DIAGNOSTIC AND FUNCTIONAL EVALUATION OF ATHEROSCLEROTIC ARTERIOPATHY

D. L. Clement, Ph. Charlier and Ch. de Meunynck

University Hospital, Department of Cardiovascular Diseases, Section of Angiology, Ghent, Belgium

Although the final mechanism of intermittent claudication is still a matter of dispute, it certainly is related to an inadequate blood flow to the muscles of the lower limbs. Blood flow measurements are therefore a logical approach to this condition.

Several studies have been devoted to this topic in the past but new data is coming to light following a significant improvement in the technical character- istics of venous occlusion plethysmography, e.g. sensitivity of the method has largely been increased, recordings are made on a semi-continuous basis because of ECG-triggering and an adaptable programme of venous occlusion and release. Also, the calculated results for flow are plotted simultaneously on a second channel (Brugmans *et al.*, 1977).

In this paper our most recent data will be reviewed as an introduction to the question "what is the actual place of plethysmography in the vascular laboratory?". All data presented in this paper were obtained with Periflow®, Janssen. In every patient, resting blood flow and reactive hyperaemia curves are recorded. In all curves, peak blood flow, time to peak flow and 50% recovery time are calculated.

Serono Symposium No. 37, "Vascular Occlusion: Epidemiological, Pathophysiological and Therapeutic Aspects", edited by M. Tesi and J. Dormandy, 1981. Academic Press, London and New York.

REPRODUCIBILITY OF THE DATA

When we want to make a functional diagnosis or evaluate follow-up of a patient using plethysmography, it is important to investigate first to what extent the results are reproducible. This was tested in a group of 16 patients having typical symptoms of intermittent claudication and positive to all clinically used criteria (Clement and Brugmans, 1979). In these patients, claudication distance and blood flow were measured twice, one month apart. The vascular state of the patients was unchanged in that period as the treadmill test remained quite constant with a correlation coefficient of 0.91 ($P < 0.001$). Flow data also appeared quite reproducible: for resting blood flow and peak blood flow the r value is 0.81 ($P < 0.001$), for the time to peak flow it is 0.84 and for the 50% recovery time it scores up to 0.89 ($P < 0.001$). Notice that even with this excellent score, time-to-peak flow appears to be quite variable in the most pathological range of the data; also the 50% recovery time is significantly shorter in the first month compared with the next month. The cause for this is not clear. It is obvious that more experiments should be done in this respect.

DIAGNOSTIC PERFORMANCE OF THE TECHNIQUE

This question was studied in a group of 83 vascular "normal" and 101 vascular "abnormal" limbs (Clement et al. 1979). Differentation between normal and abnormal was made using (1) resting and post-exercise oscillography (Schoop, 1974) and (2) the index of systolic blood pressure measured with ultrasound, accepting 96% as the lowest normal value (Clement et al., 1978).

As was previously shown (Shepherd, 1963), there is no difference in resting blood flow between both groups. By contrast, reactive hyperaemia curves show quite pronounced differences between normal and abnormal. Peak blood flow is significantly lower ($P < 0.001$) in the abnormal group; the difference becomes larger when the occluding time is longer: at 5 min, peak blood flow averages 0.300 vol % per systole in the normal group vs 0.164 in the abnormal group.

Much larger differences are found as far as the time-to-peak flow in both groups are concerned. It averages seven times longer in the group of abnormal than in the group of normal limbs at 5 min. However, the standard deviation of the means in the abnormal group is large, which causes overlapping between both groups. The same remarks apply for the 50% recovery time.

As analysis of any of these parameters results in overlapping between normals and abnormals, it was investigated whether combination of parameters could improve this differentiation. Normal limits were set-up by exploring the scattergram of the data for every parameter. This resulted in the following: normal peak blood flow; 0.250 vol % per systole or more; normal time-to-peak flow; less than 10 s 50% recovery time; less than 30 s. The best score was achieved when two abnormal parameters were required in order to consider the curve as abnormal; in that case, 78 out of 80 normal limbs are correctly classified (97%) but only 70 out of the 90 abnormal limbs are classified as abnormal (78%).

CORRELATION OF BLOOD FLOW MEASUREMENTS WITH WALKING DISTANCE

In the 16 patients studied, a remarkably good correlation was found between resting blood flow and walking distance as determined on the treadmill (r = 0.51; P = 0.039). Quite similar results are obtained for peak flow and walking distance (0.48 < r < 0.51), but no significant correlation can be found for walking distance and either time-to-peak flow or 50% recovery time. Thus, it seems that measuring resting and peak blood flow provides useful information concerning the functional aspect of the vascular lesions. It also shows that there is a correlation of flow to claudicaton but since the correlation factor is only of the order of 0.50, many other factors play a role in the symptom of claudication.

CORRELATION BETWEEN PLETHYSMOGRAPHIC DATA AND SYSTOLIC BLOOD PRESSURE IN THE SAME LIMB

Finally, it seemed important to analyse whether the two parameters (pressure and flow) that are fundamental in the regulation of the circulation through a vascular bed are linked. There is a weak but highly significant correlation between systolic blood pressure and resting blood flow (r = 0.33, P < 0.001); the correlation is only slightly better for the different parameters derived from the reactive hyperaemia curve *vs* systolic blood pressure.

COMMENTS

These data are given as an introduction to the session devoted on plethysmography in order to review the value of this old technique in the diagnosis and evaluation of patients with peripheral arterial diseases. It is clear that very large differences are found in the flow data of normals and abnormals. However, there is a certain degree of overlapping, and other methods such as systolic pressure measurements are more simple and cheaper.

In clinical practice, plethysmography is useful when the other currently available techniques cannot be used. In some cases (e.g. diabetes), blood pressure can not be measured because of hardening of the vessels – plethysmography can provide the clinician with some information in that situation. Another example is when the treadmill test cannot be performed because of local (orthopaedic) or general problems (angina pectoris, pulmonary diseases) then plethysmography still can offer some functional evaluation. Finally, when information concerning "flow" is sought, e.g. in following any form of treatment again this technique can give it, at rest and during stimulation.

268   *D. L. Clement et al.*

REFERENCES

Brugmans, J., Jageneau, A., Hörig, C. and Emanuel, M. B. (1977). *Proc. R. Soc. Med.* **1**, 6.
Clement, D. L., Claeys, R. and Pannier (1978). *Angéiologie* **30**, 303.
Clement, D. L. and Brugmans, J. (1979). *Angiology* (Accepted for publication.)
Clement, D. L., Charlier, Ph and de Meunynck, Ch, (1979). Proceedings of Cardiovascular Congress II, Scottsdale, Arizona p. 19.
Schoop, W. (1974). "Praktische Angiologie," Georg Thieme Verlag, Stuttgart.
Sheperd, J. T. (1963). W. B. Saunders

A HEMODYNAMIC ANGIOGRAPHIC AND CLINICAL STUDY OF COLD VASODILATATION IN "VIBRATION ANGIOPATHY": PRELIMINARY RESULTS

G. Giuliano, L. Iacopetti, G. P. Chiriatti, U. Cappelli and G. Nuzzaci

Departments of Occupational Medicine and Internal Medicine, Cardiovascular Unit, University of Florence, Italy

The vascular disturbances due to vibrations ("vibration angiopathy" – Giuliano *et al.* 1974, 1976) are of great importance because of their significant prevalence in subjects working with vibrating tools and of the widespread use of such instruments in several kinds of working activities.

In previous research (Giuliano, 1967; Giuliano *et al.*, 1974 a,b; Nuzzaci *et al.*, 1976) some of us investigated the thermographic, arteriographic and hemo-dynamic features of "vibration angiopathy". A high prevalence of organic lesions of the digital arteries of the hand was found, but at the same time it was pointed out that the hemodynamic significance of these lesions could be considered, at least in general, as not prominent.

In the present research, we performed a study of cold vasodilatation in "vibration angiopathy". This was done since cold vasodilatation – as a partic-ularly relevant reflection of the vasomotor tone in the distal circulation – was thought to be able to provide reliable information concerning both the presence and the degree of distal circulatory impairment in "vibration angiopathy". In addition, cold vasodilatation, having a typically local pathogenic mechanism, was thought relevant in deductions as to the physiopathology of Raynaud's phenomenon, at least in the particular field of the "vibration angiopathy".

Serono Symposium No. 37, "Vascular Occlusion: Epidemiological, Pathophysiological and Therapeutic Aspects", edited by M. Tesi and J. Dormandy, 1981. Academic Press, London and New York.

G. Giuliano et al.

MATERIALS AND METHODS

Seven male subjects working with vibrating tools (pneumatic hammer, chain saw, etc.) and affected by "vibration angiopathy" were studied. The age range was 35 to 59 years (mean 44.2 years); the length of exposure to vibration ranged between 1 and 10 years (mean 8.6 years). All subjects were affected with Raynaud's phenomenon, referred to as bilateral in five cases and unilateral in two, and involving one or more fingers. In three patients, digital trophic lesions (namely, thickening of the skin and/or small stellar scars on the fingertips) were present.

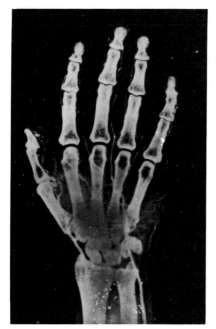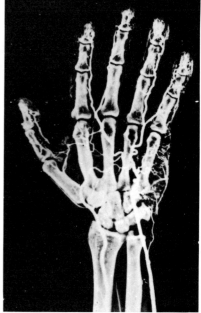

Fig. 1. Hand arteriograms of two subjects affected with "vibration angiopathy". Evident stenoses and occlusions of the digital arteries.

All patients underwent bilateral arteriography, performed under general anesthesia induced by pentothal and succinylcholine and maintained by halothane and nitrous oxide. In all the subjects, organic lesions (viz. stenoses and/or occlusions) of the digital arteries were detected (Fig. 1). Each type of lesion was given a score, according to a previously reported scale (Giuliano *et al.*, 1974a); all the lesions per finger were then summed up, and converted into a total score for each individual finger. In such a way, the most involved finger and the least involved one were identified for each hand and/or for each patient. In both fingers, the total digital flow was comparatively studied by means of strain gauge plethysmography. Digital blood flow measurements were performed initially at room temperature (20 °C) every 30 s for 15 min; then, during immersion of the hand in cold water at 10 °C every minute for

60 min; and finally at room temperature in the post-immersion period every minute for 30 min. In these experiments, electrically insulated electrodes were used in order to permit digital blood flow measurements even during the immersion of the hand in cold water.

RESULTS

The results obtained from the digital blood flow measurements carried out can be summarized as follows.

(1) In fingers with no Raynaud's phenomenon and no trophic lesions, cold vasodilatation was found to occur in all the cases studied. However, a different behavior was observed, depending on whether or not Raynaud's phenomenon was present in other fingers of the same hand. In the former case (second right finger, patient 5 – Fig. 2), cold vasodilatation behavior appeared atypical because of a delayed onset and a lessening of its cyclic course with a clear reduction of the so-called (Lewis, 1930) "hunting reaction". In the latter case, cold vasodilatation by contrast was found to have a rather normal course (second and fourth left fingers, patient 5 – Fig. 3). This was true also for blood flow measurements performed on the same subject (patient 5 – Figs 2 and 3).

COLD VASODILATION TEST

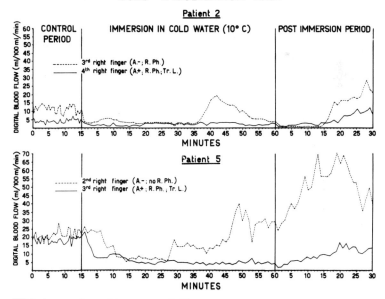

Fig. 2. Cold vasodilatation in two patients affected with "vibration angiopathy". A, arteriographic involvement (A−. minimum involvement; A+, maximum involvement); R. Ph., Raynaud's phenomenon; Tr. L., trophic lesions. Digital blood flow measurements were performed at 30 s intervals in the control period and at 1 min intervals in the immersion and post-immersion periods.

G. Giuliano et al.

COLD VASODILATION TEST

Patient 5

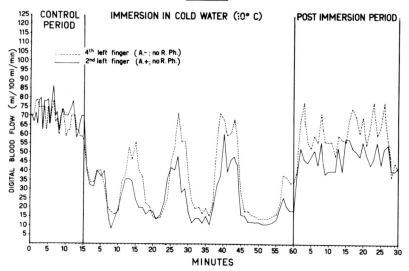

Fig. 3. Cold vasodilatation in a patient affected with "vibration angiopathy". Abbreviations as in Fig. 2.

(2) In fingers with Raynaud's phenomenon, but with no trophic lesions, cold vasodilatation was found to occur in all the cases studied; however, it appeared definitely abnormal both for onset time (> 30 min after the beginning of exposure to cold) and for behavior, which was characterized by absence of its cyclic course with disappearance of the "hunting reaction" (third right finger, patient 2 – Fig. 2).

(3) In fingers with trophic lesions, cold vasodilatation was never found to occur, since digital blood flow showed either no significant changes (fourth right finger, patient 2 – Fig. 2) or a rather uniform decrease (third right finger, patient 5 – Fig. 2) during immersion of the hand in cold water.

(4) As for the post-immersion period, the return of the digital blood flow to the control period levels was found to be clearly delayed in fingers with Raynaud's phenomenon (third right finger, patient 2 – Fig. 2), as well as in fingers with trophic lesions in which a reduction in blood flow had occurred (third right finger, patient 5 – Fig. 2).

(5) No significant differences were found either in onset time or in behavior of cold vasodilatation between the most and the least arteriographically involved finger, provided that they had comparable clinical situations (presence or absence of Raynaud's phenomenon).

CONCLUSIONS

The results obtained allow us to conclude that in subjects affected with "vibration angiopathy" there is a cold vasomotion impairment. The degree of this impairment is related to the local clinical situation: it is least pronounced in fingers without Raynaud's phenomenon and most pronounced in fingers with trophic lesions.

No evident correlation appears to exist between the severity of the cold vasomotor impairment and either the prevalence and/or the severity of digital artery lesions as revealed by arteriography. This is true, obviously, within the limits of organic lesions which do not induce significant differences in hemodynamic impairment.

The correlation found between impairment of the cold vasodilatation (which has a typically local pathogenic mechanism) and Raynaud's phenomenon seems to point to the presence of a local physiopathological mechanism for Raynaud's phenomenon also, at least with regard to "vibration angiopathy".

REFERENCES

Giuliano, G. (1967). *In*: "Atti XXX Congresso Nazionale della Società Italiana di Medicina del Lavoro" 845–850. Istituto di Medicina del Lavoro del l'Università, Palermo.

Giuliano, G. (1976) *Minerva Angiologica* 1, 35.

Giuliano, G., Cavina, C., Bartoli, V., Dorigo, B., Focardi, L. (1974a). *Lavoro Umano* 26, 161.

Giuliano, G., Cavina, C., Bartoli, V., Dorigo, B., Focardi, L., Caporale, A. (1974b). *In*: "Atti del IX Congresso Internazionale di Angiologia" 8, 95–101. Minerva Medica, Torino.

Lewis, T. (1930). *Heart* 15, 177.

Nuzzaci, G., Giuliano, G., Boccuni, M., Cupelli, V. and Arcangeli, C. (1976). *Lavoro Umano* 28, 161.

STRAIN GAUGE PLETHYSMOGRAPHIC STUDY OF THE EFFECT OF SOME SO-CALLED VASODILATING AGENTS ON PERIPHERAL HAEMODYNAMICS

S. Forconi, M. Guerrini, S. Pecchi, R. Cappelli and F. Bruni

Istituto di Patologia Speciale Medica, Università di Siena, Italy

By means of strain gauge plethysmography, we can evaluate the peripheral haemodynamics of the limbs in relation both to the arterial and to the venous behaviour. In order to investigate the activity of some so-called vasodilating drugs, we measured arterial blood flow at rest and after ischaemia, venous capacitance, tone and distensibility, arterial and venous blood pressure at calf level in patients with peripheral obliterative arterial diseases (POAD) and in normal subjects, after the administration of intravenous nitroglycerine (NTG), sublingual isosorbide dinitrate (ISD) and oral prazosin (PZ).

MATERIAL AND METHODS

For this study, we have used a strain gauge plethysmograph "Periflow", with the technique described elsewhere (Forconi *et al.*, 1979). All the subjects were studied in supine position, with their feet 15 cm above the heart level, with the strain gauge posed at the calf and the cuff for venous occlusion at the thigh.

Three groups of patients, affected by POAD in the second stage, and three groups of voluntary normal controls were studied. All the patients were selected on the basis of the defect in the hyperaemic response to ischaemia,

Serono Symposium No. 37, "Vascular Occlusion: Epidemiological, Pathophysiological and Therapeutic Aspects", edited by M. Tesi and J. Dormandy, 1981. Academic Press, London and New York.

plethysmographically demonstrated, and the diagnosis was confirmed by angiography.

The first group was composed of five patients, four male and one female, age varying from 57 to 64 years. The control group was composed of three patients, one male and two female, age varying from 27 to 63 years. In the group of patients there were three subjects with one leg completely normal from the plethysmographic and angiographic point of view, therefore the total number of legs which we studied consisted nine normal and seven pathological legs. Intravenous nitroglycerine was infused with the standard dosage of 0.35 mg in 2 min and the blood flow in the limbs (RF) was observed in a semicontinuous way until the disappearance of every effect of the drug. At the same time, heart rate (HR) and brachial systolic (SBP) and diastolic blood pressure (DBP) were recorded in the conventional manner. The same experiment was repeated in every subject the following day for the venous study. After a venous occlusion of 60 mmHg, during which basal venous capacitance (MVIV) and venous emptying (MVO) were recorded, another similar venous occlusion started simultaneously with the beginning of the infusion of NTG; and MVIV and MVO were again calculated. Owing to the short period of activity of the drug, it was not possible to investigate the post-ischaemic response in this study.

The second group was composed of nine patients (18 limbs), eight male and one female, age varying from 52 to 76 years. The second control group was composed of seven subjects (14 limbs) all male, age varying from 23 to 66 years. Sublingual ISD was administered in standard dosage of 5 mg, and the blood flow in the limbs (RF) was observed in a semicontinuous way till the action of the drug had disappeared. At the same time HR, SBP and DBP were recorded in the conventional manner. In the same experiment, local systolic blood pressure (LSBP) measured at the cuff level, was recorded. The sublingual administration of ISD was repeated in every subject for two days. The second day, before and 5 min after (maximal activity of the drug) the ISD, a venous study was performed and venous capacitance, venous distensibility (VD), venous tone (VT), venous pressure (VP) and venous emptying were calculated. The third day a study of the hyperaemic response to ischaemia (3 min) was performed before and 5 min after the ISD and peak flow (PF), time to peak flow (tPF), half time (t½) and total time (tT) were calculated.

The third group was composed of 12 patients (24 limbs), all male, age varying from 45 to 67. The third control group was composed of 12 normal subjects (24 limbs), all male, age varying from 30 to 54. Oral prazosin was administered in standard dosage of 5 mg, and the blood flow in the limbs (RF) was observed in a semicontinuous way till the 30th min (maximal activity of the drug) and in some patients till the 60th min. At the same time HR, SBP and DBP were recorded in the conventional manner. In the same study, before, 30 min after, and in some patients also 60 min after, LSBP, venous function and the post-ischaemic response were recorded in the same manner as in the ISD study (it was possible to do this in a single experiment owing to the longer period of activity of the drug).

Mean values were calculated. Statistical analysis was performed comparing basal findings with the post-treatment findings, using analysis of variance for the NTG study and Student's *t* test for paired variables in the ISD and PZ study.

RESULTS

Results are reported in Table I for the NTG study and in Table II for the ISD and the PZ study. In the NTG study, the blood flow at the calf clearly showed a rapid decrease followed at once by an increase. This phenomenon was important and highly significant from a statistical point of view in normal subjects, while it was of little account and statistically insignificant in POAD patients. This striking difference could also be seen in the three subjects with one damaged and one normal leg. The maximal decreasing activity was registered in normal subjects 45 ± 30 s (s.d.) after the onset of infusion while in POAD patients it occurred 42 ± 11 s after the same point. The maximal increasing activity was registered after 131 ± 49 s in normal subjects, after 132 ± 57 s in POAD patients, practically at the end of the infusion time which was 120 s. The activity of the drug disappeared after 197 ± 67 s in the controls and after 213 ± 78 s in POAD patients.

These differences were not statistically significant. Nor were significant differences seen in BP and HR (the slight increase in HR was not significant in the two groups). In the venous study, we noted that the curve of venous filling during venous occlusion showed a typical S shape; there was a decrease in

Table I. Action of intravenous nitroglycerine on peripheral haemodynamics.

	A	B	C	F	P
Control					
HR	65 ± 8.6	75 ± 16.3	75.1 ± 18.5	0.8877	0.4350
SBP	143.3 ± 39.3	142.5 ± 41.8	142.5 ± 39.7	0.0009	0.0463
DBP	90 ± 12.6	90.8 ± 12.8	90.8 ± 12.0	0.0089	0.1227
RF	2.7 ± 0.96	1.8 ± 0.73	4.9 ± 2.7	7.9071	0.0026[b]
MVIV	2.6 ± 0.4	3.2 ± 0.8		4.2101	0.0483[a]
MVO	68.3 ± 15.2	62.3 ± 13.7		0.6101	0.5001
AOP					
HR	66.8 ± 14.1	74.4 ± 15.3	72.8 ± 16.8	0.3339	0.6806
SBP	144 ± 23.02	138 ± 18.5	143 ± 23.8	0.1043	0.5430
DBP	90 ± 7.07	88 ± 8.3	91 ± 7.4	0.2000	0.6683
RF	3.4 ± 1.5	2.6 ± 1.9	4.04 ± 1.3	1.3341	0.2880
MVIV	2.9 ± 0.6	3.5 ± 0.7		4.2308	0.0492[a]
MVO	75.0 ± 18.3	69.9 ± 15.7		0.5303	0.4806

For legends see text. A, Before. B, Point of maximal decrease of blood flow at rest (RF). C, Point of maximal increase of blood flow at rest (RF). Analysis of variance. [a]$P < 0.05$ and [b]$P < 0.01$.

Table II. Action of sublingual ISD and oral PZ on peripheral haemodynamics.

| | CONTROL | | | ISOSORBIDE DINITRATE AOP | | |
	BEFORE	AFTER	t	BEFORE	AFTER	t
HR	81.7 ± 7.0	86.2 ± 6.4	2.488[a]	66 ± 4.1	69 ± 4.4	1.714
LSBP	152.1 ± 6.93	131 ± 4.25	6.067[b]	140 ± 8.2	122 ± 8.2	3.798[b]
SBP	139.1 ± 6.50	132.5 ± 4.42	2.390[a]	148 ± 7.7	134 ± 8.5	2.2231[a]
DBP	90.0 ± 0.0	88.33 ± 2.78	0.597	93 ± 2.6	90 ± 3.5	1.0000
RF	3.4 ± 0.48	2.5 ± 0.45	5.749[b]	3.9 ± 0.8	3.4 ± 0.9	2.511[a]
MVIV	2.2 ± 0.72	2.9 ± 0.77	3.382[b]	1.8 ± 0.1	2.6 ± 0.1	3.557[b]
VD	0.04 ± 0.01	0.04 ± 0.01	0.320	0.04 ± 0.004	0.04 ± 0.004	00000
VT	21.06 ± 5.64	22.3 ± 7.25	0.720	28.7 ± 3.8	25.2 ± 3.5	1.611
MVO	47.0 ± 12.7	43.5 ± 15.3	0.971	49.2 ± 4.5	46.7 ± 2.7	1.591
VP	16.8 ± 3.4	13.08 ± 3.75	0,464	14 ± 0.7	15 ± 1.01	0.576
PF	18.8 ± 1.2	21.1 ± 1.5	17729	12.6 ± 1.8	13.8 ± 1.9	4.323[b]
TPF	3	3		23 ± 9.7	13 ± 7.2	2.299[a]
T1/2	12 ± 1.3	10 ± 0.8	1.231	26 ± 7.3	21 ± 4.8	1.702
TT	138 ± 37	131 ± 38	0.718	221 ± 39.5	209 ± 40	1.702

Table II. Cont'd.

	CONTROL			PRAZOSIN AOP		
	BEFORE	AFTER	t	BEFORE	AFTER	t
HR	70.6 ± 1.33	73.3 ± 2.04	1.3009	71.3 ± 3.6	70.0 ± 4.9	0.8864
LSBP	147.9 ± 2.31	142.3 ± 3.54	2.2517[a]	119.5 ± 4.5	118.9 ± 5.5	0.2110
SBP	136.6 ± 2.84	126.6 ± 2.07	6.6332[b]	150.8 ± 5.1	150.0 ± 5.2	0.4114
DBP	88.3 ± 2.07	82.5 ± 2.08	3.1890[b]	91.6 ± 3.2	91.6 ± 3.2	000000
RF	2.7 ± 0.20	2.9 ± 0.29	1.1839	3.09 ± 0.15	4.17 ± 0.33	5.0470[b]
MVIV	2.49 ± 0.16	3.0 ± 0.18	3.2899	2.6 ± 0.1	3.2 ± 0.1	9.500[b]
VD	0.053 ± 0.003	0.057 ± 0.003	2.0951[a]	0.060 ± 0.002	0.064 ± 0.002	2.3565[a]
VT	20.78 ± 2.005	18.14 ± 0.875	2.5742[a]	16.8 ± 0.7	15.7 ± 0.6	2.1684[a]
MVO	55.1 ± 3.09	57.1 ± 3.38	1.8385	56.9 ± 1.3	60.5 ± 2.2	1.9851
VP	12.6 ± 0.80	10.5 ± 0.61	3.3473[a]	13.7 ± 0.4	11.4 ± 0.6	3.5889[b]
PF	19.2 ± 0.53	18.9 ± 1.03	1.5605	11.3 ± 0.9	12.9 ± 1.1	3.4822[b]
TPF	3 ± 0.0	3 ± 0.0		15.9 ± 3.2	16.7 ± 3.4	0.2504
T1/2	15.1 ± 1.17	13.3 ± 1.01	2.2233[a]	145.8 ± 27.3	144.7 ± 27.8	0.3901
TT	146.5 ± 17.5	118.7 ± 14.9	6.1495[b]	215.1 ± 16.6	160.6 ± 21.5	4.0372[a]

For legends see text. Statistical analysis was performed using Student's *t* test for paired variables were
[a] $p < 0.05$ and [b] $p < 0.01$.

venous filling and successively an increase which occurred simultaneously with the changes in arterial blood flow. This was more evident in controls than in POAD patients. On the other hand, the MVIV appeared markedly increased in comparison with the basal value, both in normal and in POAD patients, and this effect on venous function was evident also after the effect on arterial blood flow was completely over.

In the ISD study, there was a constantly significant decrease in blood flow, more evident in normal than in POAD subjects, 5 min after the sublingual administration of the drug. Subsequently, after 10 or 15 min, the phenomenon disappeared. During the maximal activity of the drug there was an increase in HR and a slight reduction in LSBP and SBP, while an important and highly significant rise was observed in venous capacitance, both in normal and in POAD subjects. The hyperaemic response to ischaemia was also modified by ISD. We noted a slight but significant increase of peak flow in POAD patients and a tendency to a reduction of the times studied (tPF, t½, tT) in both groups.

In the PZ study, the increase of blood flow was important and statistically significant in POAD patients, while the increase in the control subjects was slight. A decrease of all blood pressure values was seen in control subjects. The maximal activity of the drug was gradually reached in 30 min; in the patients who were observed till the 60th min, the drug effect was still present. What seemed very important was the effect of PZ on venous function, both in normal and in POAD patients, an increase of venous capacitance with a parallel increase of VD and decrease of VT and VP were observed in all the subjects studied. The post-ischaemic hyperaemia was also modified by PZ. There was a significant increase of PF in POAD patients, while in both groups the times were reduced.

DISCUSSION

Our results demonstrate an evident action of the compounds we studied upon the peripheral haemodynamics of the limbs, affecting both arteries and veins. They may be summarized thus.

(1) The i.v. NTG provokes a brief, fleeting effect, initially decreasing and successively increasing the blood flow, only when there is a normal circulatory state. The arterial effect in patients is inconsistent. The effect upon the venous capacitance appears to be independent of the arterial effect and it is present in normal and in pathological conditions.

(2) The s.l. IDN always provokes a reduction of the blood flow of the limbs. It reminded us of the initial decreasing effect of NTG, even if it is less rapid and not followed by the subsequent increase. Simultaneously, systolic blood pressure decreased. The arterial effect seems more important when the circulation is not damaged as in the NTG study. Venous capacitance always increases.

(3) The activity of oral PZ on blood flow seems to be different: the blood flow in the lower limbs markedly increases in POAD patients and this increase is important and prolonged. Blood pressure is not affected in patients, while

in normal controls, there is a reduction of the pressure without important changes of the flow. This different behaviour of the blood flow is difficult to explain. Many problems of clinical pharmacology arise, but our knowledge of the mechanisms regulating blood flow in pathological states does not permit any interpretation of the findings. Also PZ shows a marked and prolonged venodilating effect.

(4) The activities of ISD and PZ on post-ischaemic hyperaemia are slight but significant. Both the drugs increase the flow and shorten the times in pathological conditions and tend to improve the general pattern of the response, but while the action of ISD is of a brief duration, that of PZ is more sustained and prolonged.

(5) The venodilating effect appears to be a constant and important feature of all the three componds.

In conclusion, whereas all the three compounds show an important venodilating effect, in the arterial circulation, there are some important differences. while the nitrates showed a similar activity, evident in normal and quite negligible in pathological conditions, prazosin gives an important vasodilating effect especially when there is a clearly impaired arterial bed. This confirms a different mechanism of the drug in determining the vasodilating effect.

REFERENCE

Forconi, S., Jageneau, A., Guerrini, M., Pecchi, S., Cappelli, R. (1979). *Angiology* **30**, 487.

RECOGNITION OF IMPENDING CIRCULATION FAILURE IN CLAUDICANTS BY NON-INVASIVE HEMODYNAMICAL METHODS

M. Zicot

Hôpital de Bavière, Université de Liège, Département de Clinique et de Pathologie médicales, Institut de Médicine, Liège, Belgium

INTRODUCTION

The modern plethysmographic techniques (Brugmans *et al.*, 1977) allow accurate determination of the characteristics of segmental hyperemic flow curves. The exact interpretation of the recorded figures is still open to discussion. We used an isotope method for years (Cuypers and Merchie, 1962) to assess the severity of the distal ischemia. In our hands, circulation delays of over 100s with this technique indicate a severe ischemia. We were therefore interested in analysing the calf plethysmographic findings in the light of this test, and in comparing them to a well known hemodynamic variable: the ankle systolic pressure (P/P').

MATERIAL AND METHODS

Material

A group N of 20 normal limbs was considered. They were observed among 16 subjects (51 - 70 years-old, mean age : 59.2 ± 6.6 s.d.). A group of 33 limbs with arterial occlusive disease was examined. It was divided in two subgroups following the radio-isotope test (T shorter or longer than 100 s (see Methods). In group II_A (T < 100 s), 20 limbs (all at stage II following Fontaine) were observed among

Serono Symposium No. 37, "Vascular Occlusion: Epidemiological, Pathophysiological and Therapeutic Aspects", edited by M. Tesi and J. Dormandy, 1981. Academic Press, London and New York.

Table I. Non-invasive hemodynamical data in normal and ischemic limbs.

	Normal		T < 100 s		Ischemic	T > 100 s
P/P′	1.19 ± 0.11	t = 10.6 [a] xx[d]	0.77 ± 0.14		t = 5.08 [b] xx[d]	0.46 ± 0.21
RF (% min^{-1})	5.07 ± 2.62	t = 0.39 NS	4.76 ± 2.29	t = 11.51 [c] xx[d]	t = 1.94 NS	6.92 ± 3.70
PF (% min^{-1})	24.44 ± 5.85	t = 7.71 xx	12.97 ± 3.16	t = 1.71 NS	t = 0.86 NS	11.28 ± 5.52
PF/RF	5.12 ± 1.71	t = 2.32 x	3.44 ± 2.71	t = 6.61 xx	t = 2.71 x	1.73 ± 0.66
t_1 (s)	10.34 ± 5.05	t = 5.08 xx	32.28 ± 18.63	t = 7.87 xx	t = 1.01 NS	39.10 ± 17.96
t_2 (s)	28.08 ± 7.71	t = 4.76 xx	79.12 ± 47.31	t = 5.42 xx; t = 7.18 xx	t = 1.84 NS	108.97 ± 38.57

[a]Comparison between column 1 and 2 t = test ratio. [b]Comparison between column 2 and 3 t = test ratio. [c]Comparison between column 1 and 3 t = test ratio. [d]xx:$P < 0.001$ x:$P < 0.05$ NS: non-significant.

Table II. Non-invasive hemodynamical data following the severity of ischemia.

	Group II$_A$	t (col 1–2)	Group II$_B$	t (col 2–3)	t (col 1–3)	Group III
P/P′	0.77 ± 0.14	t = 4.49 [a] xx [d]	0.49 ± 0.19	t = 4.61 [c] xx [d]	t = 0.74 [b] NS [d]	0.40 ± 0.24
RF (% min⁻¹)	4.76 ± 2.29	t = 3.16 x	8.36 ± 3.84	t = 0.41 NS	t = 2.84 x	4.33 ± 1.37
PF (% min⁻¹)	12.97 ± 3.16	t = 0.38 NS	13.59 ± 5.58	t = 3.97 xx	t = 3.24 x	7.10 ± 1.67
PF/RF	3.44 ± 2.71	t = 2.80 x	1.68 ± 0.49	t = 2.90 x	t = 0.38 NS	1.82 ± 0.94
t$_1$ (s)	32.28 ± 18.63	t = 0.36 NS	35.10 ± 17.99	t = 1.46 NS	t = 1.10 NS	47.10 ± 17.29
t$_2$ (s)	79.12 ± 47.31	t = 1.67 NS	108.00 ± 30.95	t = 1.08 NS	t = 0.06 NS	109.45 ± 56.73

[a]Comparison between column 1 and 2 t = test ratio. [b]Comparison between column 1 and 3 t = test ratio. [c]Comparison between column 2 and 3 t = test ratio. [d] xx: $P < 0.001$ x: $P < 0.05$ NS: non-significant.

13 patients (47 – 74 years, mean age : 59.1 ± 7.9 s.d.). The third group (II_B, III) (with T > 100 s) was composed of 14 limbs observed among 14 subjects (45 – 80 years, mean age : 61.3 ± 11.6). This group was further subdivided into nine limbs without rest pain (II_B) and five limbs with rest pain and/or trophic damage (III).

Methods

The subjects were submitted to a Doppler investigation with measurement of the systolic pressure ratio between ankle and arm (P/P'). Some normal limbs and all the ischemic limbs were submitted to the radio-isotope test which is familiar to us and consists of an assessment of the foot perfusion during a reactive hyperemia, after Cuypers and Merchie (1962). This test is based on the kinetics of appearance of tagged albumin in the foot after release of a thigh tourniquet (time T in seconds).

All subjects were also submitted to a plethysmographic determination of the calf flow characteristics before and during a post-occlusive reactive hyperemia. We used an ECG- triggered venous occlusion plethysmograph (Periflow^R JSI). The strain-gauge was around the calf, the cuff at the thigh. The pressure in the venous collecting cuff was 50 mmHg.

We measured the flow at rest (RF in %/min^{-1}) and during a reactive hyperemia secondary to a 3-min arterial occlusion. We determined the peak flow (PF in %/min^{-1}). In addition, we measured the interval between the release of the occlusion and the peak flow tl (s), and t2 (s) between the end of the ischemia and the point halfway on the decreasing limb of the hyperemic flow curve.

RESULTS

Table 1 compares the normal and the ischemic limbs divided in two groups following the isotope test. The relative ankle pressure P/P' differentiates well the three groups, PF, t1, t2 and PF/RF are significantly different if we compare the normal and the pathological limbs. The two ischemic groups are significantly different on comparing PF/RF.

Table II goes further in the comparison of the ischemic limbs because we introduced a distinction between severe ischemia (T > 100 s) with rest pain (III) and without rest pain (II_B). There is a higher RF in group II_B when compared to group II_A and III. PF is lower in group III. P/P' and PF/RF are not different in II_B and III.

The time course (t1, t2) of the hyperemia does not differentiate the different groups of ischemia. We were unable to measure these features in only one case from groups III and II_B because of the very flat hyperemic curves.

DISCUSSION

We have used an isotope test for years to assess the importance of distal ischemia. When the circulatory delay (T) is longer than 100 min, the ischemia is getting severe in our experience. We demonstrated an obvious inverse relationship between

P/P' and T (Zicot, 1978). The results of calf plethysmography are not so easy to analyse. All features of the hyperemic curve are statistically and significantly different between normal and ischemic limbs. Our work demonstrates the existence of an intermediate state between moderate ischemia (group II_A) and patent circulatory failure (group III). The isotope method helped us to distinguish the group which has still PF values similar to group II_A, but where the RF is increased. PF/RF therefore is significantly lowered and close to the ratio observed in group III.

We stress the fact that these limbs are only at stage II following Fontaine (claudication). We feel, nevertheless, that such hemodynamical data call attention to impending circulatory failure, even if the walking capacity is still apparently conserved. We only have a hypothesis to explain the increased resting blood flow in the calf. We do not think that it is due to therapy (vasodilators for instance). The same therapy was applied in group II_A. These limbs are probably never in a true resting condition. The ischemia is a permanent stress for tissue, opening the small vessels and even perhaps shunts by accumulation of metabolites. The isotope test depends on the perfusion of the foot and its prolongation reveals the reduced blood flow in the extremity even if the calf flow is apparently conserved.

REFERENCES

Brugmans, J., Jageneau, A., Hörig, C. H. and Emanuel, M. (1977). *Proc. R Soc. (Lond.)* **70**, Suppl. 8, 1.
Cuypers, Y. and Merchie, G. (1962). *Acta Cardiologica* **17**, 117.
Zicot, M. (1978). *Angiology* **29**, 534.

DIAGNOSIS OF THE SUBCLAVIAN STEAL SYNDROME BY DOPPLER SONOGRAPHY

L. Urai and P. Farkas

*Department of Cardiology, Semmelweis University Medical School
and the National Institute of Cardiology and Angiology,
Budapest, Hungary*

The subclavian steal syndrome (SSS) first described by Contorni (1960) was detected in the course of the detailed analysis of the syndromes of the arcus aortae and diagnosed at that time by means of arch aortography.

The joint application of ophthalmodynamometry (ODM) and ophthalmodyna-mography (ODG) to the noninvasive diagnosis of the subclavian steal syndrome was a considerable step forward but failed to always give unequivocally reliable results. The introduction of the directional Doppler technique finally brought about the possibility of the direct recording of vertebral artery flow and of its direction. Ultrasound diagnosis of the subclavian steal syndrome is in a state of development and is a much studied problem.

MATERIAL AND METHOD

In the past year, Doppler sonographic tests were carried out in our institute on 43 patients with angiographically verified subclavian steal syndrome, using the bidirectional Parks 806 continuous wave sonograph.

Depending upon the positioning of the probe, diagnosis of the subclavian steal syndrome can be performed either by pharyngeal or by occipital recording. We used the occipital method where the probe is placed on the occipital region between the apex of the mastoid process and the transverse process of the atlas

Serono Symposium No. 37, "Vascular Occlusion: Epidemiological, Pathophysiological and Therapeutic Aspects", edited by M. Tesi and J. Dormandy, 1981. Academic Press, London and New York.

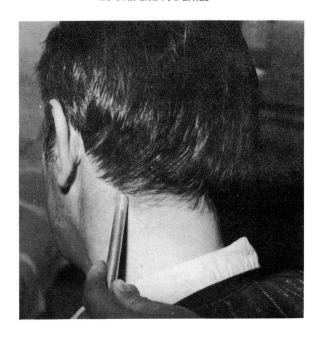

Fig. 1.

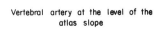

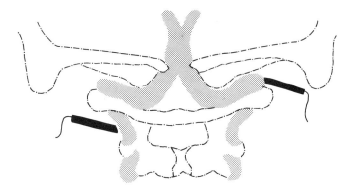

Fig. 2. Vertebral artery at the level of the atlas slope.

(Fig. 1) and is directed towards the contralateral orbit. In this way, it is possible to examine the atlas slope of the vertebral artery (Fig. 2).

RESULTS

It is obvious that by occipital recording alone the direction of flow cannot be determined reliably, since minor changes in the position of the probe will cause — (relative to the probe) — a physiological change in the direction of vertebral

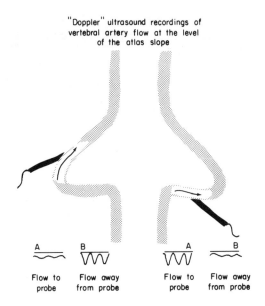

"Doppler" ultrasound recordings of
vertebral artery flow at the level
of the atlas slope

A	B		A	B
Flow to probe	Flow away from probe		Flow to probe	Flow away from probe

Fig. 3. Doppler ultrasound recordings of vertebral artery flow at the level of the atlas slope.

artery flow (Fig. 3). Thus, certain additional manoeuvres such as changing the circulation of the hypotensive (ipsilateral) upper arm are needed for the verification of the presence of a subclavian steal syndrome. When arterial flow in the upper arm is artificially reduced or augmented under normal conditions, the consequent change in flow velocity is recorded only in the arteries of the same arm, and this change will not affect the circulation of the ipsilateral vertebral artery.

The situation is, however, different in the case of the subclavian steal syndrome when the retrograde vertebral artery flow on the affected side contributes to the blood supply of the arm and will follow the flow conditions of the same. In this case, clenching of the fist or compression of the upper arm with 50–60 mmHg will cause an increase in peripheral resistance not only in the arm but also in the vertebral artery and both systolic and diastolic flow velocity will decrease (Fig. 4). This change is even more marked when the hand performs a so-called "ischaemic exercise". This observation induced us to modify the hitherto used method as follows.

During suprasystolic ischaemic compression of the upper arm (for 1 min) the patient was asked to clench his fist repeatedly. This caused a reduction of both the systolic and diastolic vertebral artery flow and the ultrasonogram was shifted towards the zero-line. After ischaemic exercise (abolishment of compression), an intense reactive hyperaemia was caused in the arm with vasodilation and a reduction of peripheral resistance, blood flow in the arm being accelerated. At this stage, the situation was similar in the ipsilateral vertebral artery which supplied the arm. The method used by us and our findings are in good agreement with J. P. Marcade's (1978) Doppler ultrasound studies.

All of this proves that the flow conditions in the arm and in the hand influence the flow conditions in the vertebral artery. The arm receives blood from the brain, thus there is a "steal mechanism" present (Fig. 5), and the generally used simple

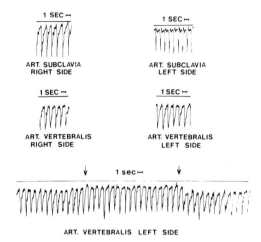

Fig. 4. Subclavian steal syndrome (left side).

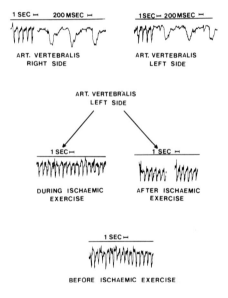

Fig. 5. Subclavian steal syndrome.

exercise of fist clenching sometimes fails to give a positive result. Also, at the beginning of the ischaemic exercise, flow velocity decreases, as during the fist clenching manoeuvre. However, this latter decrease is, as a rule, so slight (even in the case of verified steal syndromes) that it is hardly detectable. After 1 min of ischaemic work, in the phase of reactive hyperaemia, a very marked decrease in peripheral resistance and acceleration of flow takes place both in the affected arm and in the reversed vertebral artery flow. We consider this increase in flow velocity far more characteristic of the steal syndrome than the initial decrease of the same.

DISCUSSION

According to the above method, the main criterium in the diagnosis of the subclavian steal syndrome is the acceleration of vertebral artery flow after 1 min of ischaemic work. In our opinion, this modified method provides more reliable results than the recordings taken during simple fist clenching. A further advantage of our method is (and this is true for occipital recordings in general) that it permits the use of cheaper, not direction-sensitive Doppler instruments.

With respect to possible errors, we have analysed two false-negative cases which revealed the following facts. In the first false-negative case, the vertebral artery involved in the steal mechanism was also seriously stenotic and the ultrasonogram pointed to uncertain circulatory conditions whose changes were difficult to assess. In the second false-negative case, the considerable obesity of the neck hindered the adequate examination of the vertebral artery. In the one false-positive case the blood pressure difference between the two arms was only slight (20 mmHg) and rest angiography failed to verify the steal mechanism indicated by Doppler sonography (Table I).

The question now arises whether, in the case of a mild subclavian steal syndrome, reversion of the vertebral artery flow can be provoked only by exercise (e.g. ischaemic work of the arm). This, of course, is but a supposition which can be confirmed later by means of exercise angiography. Six subclavian steal syndrome patients were subjected to post-operative check-ups and normalization of the vertebral artery flow was recorded.

CONCLUSIONS

The tests carried out so far have shown that the Doppler sonographic method with occipital recording is suitable for the non-invasive diagnosis of the subclavian steal syndrome. The test can be carried out by one examiner in 15 to 20 min and the diagnostic reliability of the results surpasses that of the data obtained by other non-invasive methods. Furthermore, the test is atraumatic and can be repeated as often as required. Consequently, the method is suitable for the screening of patients to be subjected to angiography, for post-operative follow-up and for the observation of the natural course of the disease.

Table I. Subclavian steal syndrome verified by angiography.

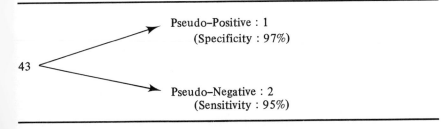

REFERENCES

Contorni, L. (1960). *Minerva Chirurgica* **15**, 68.
Farkas, P., Halmágyi, M., Istvánffy, M. and Urai, L. (1976). *Orvosi Hetilap* **117**, 2719.
Follmann, P., Littman, J., Heszberger, I. and Urai, L. (1969). *Ophtalmologica (Basel)* **159**, 363.
Grossmann, B. L., Brisman, R. and Wood, E. H. (1970). *Radiology* **94**, 1.
Káli, A., Kolonics, I., Farkas, P. and Urai, L. (1979). *Orvosi Hetilap* **120**, 689.
Kaneda, H., Irino, T., Minami, T. and Taneda, M. (1977). *Stroke* **8**, 571.
Keller, H., Meier, W. E. and Kumpl, D. A. (1976). *Stroke* **7**, 364.
Marcade, J. P. (1978). *Angeiologie* **30**, 189.
Pourcelot, L. I., Ribadeau-Dumas, Fagret, D. and Planiol, Th. (1977). *Review of Neurology* **33**, 309.
Reutern, G. M., Büdingen, H. M. and Freund, H. J. (1976). *Archiv für Psichiatrie und Nervenkrankenheiten* **222**, 209.
Urai, L. and Csákány, Gy. (1976). *Orvosi Hetilap.* **108**, 1777.

DIRECT MEASURED SYSTOLIC PRESSURE GRADIENTS ACROSS THE AORTO-ILIAC SEGMENT IN MULTIPLE LEVEL OBSTRUCTION ARTERIOSCLEROSIS

I. Noer, J. Præstholm and K. H. Tønnesen

Department of Clinical Physiology and Department of Radiology,
Bispebjerg Hospital, Denmark

INTRODUCTION

Each obstruction in the leg arteries causes a drop in systolic pressure. When only one obstruction is demonstrated on the angiogram, this lesion is responsible for the systolic pressure drop from, for example, the brachial artery to the ankle. Complete normalization of pressure and function is obtained by surgical removal of this obstruction. Useful functional information is in this case contained in the angiogram. The situation is completely different in cases of multiple level obstructions. The lesions may differ in functional importance due to the site and length of occlusions, the degree of stenosis and the number and size of collaterals.

This study presents the results of direct pressure measurements above and below different types of arterial occlusions and stenosis above the inguinal ligament in patients with multiple level lesions. This information is useful when an aorto-iliac reconstruction is considered without repair of the occluded femoral segment.

MATERIAL AND METHODS

Seventy-seven legs were examined in 47 males and 30 females with an average age of 61 years (range 36–74). Arteriograms with visualization of the pelvic and crural arteries demonstrated multiple level lesions both proximal and distal to the

Serono Symposium No. 37, "Vascular Occlusion: Epidemiological, Pathophysiological and Therapeutic Aspects", edited by M. Tesi and J. Dormandy, 1981. Academic Press, London and New York.

inguinal ligament. In most cases, both a-p and oblique exposures were made. The direct blood pressure measurements (Elema-transducers EMT 34) were carried out a few days after the aortograms. Polyethylene catheters (o.d. 1.2 mm) were inserted in a brachial artery and in the common femoral artery using the percutaneous technique. The location of the segmental obstructions and the number and the diameters of collaterals in each angiogram were noted. The degrees of stenosis were estimated as a ratio of the smaller diameter of the stenosis compared to the adjacent normal diameter. The obstructions above the groin were thereafter compared to the systolic pressure index (i.e. the ratio between common femoral systolic pressure and the brachial artery systolic pressure).

RESULTS

The results are shown in Fig. 1. It appears that an occlusion in the aorta-common iliac artery results in an average systolic pressure drop of about two-thirds of the brachial artery. The systolic pressure drop along the whole iliac, the common iliac and the external iliac amounted to about 50%. The systolic pressure drop due to aorto-common iliac artery occlusions were significantly larger than in occlusions which involved only iliac vessels ($P < 0.01$). No correlation between the pressure index and the number of collaterals could be found (Fig. 2) in total iliac occlusions.

With regard to the stenosis, it is obvious from Fig. 1 that these may cause any degree of pressure drop. When the degree of iliac stenosis is compared to the pressure drop, a significant correlation is seen ($r = -0.42, P < 0.05$) (Fig. 3), but due to the scatter, this result is useless in the single patient. Also the visualization of collaterals (Fig. 4) seems to be of no value in the judgement of limb prognosis in the individual patient. The systolic pressure in the common femoral artery

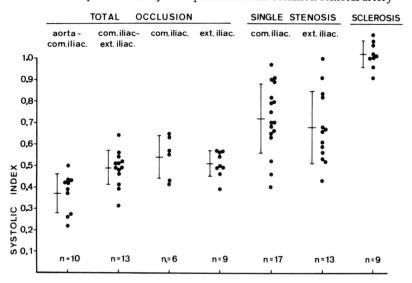

Fig. 1. The intra-arterial measured systolic pressure index in the common femoral artery is given (mean value and s.d.) in different groups of above ligament arteriographic findings (total number of legs 97).

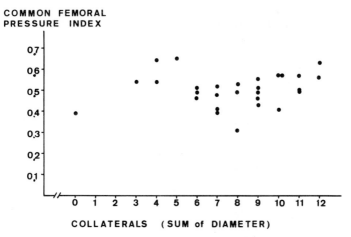

Fig. 2. In total iliac artery occlusion, the leg is supplied by collaterals. A quantitation of collaterals (given as the sum of diameters of the collaterals) is compared with the measured pressure index. No systematic tendency is noticed.

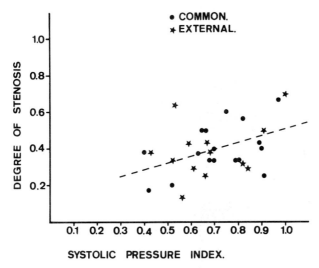

Fig. 3. Systolic pressure index in the common femoral artery is decreased distally to single, moderate to severe iliac stenosis. A positive correlation is seen between pressure index and the ratio of measured smallest diameter to expected diameter $y = 0.37x + 0.13$ ($r = 0.42$, $P < 0.05$).

distal to any roughness of the arterial wall denoted as arteriosclerosis without stenosis was equal to the arm systolic pressure (Fig. 1).

DISCUSSION

The results of the present study show that angiographic demonstration of arterial occlusions in the distal aorta and the iliac segments are useful to estimate the actual pressure drop in the resting supine position, even in cases with multiple

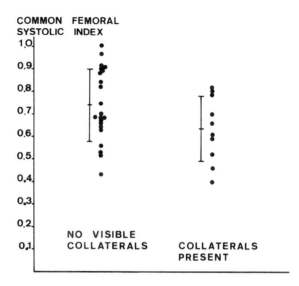

COMMON FEMORAL
SYSTOLIC INDEX

Fig. 4. In 30 legs with single iliac artery stenosis, collaterals are visible in ten legs. Even the systolic pressure index is lower (insignificant) in these legs average 0.64 mmHg as compared with legs without visible collaterals average 0.74. The information about collaterals is of poor value in the single leg in question.

level obstructions. In contrast, it is shown that angiographic visualization of stenosis, and the degree of these are useless from a functional point of view. Also, visualization of collaterals both in arterial occlusions and in stenosis are of no value in the individual patient.

The above results can be used by the vascular surgeon. According to recent findings (Noer *et al.*, 1978), ankle pressures will rise in proportion to the rise in systolic femoral artery pressure after proximal arterial reconstruction. If, for example, the systemic arterial systolic pressure is 160 mmHg, the common femoral artery systolic pressure is 80 mmHg and the ankle pressure is 50 mmHg, then after proximal reconstruction the ankle pressure will be about 100 mmHg: namely a doubling in both common femoral and ankle pressure. In such a case, it is likely that the patient will be relieved from his rest pain and/or chronic ischemic ulcer.

In contrast, if the ankle pressure in a patient with the same arm and femoral pressure pre-operatively is only 25 mmHg, it will only rise to about 50 mmHg which may be insufficient to relieve him of severe ischemia. Thus, when the surgeon has been informed of the angiogram and the ankle and toe pressure, by looking at Fig. 1, he can decide whether a proximal reconstruction is likely to relieve the resting symptoms in his patient. These arguments are valid for occlusions but not for stenosis—even tight ones. If one wishes pre-operatively to judge whether a proximal reconstruction in patients with iliac artery stenosis will suffice, then the femoral artery pressure has to be measured directly.

The abundance of collaterals at the iliac segment are discussed in great length at conferences between vascular surgeons and radiologists. As seen in Fig. 4, we found no correlation between the pressure drop and the number of collaterals (here given as the sum of diameters).

Theoretically, you could argue that a correlation between pressure index and the quantity of collaterals is positive (the better the collaterals the better the blood supply and hence a higher distal blood pressure) or you could argue a negative correlation (if the pressure gradient is small there will be less collaterals visualized).

Several other examinations could be done but we have found that in the iliac segment it is not worthwhile trying to visualize the collaterals by repeated contrast injections because it will not give any further functional information. For the same reason, the angiographic evaluation of modest to severe stenosis must be abandoned. So, beside the added information that a total iliac occlusion diminishes the systolic blood pressure by about one half, we agree with Maddison (1977) that angiography should not be performed merely to confirm a diagnosis, but only to provide the anatomical information required for a therapeutic decision.

From this functional point of view, it follows that the radiologist should only be concerned with visualization of the main vessels in the iliac segment. One can expect a doubling in the ankle pressure following recanalization of a total iliac occlusion. By contrast, in cases with an iliac stenosis and multiple level obstructions, one needs to measure the pressure drop to be able, pre-operatively, to assess the result of a proximal operation.

REFERENCES

Maddison, F. E. (1977). *In* "Vascular Surgery" (B. B. Rutherford, ed.) 251–254. W. B. Saunders, Philadelphia, London and Toronto.
Noer, I., Tønnesen, K. H. and Sager, Ph. (1978). *Annals of Surgery* **188**, 663.

NON-INVASIVE EVALUATION OF VENOUS PRESSURE
BY DOPPLER ULTRASOUND METHOD

M. Bartolo, S. Raffi, F. Rulli and A. D'Uva

Department of Angiology, S. Camillo Hospital, Rome, Italy

INTRODUCTION

Using the method described previously, we have used the Doppler ultrasound examination for non-invasive determination of venous pressure (VP) under physiological conditions and in various pathological conditions of both upper and lower limbs, standing and lying, comparing our results with invasive measurements carried out on the same patients.

When a pressure cuff is inflated and slowly deflated above a vein, the Doppler measures the resumption of venous flow as soon as the endovenous pressure is greater than the applied pressure; at that moment, the level appearing on the scale of the sphygmomanometer will indicate the VP in the vessel (Fig. 1). This condition is a function of the tonic reactivity of the veins (Condorelli's active venous hypertension) and thus, in the second part of the study, we have documented the venous pressure obtained in the same patients with the invasive method and the Doppler method. An analagous method has been used by Gaylis, who takes as the VP index the end of the sound mentioned above (Fig. 2).

MATERIALS AND METHOD

We investigated 325 normal subjects; 207 subjects with varicose veins; 59 subjects with post-varico-phlebitic syndrome; 198 subjects with post-phlebo-

Serono Symposium No. 37, "Vascular Occlusion: Epidemiological, Pathophysiological and Therapeutic Aspects", edited by M. Tesi and J. Dormandy, 1981. Academic Press, London and New York.

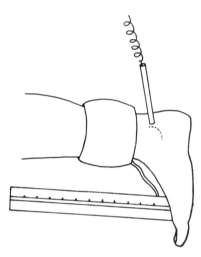

Fig. 1. Doppler registration method of posterior tibialis vein flow.

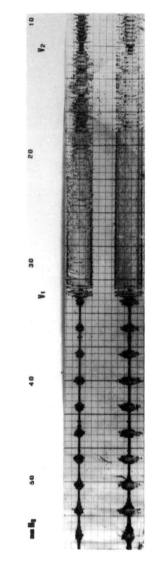

Fig. 2. The blowing noise, corresponding to venous flow, is detected by phonoangiographic apparatus.

Table I. Comparison between two methods.

Cases		Cuff pressure at which the signal were audible	Data obtained by electromanometer	Percentage of error
Arm veins	1	14	10	40
	2	12	8	50
	3	15	10	50
	4	40	40	0
	5	10	7	42.8
Leg veins	6	100	80	25
	7	100	80	25
	8	80	65	23

thrombotic syndrome; 25 with lymphoedema; 36 cases of deep phlebo-thrombosis in the lower limbs and three cases of axillary phlebothrombosis. The method has already been mentioned in the introduction and has been described sufficiently. For checking the invasive evaluation, an electromanometer, type XM 5421/00 connected to a floating "Pulmocath" catheter XM 5335/00, has been used. We did not use the invasive probes in phlebopathic patients, using instead patients affected by cardiac disturbances for which haemodynamic tests were necessary.

RESULTS

Acute venous pathology in the lower limb (tests in dorsal position); 36 subjects affected by acute phlebothrombosis: average level 35 mmHg (normal subjects: 10 mmHg); in the upper limb (tests in dorsal position): six subjects: average level 40 mmHg (normal subjects 10 mmHg).

Chronic venous pathology in the lower limb (tests in standing position)— varicosities: 307 subjects: average level 92 mmHg on great saphena, 88 mmHg on posterior tibial vein. Post-varicophlebitic syndrome: 59 tests: average level 98 mmHg on great saphena, 99 mmHg on posterior tibial vein. Post-phlebitic syndrome: 195 tests: average level 99 mmHg on great saphena, 100 mmHg on posterior tibial vein. Phlebostatic syndrome: 242 tests: average of 79 mmHg both veins. Lymphoedema: 25 tests: 62 mmHg on great saphena and 77 mmHg on posterior tibial vein. Pedrada syndrome: 79 mmHg on great saphena and 70 mmHg on posterior tibial vein (average of tests on nine subjects).

The eight tests carried out with the invasive method to confirm the Doppler test results are shown on Table I.

COMMENT

Note how in the case of acute phlebothrombosis, the VP of the affected limb is considerably higher than in the healthy limb (33 mmHg compared with 10 mmHg). It seems that such simple explorative methods could replace diagnostic examinations with radioactive fibrinogen, venography or plethysmography using venous occlusion, until now considered the most valid.

The results in post-phlebitic syndrome reached the highest levels (99 mmHg on the posterior tibial vein) on standing. It is perhaps surprising that lymphoedema does not necessarily bring about a notable VP increase.

The results obtained in the group of subjects who were to undergo cardiac catheter treatment and who underwent an electromanometer VP test of the upper limb show an increase of non-invasive levels as compared to invasive levels. This was to be anticipated since the vein reacts with an internal hypertonicity to the blocking caused by the cuff.

In three subjects, whose VP in the saphena vein was measured with a phlebograph, the average levels were 80.5 with an error of 24.3. The small difference in the readings from the lower limb on standing is probably due to the tonic anti-gravitational reaction already present, before positioning and pressurizing of the cuff.

The most important aspect for venous pathology is not so much the absolute level of pressure as the difference in the levels of the two limbs.

REFERENCES

Bartolo, M. (1977). *Folia angiologica* 25, 199.
Bartolo, M., Artizzu, G., Marchetti, M. and Pittorino, L. (1978). Atti III *Congr. Naz. S. I. S. U. M.* suppl. a Rays.
Barsotti, J., Pourcelot, L., Greco, J., Planiol, T., Kiniffo, H. V. T. and Castellani, L. (1973). *Angeiologie* 25, 153.
Gaylis, H. (1975). *British Journal of Surgery* 62, 259.
Kakkar, V. V. (1976). *Recenti Progressi in Medicina.* 60, 13.
Marcialis, A., Piegari, V., Pignatelli, C., Carrelli, B. and Del Genio, A. (1969). *Giornale Italiano di Chirurgia.* Abstr. 25, 1.
Strandness, D. E., Schultz, R. D., Sumner, D. S. and Rushmer, R. F. (1967). *American Journal of Surgery* 113, 331.
Strandness, D. E. and Sumner, D. S. (1975). Hans Huber Publishers, Bern, Stuttgart, Vienna.
Yao, J. (1975). *Angiology* 26, 528.

SEQUENTIAL ANGIOSCINTIGRAPHY OF AORTA AND
LIMB ARTERIES

P. Zaniol, D. De Maria, M. Pantusa, F. Romani and G. Tuscano

*Istituto di Radiologia e Cattedra di Anatomia Chirurgica Della Università
di Modena, Italy*

Angioscintigraphy is a technique for representing the vessels which, by means of the sequential recording with a gamma camera of an injected intravenous medium, enables us to obtain images of the radioactivity crossing the vessels.

Its fundamental features are that it: (1) is quick to perform; (2) provides immediate images and (3) is easy to repeat at short time intervals.

To carry out an angiography, the necessary equipment consists of a gamma camera-type detecting system. The gamma camera, having a large-size crystal or highly-sensitive multiple crystal system with reconstruction of the images, enables us to detect simultaneously the radioactivity distributed over a vast area. In this sense scintigraphy loses its original character of line scanning and becomes a photographic technique. With the aid of a computer, data obtained through an angioscintigraphical study can be analysed in various ways. For instance, by means of digital elaborator it is possible to evaluate the flow and capacity of various sections of the cardiocirculatory system, or it is easy to visibly determine on the screen a so-called "interesting region" and obtain data relating to that specific region.

With regard to the radioactive media, numerous considerations relating to techniques and methods, not least the search for "non-invasive" procedures, dictate the use of *non-diffusible* contrast media, such as albumin-serum labelled 99mTc, introduced intravenously, which follow the biological physiochemical principle of dilution. The selection of a short-life isotope such as technetium, which rapidly degenerates, bestows the advantage of being able to considerably increase the administered activity and therefore the activity of the apparatus in

---

Serono Symposium No. 37, "Vascular Occlusion: Epidemiological, Pathophysiological and Therapeutic Aspects", edited by M. Tesi and J. Dormandy, 1981. Academic Press, London and New York.

Table 1. Advantages and disadvantages of local perfusion.

Angioscintigraphy	Arteriography
Information regarding quantity of blood flow without upsetting physiological conditions	Information regarding only quality and interference with physiological conditions due to their introduction at high pressure and the hyperosmolarity of the contrast media
Lack of complications	
Non-invasive technique	
	Possible reactions from intolerance to the contrast medium
Poor resolution of the images	
	Invasive technique
	Accurate anatomical details even for small and average calibre vessels

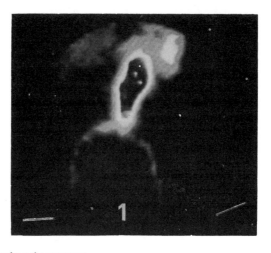

Fig. 1. Abdominal aortic aneurysm.

question, as it limits the overall dose of radioactivity absorbed by the patient.

The type of information angioscintigraphy can provide is the same as the type provided by arteriography. Therefore a comparison should be made between these two investigations. We must stress immediately that the angioscintigraphic picture at present cannot compete with arteriographic investigations in contrast or resolving capacity, and therefore in the amount of information. Isotopic angiography can be placed between traditional scintigraphic and radiological examinations on one side and angiography on the other.

As with all radio-isotopic examinations, angioscintigraphy is in fact simple to perform, totally non-traumatic and completely harmless. These features render it a screening technique to combine usefully with the more accurate,

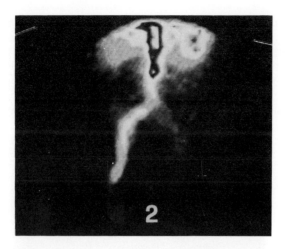

Fig. 2. Occlusion at the origin of the left, common iliac artery.

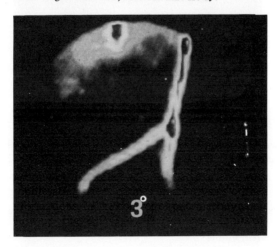

Fig. 3. Axillary bi-femoral bypass. Post-operative control.

but invasive, radiological techniques. In Table I, the advantages and disadvantages of angioscintigraphy are given.

Isotopic angiography of the aorta and of the large arterial vessels of the limbs is mainly used in obliterating arteriopathies, in aneurysms of the large vessels, in arteriovenous malformations, in the control of pharmacodynamic tests and as a post-operative follow-up (Figs 1, 2, 3, 4). The value and limits of angioscintigraphy are listed in Table II.

To conclude we would like to stress the following points.

(a) Although the technical procedure is simple the angioscintigraphic investigation provides more or less information depending upon the various organs studied and the apparatus used. Regarding the application of the investigation to the large vessels, results obtained are so far more than promising. Angioscintigraphy at present provides information which is often only inferior to that of angiography.

(b) In respect to angiography, the radio-isotopic investigation has the advantage of being easier to perform, totally non-traumatic and completely harmless.

(c) In view of these features, angioscintigraphy presents interesting prospectives: (1) as a screening investigation; (2) as an easily repeatable control investigation during the after treatment; (3) in the study of patients in poor condition.

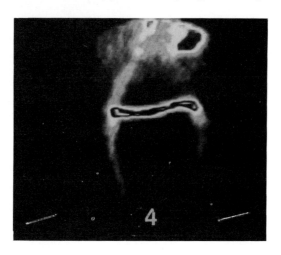

Fig. 4. Post-operative suprapubic cross-over control.

Table II. Angioscintigraphy.

Value	Limits
Simple to perform	Poor resolution of the image especially for small vessels (collateral loops)
Non-invasive technique	
Possibility of detecting pathological changes in large vessels	No direct information on alterations of the vessel walls
Lack of reactions caused by hypersensitivity to the medium	It is not in a position to replace arteriography
Possibility of carrying out numerous controls over a prolonged period	
Suitable for a study of the amount of local flow	

BIBLIOGRAPHY

Bassinghwaighte, J. B. and Holloway, G. A. Jr. (1976). *Seminars Nuclear Med.* **6**, 141.

Bergan, J. J., Yao, J. S., Henkin, R. E. *et al.* (1974). *Arch. Surg.* **109**, 80.

Dibos, P. E., Muhletaler, C. A., Natarajan, T. K. and Wagner, H. N. Jr. (1972). *Radiology* **102**, 181.

Fossati, F. and Spinelli Ressi, F. (1975). *Rad. Med.* **61**, 612–626.

Freeman, L. M., Meng, C. H., Bernstein, R. G. *et al.* (1969). *Radiology* **92**, 918.

Freeman, L. M. and Mindelzun, R. (1968). *Am. J. Surg.* **116**, 433.

Masi, R., Pelù, G., Pesciullesi, E. and Modigliani, U. (1974). *Atti Congr. Int. Angiol.* 1–4 Aprile Firenze.

Masi, R., Pesciullesi, E., Bisi, G. and Grandonico, F. (1976). *Atti II° Riunione Gruppo Chir. Vascolare*, Firenze.

Masi, R. (1978). *Atti 1° Corso sulle Indagini strum. Malattie Vasc. MedIc. Viva* 251–262.

Muroff, L. R. and Freedman, G. S. (1976). *Seminars Nucl. Med.* **6**, 217.

Siegel, M. E. and Wagner, H. N. Jr. (1976). *Seminars Nucl. Med.* **6**, 253.

Sveinsdottir, E., Larsen, B., Rommer, P. and Lassen, N. A. (1977). *J. Nucl. Med.* **18**, 168.

SECTION IV
MEDICAL THERAPY

LOCAL THROMBOLYTIC THERAPY IN VASCULAR OCCLUSIONS – EXPERIMENTAL INVESTIGATIONS

R. Gottlob

Department of Experimental Surgery, Ist Surgical Clinic, Vienna University, Austria

INTRODUCTION

For localized lesions, treatment by continous infusions of solutions of drugs is frequently attempted. The infusions may be made into the artery supplying the limb or organ and into a peripheral vein for thrombi, situated proximally. Such localized infusions were used for treatment of venous thromboses by Gottlob and May (1954). Later, the intra-arterial infusion of cytostagic drugs for malignancies became routine in many cases.

Little is known about the factors governing the local concentrations of infused drugs. The purpose of this paper is to develop a simple equation, indicating the gradient between the local concentration and the concentration in the systemic circulation.

THEORETICAL CONSIDERATIONS

The gradient between the local and the systemic circulation (G) may be defined as the quotient of the local concentration (LC) and the systemic concentration (SC).

Serono Symposium No. 37, "Vascular Occlusion: Epidemiological, Pathophysiological and Therapeutic Aspects", edited by M. Tesi and J. Dormandy, 1981. Academic Press, London and New York.

$$G = \frac{LC}{SC} \qquad \text{Equation 1.}$$

The systemic concentration of a drug, continuously infused, is dependent on the rate of infusion (I) and the total clearance of the infused drug (Cltot).

$$SC = \frac{I}{Cltot} \qquad \text{Equation 2.}$$

Equation 2 indicates that the concentration in the systemic circulation is dependent on the rate of infusion and inversely correlated to the total clearance, (the volume of plasma, cleared of the infused drugs per minute in the steady state). This is not only the renal clearance since the hepatic clearance may be important as may all other paths of elimination or inactivation of the infused drug (Dost, 1958).

The local concentration of the infused drug consists of the concentration recirculating from the systemic circulation plus the concentration induced by the local application of the drug. The latter is dependent on the local blood flow (Lbfl) at the site of infusion:

$$LC = \frac{I}{Lbfl} + \frac{I}{Cltot} \qquad \text{Equation 3.}$$

By combining equations 2 and 3 with equation 1 we obtain:

$$G = \frac{Cltot}{Lbfl} + 1 \qquad \text{Equation 4.}$$

Equation 4 indicates that the gradient between the local and the systemic circulation is dependent on the total clearance of the infused drug and inversely dependent on the blood flow at the site of infusion.

Drugs cleared very rapidly from the circulation, e.g. acetylcholine (which is destroyed within a short time by the acetylcholinesterase), will create only a local concentration, the systemic concentration being practically zero. The gradient G is consequently very high. Conversely, if the total clearance is negligible, most of the infused drugs will recirculate, so that the gradient G will be very low. If the total clearance and the local blood flow are equal, then the gradient will become 2, indicating that the local concentration will be twice the systemic concentration.

In previous investigations, we attempted to increase the gradient by increasing the total clearance of the infused drugs. Using local infusions of heparin into the femoral artery of an animal and by infusion of protamine solution into systemic circulation, we succeeded in rendering the blood of the extremity anti-coagulated, whereas the coagulation in the rest of the body remained unchanged (Gottlob and May, 1954). If only heparin was infused locally, no clear-cut gradient developed. Benzer et al. (1963) carried out similar experiments

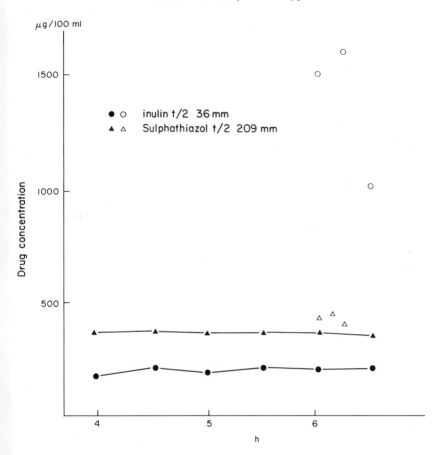

Fig. 1. Local and systemic concentrations of inulin and sulphathiazol after local infusion. The symbols connected with straight lines indicates the systemic concentrations. 16 mg/min inulin and 0.42 mg/min. Sulphathiazol were infused simultaneously. Note the insignificant differences between the local and the systemic concentrations of sulphathiazol, the slower excreted drug.

by local infusions of streptokinase and simultaneous systemic application of the fibrinolytic inhibitor aprotinin (Trasylol®, Bayer). Great differences between the local and the systemic fibrinolytic activity were thus obtained.

The importance of the total clearance could also be demonstrated by infusing two drugs with different clearance conditions. If, for instance, sulphathiazol and inulin were infused simultaneously, during the steady state, a comparatively low gradient for sulphathiazol was found (half-life of 209 min), whereas for the readily excreted inulin (half-life of 36 min) a very high gradient was obtained (Fig. 1).

The following experiments were carried out to demonstrate the influence of the local blood flow on the gradient with special reference to those clinical conditions where the local blood flow is reduced by arterial obliterations.

MATERIAL AND METHODS

In dogs, the femoral vessels of a leg were dissected and a square-wave flow-meter was applied to the artery. At the same level on the proximal thigh, a tourniquet was applied to the extremity in such a manner that the dorsal part of the thigh could be compressed without interfering with the blood flow in the femoral artery and the femoral vein.* The infusion of the drugs was per-formed after cannulation of branches of the femoral artery by thin plastic catheters so that the tip of the catheter was situated inside the artery. Similarly, a branch of the femoral vein was cannulated so that venous blood samples could be easily obtained (Fig. 2).

For infusion, an antibiotic and streptokinase, both dissolved in Ringer solution, were used. ^{14}C-labelled cephazolin sodium was used as the antibiotic. The specific activity was 8.73 mCi/mg. We made up 45 μCi of the labelled cephazolin plus 1.0 g unlabelled cephazolin and 250 000 units of streptokinase (Streptase, Behringwerke) with Ringer solution to a final volume of 150 ml. The solution was kept refrigerated during infusion. We injected 10 ml of the solution as a priming dose, the rest was infused through a Harvard pump at a speed of 3.8 ml/min. Every 10 min., blood was sampled from the femoral

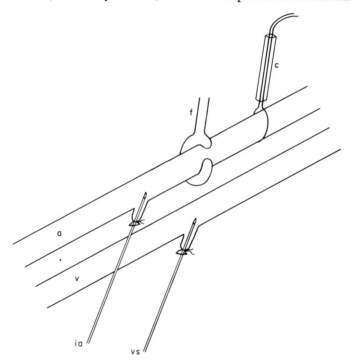

Fig. 2. The situation at the site of infusion. a: Femoral artery of the dog. v: Femoral vein ia: Plastic tube for infusion into the artery vs: Plastic tube for venous blood sampling. f: Flowmeter® c: Thread for constriction of the artery.

*This tourniquet served to compress the gluteal artery, fairly well developed in the dog, thus confining the arterial supply to the femoral vessel.

artery (= local blood flow) and from one of the jugular veins of the animal (= systemic blood flow). After clotting of the blood and clot retraction, the serum was separated.

Fibrinolysis

The fibrinolytic activity in the serum was assessed in small tubes, containing 1 ml of human fibrin clotted by the addition of thrombin. After clotting, the upper level of the fibrin was marked on the outside of the tube. Forty hours after application of the serum (200 μl) on top of this fibrin all liquid was poured out so that only unlysed fibrin remained in the tubes. Water was added by pipette to the mark outside the tube. The amount of water required equalled the amount of fibrin lysed.

Cephazolin Sodium Concentration

From the blood samples, 200 μl of serum was added to 15 ml Instagel (Packard). The activity was measured in a Beckmann LS 7000 Beta-Counter.

RESULTS

The results are displayed in Fig. 3a. The abscissa indicates the time in hours. The ordinate indicates the activity of the blood samples in counts X 1000/minute (minus background). The systemic concentration is found at the lower end of the bars, where a steady state is seen with minor deviations of the concentration. The local concentration, however, shows great differences (top of the vertical bars). The longer bars, indicating great differences between the local and systemic concentration, are found only during periods of constriction of the femoral artery. These periods are indicated by the horizontal bars, also representing the flow measured in the femoral artery. In Fig. 3b the fibrinolytic activity is displayed. There was no fibrinolytic activity in the serum from the systemic circulation. In the local circulation there was no fibrinolytic activity unless the femoral artery was constricted. Only when the blood flow was reduced did the serum from the femoral artery exhibit strong fibrinolytic activity.

DISCUSSION

Our investigations demonstrated the validity of the equations outlined above for the gradient between the local and the systemic concentration of the locally infused drugs. Figure 3 especially demonstrates the inverse relation between the local concentration and the blood flow. As both of the drugs (streptokinase and cephazolin) are comparatively slowly eliminated, a considerable gradient only was achieved when the local blood flow was reduced by the constriction of the artery.

What is the clinical relevance of our findings? Some drugs, like antibiotics or fibrinolytic agents which are slowly eliminated, should be applied systemically if the local blood flow is normal, since under these conditions, the gradient will not be considerable. A local infusion, however, might be advantageously applied if the blood flow is impaired. For example, if the arterial circulation is

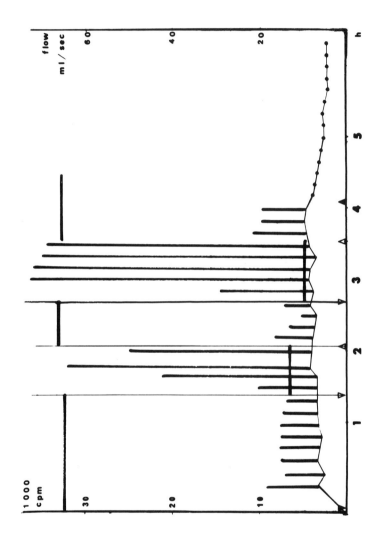

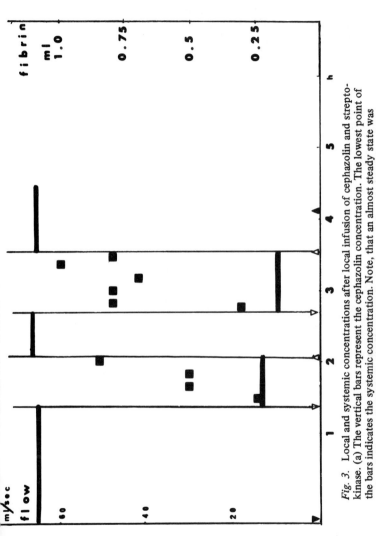

Fig. 3. Local and systemic concentrations after local infusion of cephazolin and strepto-kinase. (a) The vertical bars represent the cephazolin concentration. The lowest point of the bars indicates the systemic concentration. Note, that an almost steady state was achieved. The vertical thin lines indicate the beginning and the release of the arterial con-striction. The thick horizontal bars indicate the blood flow in the femoral artery. Great differences between local and systemic concentrations are seen only during the reduction of the femoral blood flow. Note the slow decrease of activity after stopping the infusion. (b) The same experiments as in Fig. 3a, the black squares indicate the fibrinolytic activity in the serum. Note that such activity was seen only during constriction of the femoral artery and only in the local circulation.

obstructed by thrombi or emboli, the local application of fibrinolytic agents may induce a high local fibrinolytic activity in the infused extremity even when rather small doses of the fibrinolytic agents are applied. In the systemic circulation, however, the fibrinolytic activity may remain sufficiently low to prevent side effects such as haemorrhage. The same applies to the antibiotic treatment of gangrene. The extremely reduced blood flow in these extremeties will allow the use of a rather high concentration of the antibiotics. (First clinical experiences with this method will be published elsewhere.)

REFERENCES

Benzer, H., Blümel, G., Gottlob, R. and Piza, F. (1963). *Langenbecks Archiv und Deutsche Zeit-schrift für Chirurgie* **304**, 775.

Dost, F. H. (1953). Thieme, Leipzig.

Gottlob, R. (1954). *In* "Thrombose und Embolie", I. Internationale Tagung, Basel 1954 (Benno Schwabe & Co., ed. Basel, 1955).

Gottlob, R. and May, R. (1954). *In* "Thrombose und Embolie", 1. Internationale Tagung, Basel 1954 (Benno Schwabe & Co., ed. Basel, 1955).

Gottlob, R. and Zinner, G. (1957). *Journal of International College of Surgeons* **28**, 575.

May, R. (1954). *In* "Thrombose und Embolie", I. Internationale Tagung, Basel 1954 (Benno Schwabe & Co., ed. Basel, 1955).

STREPTOKINASE AND SURGERY IN THE TREATMENT OF ACUTE ISCHEMIA IN PATHOLOGICAL ARTERIES

Cl. Olivier, J. B. Levy, J. Conard and M. Samama

Hôtel-Dieu de Paris, 1 Place du Parvis de Notre-Dame, Paris

Acute ischemia in pathological arteries still gives rise to extremely severe consequences despite the various available treatments, both medical and surgical. Thrombolysis by streptokinase now offers another alternative treatment to surgery. These two methods each have their own indications and can be used in association.

METHODS AND MATERIALS

We have studied a group of 169 patients presenting with acute ischemia due to pathological arteries: 120 of them were treated by surgery alone and 49 by fibrinolysis with streptokinase (SK). The following is an analysis of this retrospective study which is intended to provide a more precise understanding of the therapeutic indications.

Group Treated by Surgery Alone

The group of patients undergoing surgery alone was formed of 120 subjects. It is unnecessary to discuss these patients' previous case histories except to mention the fact that more than 60% of them were aware that they were affected by an arteriopathy. The importance of the functional symptoms did not seem to correlate with the risk of acute ischemia, since only 15–20% of the subjects had rest pain or trophic disturbance (dysfunction, alterations). (Table I.)

We have observed (including relapses) 132 ischemic episodes in 120 patients.

Serono Symposium No. 37, "Vascular Occlusion: Epidemiological, Pathophysiological and Therapeutic Aspects", edited by M. Tesi and J. Dormandy, 1981. Academic Press, London and New York.

Table I. Previous history of patients.

No previous history	25%
Untreated intermitten claudication	35%
Arteriopathy undergoing treatment	15%
Aneurism or aortitis	5%
Unclassified	20%

Table II. Results of surgical treatment.

Procedure	No.	Successes	Amputations	Deaths
Isolated thrombectomy	24	9	8	7
Thrombectomy + sympathectomy	12 (14)	7	2[a]	3[a]
Sympathectomy	26 (30)	18	7[a]	1[a]
Aorto-iliac revascularization	30 (34)	16	6[b]	8[b]
Femoro-popliteal or leg revascularization	28 (30)	15	8[a]	5[a]
Total	120 (132)	65 (54.2%)	31 (25.8%)	24 (20%)

[a] 1 After relapse; [b] 2 after relapse.

Table III. Causes of death after surgery.

Cause of death	Surgery (%)	SK (%)
Kidney failure	28	31.5
Cardiac arrest	26	25
Pulmonary emboli	15	12.5
Hemorrhaging	–	12.5

The 12 relapses led to 5 deaths, 5 amputations and only 2 successes. Considering the 120 patients, we have observed a total of 54.2% successes, 25.8% amputations and 20% deaths (Table II). Without going into detail concerning these figures we can make the following observations.

1. Isolated thrombectomy is a very mediocre operation because it can at the most repair the precarious vascular bed to the state preceding the incident (we shall see that this reproach can also be made regarding streptokinase).

2. Emergency direct aorto-iliac repair has a very high mortality rate; for this reason we more and more often perform axillo-femoral bypass or crossed bypass for acute thrombosis of the proximal areas.

3. Isolated sympathectomy is performed only in moderate distal ischemia, and this explains the relatively satisfying results obtained.

4. Causes of death are not unusual: 28% for kidney failure, 26% for cardiac failure and 15% for pulmonary emboli. The importance of the risk of cardiac or kidney failure is often a reason for the surgeon to forego revascularization and to prefer immediate amputation (Table III).

Group of Patients Treated with Streptokinase

This group includes 49 patients, 41 men and 8 women with an average age of 63 for the men and 72 for the women, with extremes of 20 and 87 years of age. All of these had been declared inoperable by the surgeon. Among these 49 patients, 15 had no history of peripheral arterial disease. These patients received doses of streptokinase considered quite high; 500 000 units as an initial dose i.v. in 30 min; then 150 000 units an hour for 48/72 h. Heparin was given in addition to streptokinase when the fibrinogen level rose to more than 1.50 g/l, a condition which can be observed after hour 36 of treatment.

Table IV. Comparison between results of surgery and of SK treatment.

	No.	Successes	Amputations	Deaths
Surgery	120	65 (54%)	31 (26%)	24 (20%)
SK	49	18 + 8[a] (53%)	15 (31%)	8 (16%)
Total	169	91 (54%)	46 (27%)	32 (19%)

[a]SK + Surgery.

The results obtained with streptokinase are in general comparable to those obtained by surgery (Table IV), if we take into account the eight successes obtained after complementary surgery. Results obtained with streptokinase showed that in a total of 49 patients, 26 obtained relief of rest pain, but five kept a limited perimeter of movement. Negative results include eight deaths, three of them being treated with SK (two incidences of hemorrhaging).

SK can moreover be held responsible for 15 incidents or complications. Two incidents were due to contraindications which were not respected: acute hemorrhaging after Seldinger and from a recent operation wound required transfusion. It is useful to stress that when fibrinolytic treatment is considered, only femoral arteriograms using a fine needle can be performed. Other complications include six intolerance reactions, two peripheral emboli, two transitory neurological incidents and some minor hemorrhage.

The frequency of these occurrences makes it imperative to take necessary precautions including the study of contraindications (neurological antecedents, HTA . . .), very attentive clinical care, and the suspension of the treatment whenever there is the slightest suspicion of complications.

ANALYSIS AND COMMENTS ON RESULTS

The Delay in Treatment

The duration of the obliteration is one of the basic factors in prognosis. In the SK group (Table V) we have observed that, after ten days, there were ten negative results in ten patients. In the first 48 hours, 13 good results were obtained, in 20 patients treated, ten of them with SK alone. In the 19 ischemic episodes occurring

Table V. Results according to interval elapsed before SK treatment.

Period	No.	Successes	Failures
0–2 days	20	10 + 3[a]	7
3–10 days	19	4 + 4[a]	11
> 10 days	10	0	10
Total	49	14 + 7[a]	28

[a] After surgery.

3–10 days previously, we had eight good results, four of them using SK alone. Thus it seems that in the case of long-standing obliterations, it is better to operate instead of prolonging the delay with fibrinolytic treatment.

The Mechanism

In this study, we have examined only patients having pathological arteries. Thrombosis *in situ* is therefore by far the most frequent mechanism. Emboli can certainly occur in such arteries, but demonstration of this is not always possible. In ten patients treated with SK, in whom emboli was probable, we obtained five successes. One of them, after failure of treatment with SK, was a surgical success. SK was used only in distal emboli involving only partial ischemia. It is, however, the logical procedure when embolism is certain, since surgery is unnecessary if the SK treatment obtains complete repair of the vascular bed. Prevention of repeat emboli may be sufficient to avoid further ischemia. In this study, no patient presenting with thrombosis *in situ* caused by shock (trauma) or low flow, was treated with SK.

Site of the Obstruction

It seems that the higher the site of the obstruction the more favorable is the prognosis. Localized thrombosis is preferable to diffuse or wide-spread thrombosis. Paradoxically, it is for the distal and diffuse thrombosis that treatment with fibrinolytics is the first choice, since surgery in these cases is ineffective and difficult.

In this short series, surgery was possible and successful in five cases after fibrinolytics. It may perhaps be interesting in these diffuse forms to try to improve the vascular bed downstream by fibrinolytic treatment before performing surgical revascularization.

Long-term Results

The 21 patients showing good results after SK, whether followed by surgery or not, have undergone regular follow-up: four patients were followed for 4 months to 1 year, six patients for 1 to 3 years and 11 patients for more than 3 years. The results obtained appear to be relatively stable.

Degree of Ischemia

Because of its slow action, treatment by fibrinolysis is not to be considered in patients presenting with sensomotor disturbances likely to become irreversible. SK improved the condition of only one of the five patients with little or no rest pain; it achieved 20 successes in the 44 cases of permanent pain and halted deterioration in five.

Lastly, there were four successes in 44 cases presenting some neurological disturbance (paresis, hypoasthesia etc.). Thus, given the risk of hemorrhage it seems useless to treat those with well-established ischemia with SK. On the other hand, ischemia with permanent pain or even minor paresis are good indications for such treatment.

Other Observations

1. The use of SK with obstructed bypasses seems to complement surgery, even if it has not been efficacious alone. In several patients, who had thrombosed prostheses, we have noted the existence of non-adherent thrombus partially lysed by SK. Fibrinolysis facilitates surgical relief of obstruction by balloon catheter and makes it possible, in certain cases, to avoid replacing the prosthesis completely.

2. The impression of clinical improvement felt by patients under treatment with SK is not always a sign of the efficacy of the therapy; but may be due to better collateral circulation.

Similarly, a transitory worsening of the condition may result from the migration of a fragment detached from the thrombus, a fragment which is destined to undergo eventual lysis.

3. The best method for following these patients seems to be that of regular Doppler control. Upon suspension of the SK treatment an arteriogram will make it possible to evaluate precisely the results obtained and to decide whether or not it is necessary to perform immediate surgery to avoid the formation of a new thrombosis after a good result.

CONCLUSIONS

Our study is retrospective. It is almost impossible to set up a prospective randomized study in this field. There is no question of demonstrating the technical superiority of one method over another. We can however, cautiously advance a certain number of proposals.

When the ischemia is massive with sensomotor disturbances, the use of SK is not to be advised, as it is too slow in its action.

If the ischemia is progressive, or if the lesions are diffuse, SK treatment may usefully precede surgery by improving the distal vascular bed.

When the obstruction involves an aorto-iliac prosthesis or even a pathological artery without imminent risk of irreversibility, SK can make possible a simpler alternative.

SK alone can have little use for emboli in arteries which are pathological or thrombosed due to shock; in such cases, a new thrombosis is probable if hemo-dynamic conditions are not modified; this can be done only by the surgeon. It is not necessary to have available a highly-sophisticated laboratory in order to put into practice SK therapy, but for rapid correction of fibrinolysis, if surgery becomes necessary, there must be excellent co-operation between the laboratory and the surgical team.

The indication for SK must therefore be established together, after careful evaluation of the risks, while control must be continuous and shared, judging from the tolerance and result, the necessity for continuing or interrupting the treatment. On this basis the contribution of SK is of interest in facilitating surgery and in making it possible to avoid an operation in some cases of acute ischemia with pathological arteries.

BIBLIOGRAPHY

Conard, J. and Samama, M. (1973). *Thromb. Diath. Haem.* Suppl. 56, 191–198.
Conard, J. *et al.* (1981). *Press. Med.* (Accepted for publication.)
Fiessinger, J. M., Aiach, M., Lagneau, P., Cormier, J. M. and Housset, E. (1975). *Sem. Hôp. (Paris)* 51, 1291–1295.
Jue-Denis, P. *et al.* (1981). *Chirurgie* (Accepted for publication.)
Olivier, Cl., Samama, M., Conard, J., Rettori, R. and Levy, J. B. (1974). *J. Chir. (Paris)* 108, 501–508.
Olivier, Cl., Samama, M. and Bilski-Pasquier, G. (1974). *Chirurgie* 100, 33–38.
Olivier, Cl., Rettori, R. and Levy, J. B. (1977). *Chirurgie* 103, 544–551.
Olivier, Cl., Samama, M., Chabrun, B., Conard, J. and Horellou, M-H. (1978). *Chirurgie* 104, 517–524.
Persson, A. V., Thompson, J. E. and Patman, R. D. (1973). *Arch. Surg.* 107, 779–784.
Poliwoda, H., Alexander, K., Buhl, V., Holsten, D. and Wagner, H. H. (1969). *New Engl. J. Med.* 280, 689–692.
Samama, M. (1968). La thombolyse. Etude experimentale et clinique. A propos de 66 cas traites par la streptokinase. p. 203. *These Doctorat Med., Paris.*
Schmutzler, R. (1975). Indications and results of fibrinolytic treatment with streptokinase in chronic arterial stenoses and occlusions. A multicentre trial of 708 patients. *Vth Cong. Int. Soc. Thromb. Haemost. Paris.* Abstract p.240.

INTRA-ARTERIAL UROKINASE IN ACUTE ARTERIAL OCCLUSION

M. Vayssaitat,[1] J.-N. Fiessinger, Y. Juillet,[1] M. Aiach,[2], J.-M. Cormier[3]
and E. Housset[1]

[1] *Chaire de Clinique Médicale et de Pathologie Vasculaire Hôpital Broussais, Paris, France*
[2] *Département d'Hémostase, Laboratoire Centre de Biochimie Hôpital Broussais, Paris, France*
[3] *Service de Chirurgie Vasculaire Hôpital Saint-Joseph, Paris, France*

INTRODUCTION

Systemic administration of streptokinase (SK) has been proved to be very efficient for lysing arterial thrombi in man (Martin *et al.*, 1970; Poliwoda, 1972; Reichle *et al.*, 1977; Fiessinger *et al.*, 1978a). Therefore since 1973 we have treated 194 patients suffering from arterial occlusions with high doses of streptokinase (Fiessinger *et al.*, 1978a) administered intravenously. Thrombolysis was achieved for 57 (29.5%) of these patients. The use of systemic SK was limited because of its antigenicity and embolic or bleeding complications (Ness *et al.*, 1974; Reichle *et al.*, 1977). Six out of our 194 patients died from intracerebral embolism or hemorrhage (Fiessinger *et al.*, 1978a). Local intra-arterial thrombolytic therapy might circumvent these problems (Dotter *et al.*, 1974; Edwards, 1977; Stankowiak *et al.*, 1978; Sautot *et al.*, 1979), low dose administration of urokinase (UK) allowing thrombolysis without production of a systemic hyperlytic state (Michaud *et al.*, 1978). This report summarizes our experiment on 52 patients with acute arterial occlusion by selective intra-arterial urokinase.

Serono Symposium No. 37, "Vascular Occlusion: Epidemiological, Pathophysiological and Therapeutic Aspects", edited by M. Tesi and J. Dormandy, 1981. Academic Press, London and New York.

PATIENTS AND METHODS

Patients

Fifty-two patients were treated, 36 males and sixteen females. The average age of the patients was 67 years (range 37 - 87). In all cases, the acute arterial occlusion of the lower limbs was under two months : 19 under 10 days, 25 between 10 and 30 days, 8 over 30 days. The arteriography showed 30 superficial femoral artery occlusions, 22 popliteal occlusions. Each one had poor leg arteries and good filling of aortic and iliac arteries.

Thirty patients suffered from thrombosis on arteriosclerosis obliterans; 22 from arterial embolism. All patients had severe peripheral ischemia; ten had acute ischemia with complete neuromuscular paralysis; 25 had subacute ischemia with partial neuromuscular paralysis; 13 had pain at rest; only four patients had intermittient claudication before 50 metres. The severity of ischemia was shown by Doppler ankle pressure. The mean ankle pressure was 5.2 mmHg and 32 patients had no pressure in their ankle arteries.

Methods

Under local or general anaesthesia, the common femoral artery of the ischemic leg was exposed. A thin Teflon® catheter was slipped into a collateral artery, then the tip of the perfusion catheter was placed just above the thrombus. Afterward, a loading dose of 75 000 UCTA Urokinase (Urokinase Choay) was infused through the arterial catheter at a dose of 37 500 UCTA/hour. Continuous intravenous administration of heparin was started simultaneously. Its flow was adjusted to maintain the plasma heparin concentration between 0·10 and 0·25 IU.

The occurrence and progress of lysis was evaluated clinically by ultrasound and daily arteriography (injection via the perfusion catheter). The treatment was stopped and the catheter removed when lysis occurred or after four days of treatment. Blood samples were drawn before treatment, at the fourth hour of treatment, then daily for the determination of plasminogen, fibrogen, fibrinogen's degradation products (FDP), thrombin time and activated partial thromboplastin time.

RESULTS

Thrombolysis was achieved for 23 (45%) patients, total thrombolysis for 6 of them, partial for 9 as shown on arteriography; 8 patients with no change on their arteriographic findings had dramatic improvement of their ankle pressure (more than 500 mmHg) very likely by leg arteries recanalizing and thrombolysis of associated venous thrombosis.

Eight patients had a recurrent thrombosis a few days or a week after the treatment. Twenty-nine patients (55%) had no thrombolysis at all. No patients died during the treatment period; three bleeding from the scar made us stop the treatment, one patient had a distal embolus, with aggravating effects during treatment.

Table I. Results of attempted limb salvage using intra-arterial urokinase.

	Healing	Amputations
Persistant arterial patency n = 15	n = 14 93%	n = 1 (distal embolus) 7%
Recurrent thrombosis n = 8	n = 5 63%	n = 3 37%
No thrombolysis n = 29	n = 13 45%	n = 16 55%

The clinical results were judged according to three possibilities: a persistant thrombolysis, a recurrent thrombosis after a thrombolysis success, no thrombolysis (Table I). In the group of no thrombolysis at all (n = 29), the results were very poor and amputation was required in 16 cases (55%). In the group with recurrent thrombosis (n = 8), amputation was required in three cases (37%). In the group with persistant thrombolysis, the results were very good. Only one patient (7%) required an amputation (distal embolus).

DISCUSSION

The practice of intra-arterial thrombolysis is difficult; it needs a vascular surgeon with arteriographic facilities and very careful clinical, hemodynamic and laboratory controls.

The risk is very low (0% death) in comparision with 3% of mortality with high intravenous doses of fibrinolytic agents (SK).

The safety of intra-arterial UK allows the addition of intravenous heparin at therapeutic doses and extends the use of this treatment to patients undergoing surgery (Sautot *et al.*, 1979; Fiessinger *et al.*, 1978b), the catheter being positioned at the end of the procedure.

However, due to the difficulties of the methodology, we are compelled to use this treatment only in cases of severe ischemia with no change of revascularization or when surgery is not sufficient for the limb salvage.

CONCLUSIONS

Selective intra-arterial urokinase is effective in the treatment of recent arterial thromboembolism. However, usually only partial lysis is achieved, but it is enough for limb salvage. At the dose of 37 500 UCTA/h it does not produce systemic fibrinolysis. This method offers a substantial reduction of the risk of systemic bleeding and embolism and allows its application to operative patients. The association of surgery and UK seems particularly promising in atherosclerotic arterial thrombosis.

REFERENCES

Dotter, C. T., Rosch, J. and Seaman, A. J. (1974). *Radiology* **111**, 31.
Edwards, I. R. (1977). *In* "Thrombosis and Urokinase" (R. Paoletti, and S. Sherry, Eds.) 169–179. Academic Press, London, New York and San Francisco.
Fiessinger. J. N., Aiach, M., Vayssairat, M., Juilet, Y., Cormier, J. M. and Housset, E. (1978a). *Annales de l'Anesthèsiologie Française* **19**, 739.
Fiessinger, J. N., Vayssairat, M., Juillet, Y., Janneau, D., Aiach, M., Cormier, J. M. and Housset, E. (1979b). *Annales de Médecine Interne* **130**, 215.
Martin, M., Schoop, W. and Zeitler E. (1970). *Journal of the American Medical Association* **211**, 1169.
Michaud, A., Aiach, M., Fiessinger, J. N., Vaussairat, M. and Juillet, Y. (1978). *La Nouvelle Presse Médicale* **35**, 3151.
Ness, P. M., Simon, T. L., Cole, C. and Walston, A. (1974). *American Heart Journal* **88**, 705.
Poliwoda, H. (1972). *Journal of Clinical Pathology* **25**, 642.
Reichle, F., Rao, N., Chang, K., Marder, V. and Algazy, K. (1977). *Journal of Surgical Research* **22**, 202.
Sautot, J., Demerciere, J. and Sautot, M. (1979). *Lyon Chirurgical.* **75**, 92.
Stankowiak, C., Soots, G., Espriet, G. and Wattel, A. (1978). *Journal des Maladies Vasculaires* **3**, 43.

CLINICAL EFFECTS OF UROKINASE IN CHRONIC OBLITERATING ARTERIOPATHY OF THE LOWER LIMBS

M. Tesi, A. Carini, F. Torrini, S. Cinotti and M. Morfini

Department of Angiology and Department of Haematology, Main Regional Hospital of S. Maria Nuova, Firenze, Italy

INTRODUCTION

Administration of elevated doses of urokinase (UK) in the treatment of acute vascular occlusions — both in obliterating arteriopathy and in deep venous thrombosis — has been used by several authors. The theoretical basis is that of thrombolytic therapy: in the recent thrombus, lysable fibrin is present, and the administration of UK can induce vascular recanalization in a certain number of cases.

In chronic forms (and particularly in chronic atherosclerotic arteriopathy) the vascular occlusions have been present for a long time. The disease shows clinical symptoms when the thrombi, no longer recent but old, in the majority of cases, are by now organized and do not contain lysable fibrin. For this reason, thrombolytic therapy in the chronic forms can induce recanalization of blood vessels only in a quite modest percentage of cases.

In this study, we have administered UK in chronic obliterating arteriopathy of the lower limbs, not to obtain pharmacological disobliteration of the occluded arteries, but with the intention of inducing (through the potentiation of a physiological activity such as that of fibrinolysis) an improvement in clinical conditions in cases of arteriopathy progressing toward gangrene or already gangrenous.

The dosage of UK chosen by our group may be defined as an intermediate dosage. The mode of administration, a daily arterial perfusion lasting 30 min,

Serono Symposium No. 37, "Vascular Occlusion: Epidemiological, Pathophysiological and Therapeutic Aspects", edited by M. Tesi and J. Dormandy, 1981. Academic Press, London and New York.

was established near the peripheral site of the arterial obliteration. The duration of the treatment (20 days) was related to the degree of chronic arteriopathy; the fibronolytic activation, in order to become effective in this condition, must arrive repeatedly at the affected region.

MATERIALS AND METHODS

The research was conducted on 40 cases of arteriopathy with chronic occlusions of femoral, popliteal, or tibial arteries, with rest pain, and in some cases with gangrene either early or at a more advanced stage. The disease had been present 3-12 years.

The UK was administered thus. Drug: 200 000 IU/day. Method: 30 min perfusion in the femoral artery. Period: 1 perfusion per day for 20 days. The following data were collected: haematological data, angiographic data, clinical data.

Haematological Data

The following tests were carried out: euglobulin lysis time (Buckell, 1958); plasminogen (Mancini et al., 1965); antiplasmin (Tager-Nilsson, 1977); fibrinogen (Clauss, 1957); FDP (Merskey et al., 1969); PTT (Proctor and Rapaport, 1961); prothrombin time (Quick, 1966); thrombin time (Austen and Rhymes, 1975); procoagulating factor VIII (Egeberg, 1961); immunological factor VIII (Laurell, 1966); antithrombin III (Scully and Kakkar, 1975); platelet count (Brecher and Cronkite, 1950); platelet aggregation ADP, adrenalin, ristocetin (Born, 1962).

Tests were carried out on blood samples taken from the following regions.

(1) Affected region: on arterial and venous femoral blood of the lower limbs, prior to and after UK perfusion in the femoral artery.

(2) Unaffected region: arterial and venous blood of the upper limb, after UK perfusion in the femoral artery. All data were collected at the first and twentieth UK perfusion.

Angiographic Data

Femoral angiography or translumbar aortography was carried out on 40 patients before the series of arterial UK perfusions. The same angiographic tests were repeated within 7 days of the last administration of the drug.

Any progression which may have occurred in the arterial occlusions was assessed.

Clinical Data

Clinical data were collected before and after therapy with UK. Evaluation was performed on the basis of the changes in rest pain, which was present in all patients, and on the basis of the progress of the gangrene in five patients.

RESULTS

Haematological Data

The *euglobulin lysis time* at the first arterial perfusion of UK was reduced, although not to a very high degree (Fig. 1). The average of the samples of blood taken from the femoral artery to the affected region went from 410 (± 20) min before the UK injection, to 280 (± 10) min after UK. In samples of femoral venous blood, lysis went from 400 (± 20) min to 230 (± 40) min. In samples of humeral venous blood (non-affected and non-injected zone), time of lysis changed from 400 (± 20) min to 250 (± 50) min.

At the twentieth perfusion of UK, lysis was observed to be still activated with values quite similar to the preceding ones (Fig. 1). In samples taken from the femoral artery, the average values passed from 400 (± 60) min to 290 (± 30) min and in samples of femoral venous blood, from 390 (± 20) min to 210 (± 90) min. In samples from the upper limb, values changed from 390 (± 100) min to 290 (± 90) min.

Plasminogen measured before and after the first UK perfusion was observed to be lowered (Fig. 2). The average values calculated in the samples taken from the femoral artery with the lower limb obliterated and perfused with UK, was

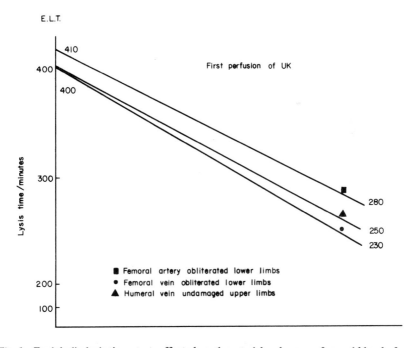

Fig. 1. Euglobulin lysis time: tests effected on the arterial and venous femoral blood of the lower occluded limbs, and on the venous humeral blood of the undamaged upper limbs. Differences between before and after the first perfusion of UK. Mean values.

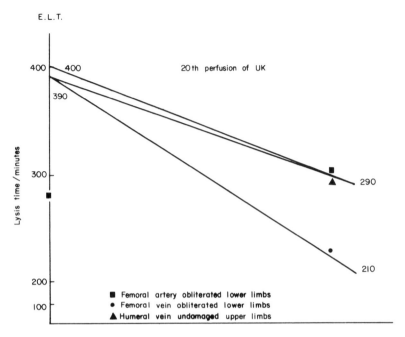

Fig. 2. Euglobulin lysis time: tests effected on the arterial and venous femoral blood of the lower occluded limbs and on the venous humeral blood of the undamaged upper limbs. Differences between before and after the 20th arterial perfusion of UK. Mean values.

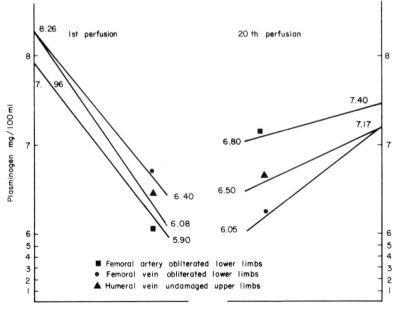

Fig. 3. Plasminogen: tests effectuated on the arterial and venous femoral blood of the lower occluded limbs and on the venous humeral blood of the undamaged upper limbs. Differences between before and after the first and the 20th arterial perfusion of UK. Mean values.

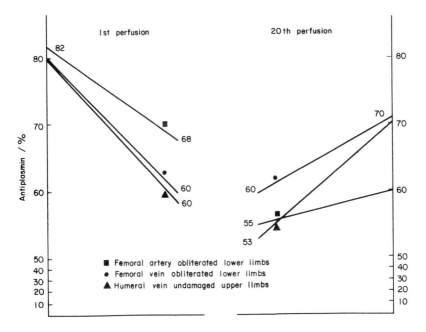

Fig. 4. Antiplasmin: tests effectuated on the arterial and venous femoral blood of the lower occluded limbs, and on the venous humeral blood of the undamaged upper limbs. Differences between before and after the first and the 20th perfusion of UK. Mean values.

7.96 (± 0.30) mg in basal conditions and 5.90 (± 1) mg after UK. The values found in the femoral venous blood, were respectively 8.26 (± 0.10) mg and 6.40 (± 0.30) mg. Those of the humeral venous blood (non-affected and non-injected upper limb), were 8.26 (± 0.60) mg before and 6.08 (± 0.20) mg after UK.

At the twentieth perfusion, the basal values (after UK) appeared reduced (Fig. 2). The values for the femoral artery of the obliterated lower limb went from 7.40 (± 0.30) mg before to 6.80 (± 0.10) after UK and for the femoral vein from 7.17 (± 0.20) mg to 6.05 (± 0.20) mg. Those of the upper limb changed from 7.17 (± 0.60) mg to 6.50 (± 0.10) mg.

Antiplasmin at the first perfusion of UK (Fig. 3) the values for the femoral artery were 82 (± 5) % before and 68 (± 10) % after UK. The values from the femoral venous blood were respectively 80 (± 3) % and 60 (± 8) %. Those of the humeral venous blood were 60 (± 10) % before UK and 60 (± 2) % after UK.

At the twentieth perfusion of UK, the basal values (after UK) appeared reduced (Fig. 3). The values of the femoral artery passed from 60 (± 3) % to 55 (± 10) % and the femoral vein from 70 (± 2) % to 60 (± 5) %. Those of the upper limb changed from 70 (± 1) % to 53 (± 2) %.

Fibrinogen remained practically unchanged at the first administration of UK (Fig. 4). In the femoral artery, values before and after UK passed from 366 (± 20) mg to 298 (± 20) mg and in the femoral vein from 355 (± 80) mg to 318 (± 60) mg. In the humeral vein values changed from 355 (± 40) mg to 330 (± 80) mg after UK.

At the twentieth perfusion of UK, a slight drop in the level of fibrinogen occurred after drug administration (Fig. 4). In the femoral artery, the values

passed from 342 (± 20) mg to 276 (± 20) mg. In the femoral vein, the values
were respectively 365 (± 1) mg and 249 (± 50) mg. In the upper limb, they
were 365 (± 30) mg before UK and 222 (± 10) mg after the perfusion.

Other Haematological Tests

In regard to FDP, PTT, prothrombin time, thrombin time, procoagulant
factor VIII, immunological factor VIII, antithrombin III, platelet count, platelet
aggregation from ADP adrenaline and ristocetin, the results were as follows. The
averages calculated on samples taken from femoral arteries, femoral veins, and
humeral veins showed either no variations, or insignificant changes.

Angiographic Data

Angiographies of the lower limbs, performed by translumbar aortography or
femoral angiography before the treatment with UK, revealed the existence of
arterial obliterations at various levels (Fig. 5). These were most frequently
femoral, in the adductor canal or at the origin of the deep femoral artery, but
also popliteal or tibial (both anterior and posterior).

Tests carried out after the twentieth perfusion of UK have not demonstrated
the appearance of recanalization (Fig. 6). Evidently, given the chronic state of
arteriopathy with long-standing thrombi, the relatively modest doses of UK

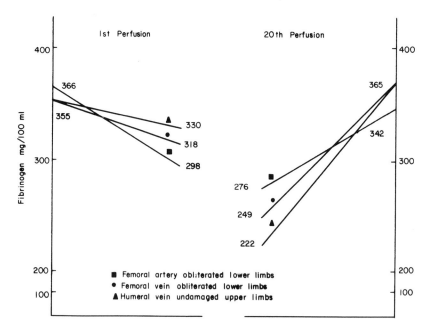

Fig. 5. Fibrinogen: tests effectuated the arterial and venous femoral blood of the lower
occluded limbs, and on the venous humeral blood of the undamaged upper limbs. Differences between before and after the first and the 20th arterial perfusion of UK. Mean
values.

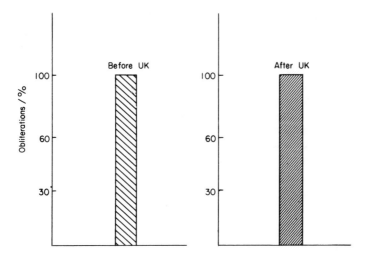

Fig. 6. Angiographies of lower limbs. Percentages of arterial obliterations: femoral popliteal and tibial, before and after the series of arterial perfusions of UK.

have not been able to modify the existing occlusive conditions by producing vascular recanalization.

Clinical Data

Clinical results were evaluated on the basis of rest pain present in all 40 patients studied, and on the basis of gangrene of the limbs – either early or established – present in 5 patients.

In regard to rest pain, which was the dominant symptom for our choice of patients to be treated with UK, the results were excellent (Table I). These were patients who had been treated with other therapies, including arterial perfusion of other drugs, and who had shown little improvement with these treatments. With arterial perfusion of UK, their symptoms gradually reduced to the point of disappearing entirely. In all of the 40 patients suffering from rest pain and treated with UK, regression of the symptomology was observed after the twentieth perfusion.

Table I. Clinical data. Evolution of main clinical symptoms in patients with chronic obliterating arteriopathy of the lower limbs, following treatment with UK.

Symptoms	Number of cases	
	Reduction	Disappearance
Rest pain patients : 40	–	40
Gangrene patients : 5	1	4

Regarding arterial gangrene, results were good, although not as excellent as the preceding ones (Table I). Gangrene was present in five patients, with two cases of early gangrene and three cases of established gangrene. These patients had previously undergone various treatments with no satisfactory results. They had also been treated with arterial perfusion of acetylcholine, which is the usual procedure for the treatment of this clinical condition in our angiological department. The perfusions with UK-induced regression of the gangrene in four cases, disappearance of symptoms in the cases with early gangrene, and demarcation in the established cases. In the fifth case with established gangrene, there was only slight demarcation and the pain was only reduced but did not disappear.

CONCLUSIONS

On the basis of this study, we can state that the perfusion of medium doses of UK into the femoral artery in atherosclerotic obliterating arteriopathy of the lower limbs in the evolving chronic stage or in gangrene is to be advised. Rest pain and distal gangrene are favourably influenced by this treatment.

We have observed that fibrinolytic activation is present, that the consumption of plasminogen at the end of the treatment is slight and that fibrinogen during the whole course of the treatment diminished a little. The other tests for investigating certain coagulation fibrinolysis and platelet activities do not show appreciable variations. No clinical or laboratory evidence of haemorrhage was found.

Angiographic data demonstrate the continuation of a static morphological condition as the arterial obliterations remain even after the treatment. This had already been anticipated, given the chronicity of the occlusions (3–12 years), the consequent lack of lysable fibrin in the thrombi and the medium doses of UK employed in this study. We should like to point out that in Bell's trials (1977) on pulmonary embolism, the angiographic disobliterations were only 58%, notwithstanding the recent origin of the occlusions and the full dosage of the drug (4 000 000 IU/12 h or 8 000 000 IU/24 h). The study showed, however, that the usual mortality rate from pulmonary embolism (35–45%) was reduced by 9%.

Similarly in our case, the clinical results were good even without the disappearance of the vascular occlusions and with limited fibrinolytic activation. It is probable that in treatment with UK, a natural activator of the fibrinolytic system, other functions may be involved in addition to the classic function of thrombolysis. And it is precisely for this reason, and not in the hope of an improbable recanalization, that we have established our therapy using intermediate doses of UK, administered daily via arterial perfusion, for a period of 20 days.

REFERENCES

Austen, D.E.G. and Rhymes, I. L. (1975). *In* "A Laboratory Manual of Blood Coagulation", p. 118 Blackwell Scientific Publications, Oxford.

Bell, R. W. (1977). *In* "Thrombosis and Urokinase", p. 153. Academic Press, London, New York, San Francisco.
Born, G.V.R. (1962). *J. Physiol.* **162**, 927.
Brecher, G. and Cronkite, E. P. (1950). *J. Appl. Physiol.* **3**, 365.
Buckell, M. (1958). *J. Clin. Pathol.* **11**, 403.
Clauss, A. (1957). *Acta Haemat.* **17**, 237.
Egeberg, O. (1961). *Scand. J. Lab. Invest.* **13**, 140.
Laurell, C. B. (1966). *Analyt. Biochem.* **15**, 45.
Mancini, G., Carbonara, A. O. and Heremans, J. F. (1965). *Immunochem.* **2**, 235.
Merskey, C., Lalezari, P. and Johnson, A. J. (1969). *Proc. Soc. Exp. Biol. Med.* **131**, 871.
Proctor, R. R. and Rapaport, S. I. (1961). *Am. J. Clin. Path.* **36**, 212.
Quick, A. J. (1966). *In* "Haemorrhagic Disease and Thrombolysis" p. 219, Lea & Febiger, Philadelphia.
Scully, M. F. and Kakkar, V. V. (1977). *Clinica Chimica Acta* **79**, 595.
Tager-Nilsson, A. C. (1977). *Scand. J. Clin. Lab. Invest.* **37**, 403.

HEPARIN-UROKINASE TREATMENT IN MASSIVE CEREBRAL VENOUS SINUS THROMBOSIS

G. Leone, M. Moschini, R. Landolfi and B. Bizzi

Istituto di Clinica Medica, Istituto di Semeiotica Medica, Istituto di Radiologia Medica, Università Cattolica del Sacro Cuore, Rome, Italy

INTRODUCTION

Thrombolytic treatment of acute cerebral infarction is not universally accepted. Prompt and exact diagnosis, essential for successful thrombolytic therapy, is not always attained. Fatal haemorrhages may easily occur during thrombolytic therapy in patients with cerebral vessels injured by atherosclerosis, hypertension and further damaged by hypoxia (Breda and Bizzi, 1972; Fletcher and Alkjaersig, 1977). These considerations have led us (Bizzi *et al.*, 1978) to use this treatment only in young patients, when vessel occlusion was likely to be due to thromboembolism (i.e. in patients with mitral stenosis and atrial fibrillation).

Conversely, we think that thrombolytic agents are often indicated in cerebral vein thrombosis (CVT). In this case, the beginning of therapy may wait for angiographic evidence of thrombosis and the risk of local haemorrhage is lower. Furthermore, the poor prognosis of patients treated with the usual therapy largely justified the risks of thrombolytic therapy (Rusu *et al.*, 1978).

At present, few data are available about this therapy in CVT patients. Very good results have been reported with streptokinase by some authors and more recently with urokinase at various dosage schedules (Friedman, 1971; Abastada, 1974; Fletcher and Alkjaersig, 1977).

Serono Symposium No. 37, "Vascular Occlusion: Epidemiological, Pathophysiological and Therapeutic Aspects", edited by M. Tesi and J. Dormandy, 1981. Academic Press, London and New York.

Table I. Clinical and radiological findings. Heparin-urokinase dosage schedules.

| | UK Dosage | | Clinical | Radiological |
	Continuous	Intermittent	Response	Response
1. R.C.–18 y.o.F.	$1,2 \times 10^6/6h$	$2 \times 10^6/3$ days	excellent	good
2. M.P.–26 y.o.F.	$2,4 \times 10^6/12h$	$1,2 \times 10^6/2$ days	excellent	good
3. M.M.–58 y.o.M.	$1,2 \times 10^6/9h$	$3 \times 10^6/5$ days	excellent	not demonstrated
4. M.G.–50 y.o.F.	—	$4,5 \times 10^6/6$ days	excellent	not demonstrated

1. Infectious thrombophlebitis of cavernous sinus.
2. Thrombosis of superior sagittal sinus "post partum".
3. Thrombosis of sagittal and cavernous sinuses (idiopathic).
4. Thrombosis of longitudinal sinus post lymphoangiography.

METHODS

Four patients with massive cerebral venous sinus thrombosis have been treated with urokinase and heparin (Table I). The clinical picture was very serious in all patients. Patient 1 (Fig. 1) presented with typical signs of thrombophlebitis of the cavernous sinus: fever, ocular pains, palpebral oedema, exophthalmus, papilloedema, ocular palsies and purulent meningitis. The patients 2 and 4 presented with headache, papilloedema, confusional state and hemiparesis *en bascule*. For patient 3, the predominant clinical signs were a confusional state, papilloedema and palpebral oedema.

In all cases, the diagnosis of massive cerebral venous sinus thrombosis was confirmed by cerebral angiography (Figs 2, 3, 4a and 4b). In three patients,

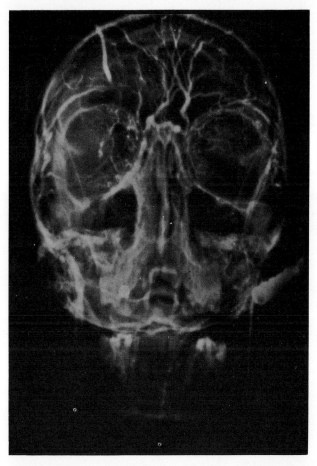

Fig. 1. Case 1. Orbital phlebography. Semi-axial view. Inadequate filling of the cavernous sinus.

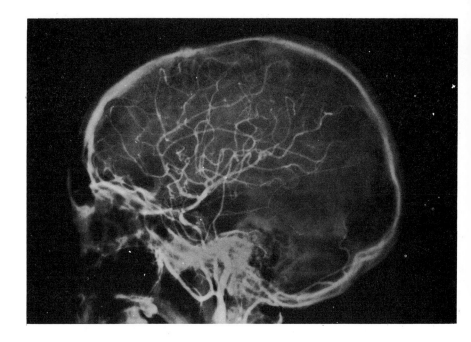

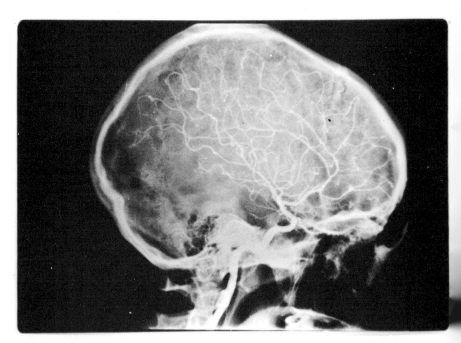

Fig. 2. Case 1. Carotid angiography. Lateral view. (Above). Pre-treatment study. Narrowing of the left cranial carotid lumen. (Below). Post-treatment study. Complete restoration of vessel lumen.

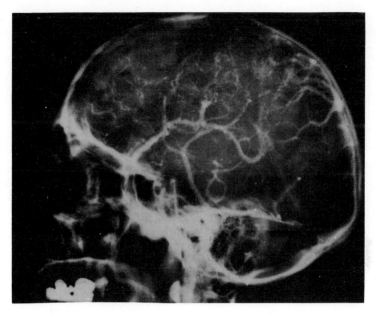

Fig. 3. Case 2. Carotid angiography, cerebral venous filling phase. Lateral view. Inadequate filling of superior sagittal sinus.

UK has been used according to our schedule (Bizzi *et al.*, 1976): after heparin pre-treatment 7500 units.i.v.) UK was administered by continuous venous infusion (250 0000 units CTA for 6–12 hours). Afterwards heparin-UK therapy was continued for 2–6 days (heparin 35 000 U/day by continuous infusion UK 200 000 units i.v. every 6–8 hours). In one patient, only the latter dosage schedule was used. Two months' anticoagulant therapy with heparin or oral anticoagulant was finally administered in all patients.

RESULTS

Clinical results were excellent with complete recovery in all cases. Clinical improvement was rapid in the patient 2 but slower in the other patients. All patients were considerably improved 1–2 days after the start of treatment. Post-treatment control angiography was performed in two patients within three weeks of therapy. In both cases, complete thrombus dissolution was observed (Figs 2 and 4). No severe haemorrhage occurred. In one patient, after four days of heparin-UK therapy, a haemorrhagic complication at the puncture site of angiography required UK suspension and heparin reduction.

CONCLUSION

Our report emphasizes the usefulness of thrombolytic treatment which, in some cases, appears lifesaving. The haemorrhagic risk is dependent on invasive but necessary diagnostic procedures.

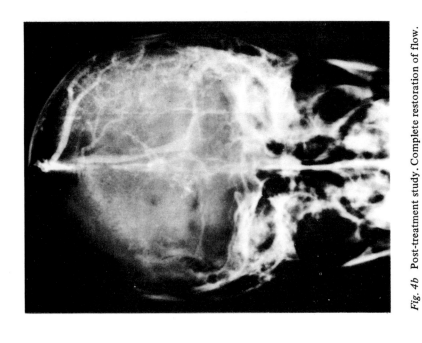

Fig. 4b Post-treatment study. Complete restoration of flow.

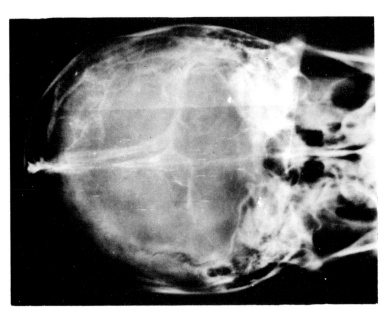

Fig. 4. Case 2. Carotid angiography, cerebral venous filling phase. Frontal view. *4a*: Pre-treatment study. Incomplete filling of sagittal sinus.

REFERENCES

Abastado, M. (1974). *Gazette Med.* **25**, 33.

Bizzi, B., Leone, G. and Accorrà, F. (1976). *Haemostasis* **5**, 147.

Bizzi, B., Leone, G., Tutinelli, F. and Llandolfi, R. (1978). *Clin. Therapeut.* **86**, 419.

Breda, R. and Bizzi, B. (1972). *In* "La Fibrinolisi in Medicina Interna". Pozzi Ed. Roma.

Fletcher, P. and Alkjaersig, N. (1977). *In* "Use of Urokinase Therapy in Cerebrovascular Disease (Paoletti and Sherry, eds) p.203. Academic Press, New York.

Friedmann, D. G. (1971). *Radiologue* **11**, 424.

Rusu, M., Cozma, V., Costachescu, G., Tetraru, C. and Anghel, M. (1978). *Rev. Roum. Med. Neurol. Psychiat.* **16**, 1.

COMPARISON BETWEEN LUNG SCANS AND PULMONARY ANGIOGRAMS IN THE EVALUATION OF THE PERFUSION DEFECT IN MASSIVE AND SUBMASSIVE PULMONARY EMBOLISM

M. Brochier,[1] Ph. Raynaud,[1] J. P. Fauchier,[1] B. Charbonnier,[1] F. Latour,[1] D. Alison,[1] A. Pellois[2] and T. Planiol[2]

Clinique Cardiologique,[1] *Service de Médicine Nucléaire,*[2]
University of Tours, France

INTRODUCTION

Selective pulmonary angiography has proven to be a readily available and accurate procedure in the diagnosis of pulmonary embolism (Dalen *et al.*, 1971). The procedure is sometimes hazardous for patients with a severe disease and the use of serial angiograms for the follow-up period of treatment is rather difficult.

Pulmonary perfusion imaging with radiolabelled albumin macroaggregates is considered to be less specific and less accurate than angiograms (Brochier, 1976). Nevertheless, in the diagnosis and follow-up of the disease, serial scans are safe, reproducible, speedy and simple to perform at frequent intervals (Moser *et al.*, 1973).

The purpose of this work is to compare the value of lung scanning and of pulmonary angiography performed within the same day, on patients treated for massive or submassive pulmonary embolism (PE) in the intensive care unit and to compare both methods in the evaluation of the initial perfusion defect before treatment and the pulmonary reperfusion after thrombolytic therapy.

Serono Symposium No. 37, "Vascular Occlusion: Epidemiological, Pathophysiological and Therapeutic Aspects", edited by M. Tesi and J. Dormandy, 1981. Academic Press, London and New York.

MATERIALS AND METHODS

Out of a total of 200 severe PEs treated in the intensive care unit from 1973 to 1977, 53 patients, 27 men and 26 women, 43 years-old on average, were investigated.

One-hundred-and-nine lung scans were compared to 109 pulmonary angiograms (52 before treatment and 57 after urokinase perfusion). Forty-two patients have been studied both before and after thrombolytic therapy.

Pulmonary scan (PS) is performed by means of intravenous injection of 1 millicurie (1 mCi) of technetium-labelled macroaggregates (MAA 99 m Tc) with a diameter of 35 microns. These aggregates are arrested in the pulmonary capillary bed. The particles are injected intravenously with the patient in the supine position. Four views are recorded: anterior, posterior, left and right lateral views. For each view 400 000 counts are recorded on polaroid film using a gamma camera fitted with a parallel collimator.

The panelist qualitatively expressed the degree of perfusion, noting particularly a lacunar zona or an irregular pattern; he gave a semi-quantitative value to each pulmonary lobe, as a percentage of the total pulmonary vascularization (right superior lobe 18%, right middle lobe 12%, right inferior lobe 25%, left superior lobe 13%, lingula 12%, left inferior lobe 20%). By definition, this is known as isotopic evaluation of the perfusion defect (IPD).

A pulmonary angiogram (PA) was performed less than 24 h after the isotopic investigation. Telebrix 38 (1 mg/kg at a rate of 20 to 30 ml/s) was injected into the main pulmonary artery, if necessary an additional quantity was injected in the right or left one. Films were taken every 2 or 3 s for at least 10 s in the antero-posterior view and if necessary in the lateral one.

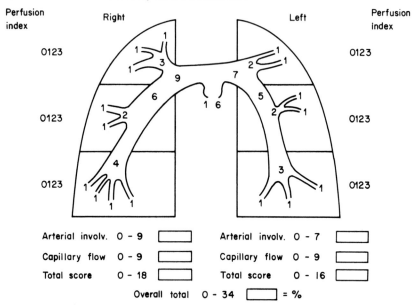

Fig. 1. Angiographic Miller's Index.

The quantitative assessment of the angiograms was performed according to the angiographic Miller's Index (AMI) (Fig. 1) with a total score from 0 to 34. For each lung, AMI appreciates both the arterial involvement (AI) with a score from 0 to 16, and the reduction of capillary flow (ACF) with a score from 0 to 18. For the whole population studied, the following data were compared: AMI, ACF and IPD. The score assessment of LS and PA was made by two observers working independently.

Table I. Compared: pre- and post-urokinase infusion lung scans and pulmonary angiograms, quantification of PE (n 109).

	Angio. Miller's Index	: 50.4% ± 21.7
$P < 0.001$	Isotopic perfusion defect	: 40.7% ± 16.2
	Angio. capillary flow	: 41.1% ± 17.6

$P < 0.001$ NS

Table II. Compared: pre-UK infusion lung scans and pulmonary angiograms (n = 52).

	Angio. Miller's Index	: 60.5% ± 16.3
$P < 0.001$	Isotopic perfusion defect	: 48.1% ± 12.2
	Angio. capillary flow	: 48.7% ± 14.2

$P < 0.001$ NS

Table III. Compared: post-UK infusion lung scans and pulmonary angiograms (n = 57).

	Angio. Miller's Index	: 41.2% ± 20.8
	Isotopic perfusion defect	: 34.1% ± 17.3
	Angio. capillary flow	: 34.1% ± 16.3

$P < 0.005$ NS

Table IV. Compared: pulmonary vascularization changes in 42 patients.

	Before UK	After UK	Revascularization (%)
Angio Miller's Index	62% ± 14.9	46% ± 20.6	28.1% ± 27.6
	$P < 10^{-5}$	$P < 0.03$	
Angio. capillary flow	49.4% ± 12.4	36.2% ± 17.8	28% ± 30.2- - - -NS
	NS	NS	
IPD	48.3% ± 11.1	36.1% ± 16.3	27.4% ± 25.1

RESULTS

For the global data, 109 lung scans and pulmonary angiograms were performed before and after treatment, there is a significant difference between AMI and IPD (with a correlation coefficient $r = 0.81$) and also between AMI and ACF (with a correlation coefficient $r = 0.88$). On the contrary, there is no difference between the IPD and ACF (Table I).

If we compare the pre-infusion lung scans and pulmonary angiograms, the same results are observed, the correlation between IPD and ACF is $r = 0.82$, there is an obvious lack of correlation if we compare each of these values to the AMI (Table II).

After thrombolysis, there is less of a difference between AMI and IPD and there is a good agreement between both IPD and ACF (Table III) ($r = 0.83$ between AMI and IPD, $r = 0.87$ between IPD and ACF).

Moreover, in the group of 42 patients examined by both pre- and post-infusion methods, there is a good agreement in each group ($r = 0.84$ between AMI and ACF, $r = 0.89$ between IPD and ACF). In this population, the revascularization percentage (RP) obtained by subtracting the percentage of vascularization defect before and after UK infusion is the same whatever the index taken into account (Table IV).

DISCUSSION

The discrepancies between lung scan and pulmonary angiography could be related to several factors:

(1) A "technical" problem: with angiography, a large volume (30 to 80 ml) of contrast material injected under high pressure is less physiological than the isotopic investigation in which a bolus of 1 ml is injected intravenously.

(2) The injection of contrast material performed by pressure injector can reduce the bronchospasm induced by embolism. These vasomotor disturbances may increase the IPD.

(3) Pulmonary scans made from several angles evaluate the perfusion defect better than the pulmonary angiogram recorded only in the anterior view, especially for the posterior capillary bed.

(4) Miller's index reflects both the vascular obstruction and the lack of blood flow in the pulmonary capillary bed. Scintigraphic estimation takes into account only the perfusion defect.

(5) Moreover, the crumbling of a large, partially obstructive clot could improve the Miller's index without changing the capillary perfusion.

CONCLUSIONS

Both investigations, isotopic investigation and pulmonary angiography, correlate well in appreciating the vascularization defect due to a severe pulmonary embolism. Pulmonary angiography quantifies the whole pulmonary vascularization,

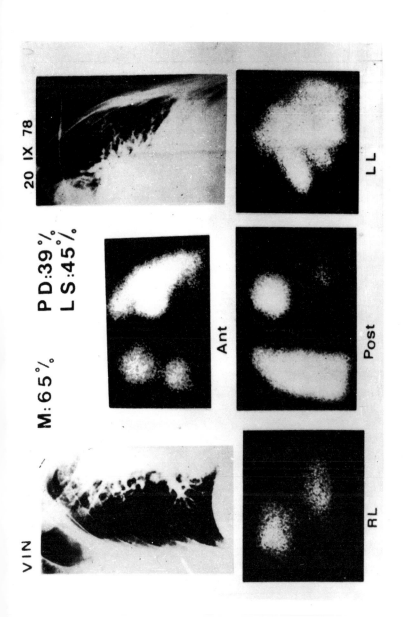

Fig. 2. Massive pulmonary embolism before treatment. AMI: angiographic Miller's Index; ACF: angiographic capillary flow; IPD: isotopic perfusion defect.

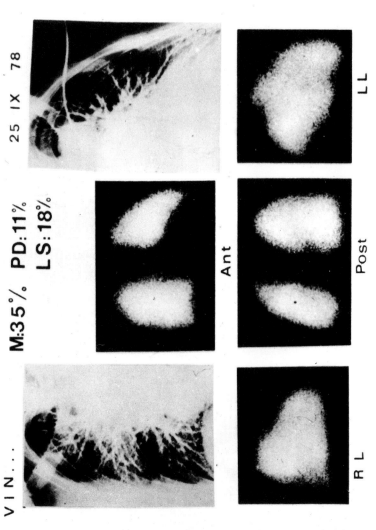

Fig. 3. Massive pulmonary embolism after UK infusion.

while lung scan merely estimates the capillary perfusion. There is a good correlation between lung scan and angiographic perfusion defect before treatment as well as after urokinase infusion.

After a total or partial clot resolution, there is a complete agreement between both lung scan and pulmonary angiogram (Figs 2 and 3). Though the emphasis has been placed upon the fact that a variety of conditions, besides pulmonary embolism, cause perfusion defects on the lung scan, the isotopic examination with macroaggregates injection is rather useful in following the treatment of pulmonary embolism.

REFERENCES

Brochier, M. (1976). *Concours medical.* Suppl. 17.

Dalen, J. E., Brooks, H. L., Johnson, L. W., Mesiter, S. G., Szucs, M. M. and Dexter, I. (1971). *Am. Heart. J.* 81, 175–185.

Miller, G. A. H., Sutton, G. C., Kerr, I. H., Gibson, R. U. and Koney, M. (1971). *Br. Med. J.* 2, 681–684.

Moser, K. N., Longo, A. M., Ashburn, N. L. and Guisan, M. (1973). *Am. J. Med.* 55, 434–441.

RESULTS OF FIBRINOLYTIC THERAPY IN ACUTE AND ESTABLISHED DEEP VEIN THROMBOSIS

G. Trübestein, Th. Brecht, D. Klingmüller, J. Hüls and F. Etzel

Medizinische Poliklinik, Medizinische Klinik, Radiologische Klinik der Universität Bonn, Institut für experimentelle Hämatologie und Bluttransfussionswesen der Universität Bonn, W. Germany

INTRODUCTION

Fibrinolytic therapy can be performed by streptokinase or urokinase. So far there is no agreement as to the dosage and duration of fibrinolytic treatment in vascular occlusion. Moreover, this form of therapy has seemed to be restricted to the 6 days after the beginning of a thrombosis. Today we know that some cases of deep vein thrombosis older than 6 days, can be treated successfully with a fibrinolytic agent (Tilsner, 1974; Widmer et al., 1977). With these older venous thromboses, fibrinolytic therapy provides the only method of treatment aimed at re-opening the occluded veins (May, 1974).

The following is a report on 72 patients with acute and established deep vein thromboses which were treated with a standardized therapeutic scheme for streptokinase and urokinase.

INDICATION

The indication for fibrinolytic therapy was occlusion of the iliac, femoral and popliteal veins or the subclavian vein up to an age of 6 days. Patients with complete occlusions of the tibial veins were also treated in this way. We also tried fibrinolytic therapy in younger patients with extensive 1 - 6-week-old venous occlusion.

Serono Symposium No. 37, "Vascular Occlusion: Epidemiological, Pathophysiological and Therapeutic Aspects", edited by M. Tesi and J. Dormandy, 1981. Academic Press, London and New York.

On account of its lower cost, streptokinase was generally used in our medical department. Urokinase was given only if there were contra-indications against streptokinase as a fibrinolytic agent; particularly if streptokinase treatment had been performed shortly before or if the anti-streptokinase titre was over one million units. Urokinase was also used for continuing fibrinolytic therapy if previous streptokinase treatment had not been successful and if the phlebogram indicated a developing severe post-thrombotic syndrome.

CONTRAINDICATIONS

Included among the absolute contra-indications for fibrinolytic therapy are a haemorrhagic diathesis, gastroduodenal ulcers, haematuria, persistent hypertension with diastolic pressure over 100 mmHg, history of stroke, atrial fibrillation with mitral valve defect, malignant tumours, recent surgery, diagnostic procedures like arteriographies 7 to 14 days previously and pregnancy within the first 3 months.

Among the relative contra-indications to which less attention is paid we include, on the basis of our own experience, intramuscular injections up to 7 days previously. Here it has to be decided in each patient whether fibrinolytic therapy can be carried out.

STREPTOKINASE DOSAGE SCHEME

We used a standardized streptokinase-heparin scheme. As an initial dose, we gave 250 000 IU SK in 20 min, as a maintenance dose 100 000 IU SK/h. After 16 - 18 h of streptokinase therapy we added heparin starting with a dose of 500 IU/h.

UROKINASE DOSAGE SCHEME

In the same way, we used a standardized urokinase scheme. As an initial dose, we have 100 000 IU UK within 10 min, as a maintenance dose 1 000 000 IU/24 h, that means approximately 40 000 IU/h. Five overweight patients received a maintenance dose of 2 000 000 IU UK/24 h. From the very beginning, heparin was given in a dosage of 1 000 IU/h and in the further course of therapy adjusted so that the thrombin time lay between 30 and 60 s (normal value: 10 - 12 s). In five patients, urokinase was given immediately after streptokinase therapy because the control phlebographies did not show an improvement after this treatment. At the end of each fibrinolytic therapy, anticoagulation with phenprocoumon was started, overlapping with heparin.

LABORATORY CONTROLS

Apart from the daily controls of the blood count and urinalysis, the fibrinogen was determined to check fibrinolysis and the thrombin time to regulate the heparin administration. To obtain an easily determinable, non-heparin influenced, parameter of the fibrinogen- and fibrin-degradation products, the reptilase time was determined (Wenzel *et al.*, 1974). Additional haemostaseological examinations determining plasminogen, antiplasmin and the fibrinogen- and fibrin-degradation products were performed at a later date.

THERAPY CONTROLS AND DURATION OF TREATMENT

In the beginning and at the end of the fibrinolytic therapy phlebography was carried out on all patients. Control phlebographies were performed between the third and fifth day depending on the clinical findings and the Doppler-ultrasound examination. The streptokinase treatment was performed mostly for 4 - 6 days, the urokinase treatment 3 - 6 days in acute deep vein thromboses, and in established deep vein thromboses, depending on the clinical and phlebographic findings, generally 7 - 14 days.

SIDE-EFFECTS OF STREPTOKINASE TREATMENT

Five patients had bleeding (haemoglobin decrease greater than 2 g%) and three of them showed a macro- rather than a micro-haematuria, which led to a short-lasting anuria in one of the patients. The most severe bleeding occurred in a patient with preceding lung embolism who developed a haematothorax. Fifteen patients showed a rise in temperature which responded well to pyrazolone. Twelve patients showed a temporary rise of the transaminases.

SIDE-EFFECTS OF UROKINASE TREATMENT

Two patients had bleeding (haemoglobin decrease greater than 2 g%) which required discontinuation of fibrinolytic therapy in one of the patients and a dose reduction in the other patient. Two of three patients developed painful gluteal haematoma after previous intramuscular injections which required an interruption of the urokinase treatment with one of the patients and a temporary dose reduction with the other patient. One patient with a 3-week-old femoral thrombosis died of pulmonary embolism on the second day of urokinase treatment. Systemic reactions, as occurred with streptokinase treatment, were not observed, with the exception of two patients who showed a temperature rise under the urokinase treatment.

PATIENTS

Seventy-two patients with acute and older deep vein thromboses were treated with streptokinase or urokinase, including five patients who received streptokinase as well as urokinase during the therapeutic course. Thirty patients were treated with streptokinase; 23 of these patients had 1 - 6-day-old occlusions and seven patients had 1 - 6-week-old occlusions. Forty-two patients were treated with urokinase; seven of these patients had 1 - 6-day-old occlusions and 35 patients had 1 - 6-week-old occlusions.

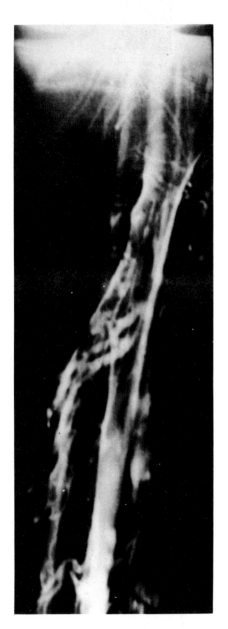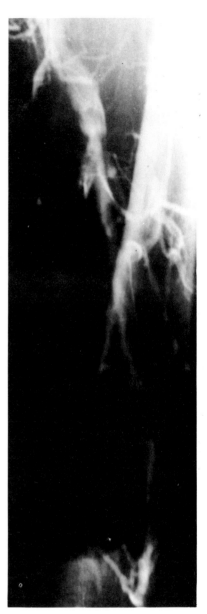

Fig. 1. Phlebographies of an 18-year-old patient with a 9-day-old occlusion of the iliac, femoral and popliteal vein and fresh thromboses in the tibial veins treated with streptokinase. (a) before fibrinolytic treatment; (b) after 7 days of streptokinase treatment complete recanalization of the occluded veins.

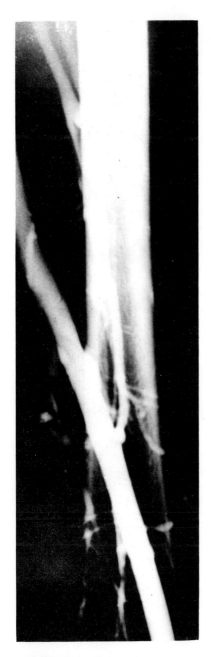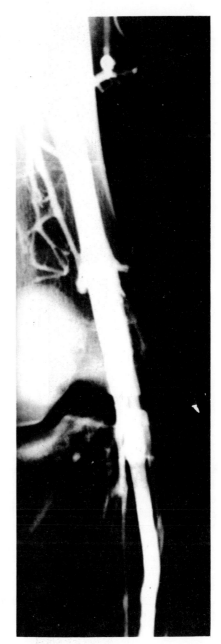

Fig. 1b.

Table I. Urokinase therapy in established deep vein thrombosis (n = 35).

Age (weeks)	Patient	Complete	Partial	Unchanged
1	10	3	5	2
1–2	11	2	6	3
2–3	5	1	3	1
3–4	3		2	+
4–5	3		2	1
5–6	1			1
6	1	1		
>6	1		1	
TOTAL	35	7	19	9

RESULTS OF STREPTOKINASE TREATMENT

In 17 of the 23 patients with 1 - 6-day-old venous occlusions, the thromboses could be dissolved completely with streptokinase therapy and one patient showed a partial recanalization. Five patients showed no amelioration in the phlebogram. In three of the seven patients with 1 - 6-week-old venous occlusions, the thromboses could be dissolved completely (Fig. 1a and b), whereas the remaining four patients showed no amelioration in the phlebograms.

RESULTS OF THE UROKINASE TREATMENT

Only in one of the seven patients with 1 - 6-day-old venous occlusions could the thromboses be dissolved completely with urokinase therapy and six patients showed no amelioration in the phlebograms. In seven of the 35 patients with 1 - 6-week-old venous occlusions, the thromboses could be dissolved completely during 7 - 20 days of urokinase therapy. With 19 patients, a partial recanalization could be achieved with patency of the iliac or the femoral veins respectively. Nine patients showed no amelioration in the phlebograms.

The analysis of the results obtained from the 35 patients with 1 - 6-week-old occlusions showed increasing age of the thromboses with a declining success (Table I). Whereas 23% of 26 patients with 1 - 3-week-old venous occlusions showed a complete dissolution of the thrombosis, we found only in 9% of the remaining nine patients with 3 - 6-week-old occlusions developed patency of the occluded veins.

EVALUATION OF THE HAEMOSTASEOLOGICAL PARAMETERS

The evaluation of the haemostaseological parameters showed a sharp drop of the fibrinogen below 1.0 g/l in the first days of the streptokinase therapy, whereas under the urokinase therapy, the fibrinogen usually showed a slow decrease and very seldom fell below 1.0 g/l. Accordingly, the reptilase times were much more prolonged under the streptokinase therapy than under the urokinase therapy (Figs 2 and 3). Moreover, both the fibrinogen and the reptilase times varied considerably with the two therapeutic schemes. Most remarkable was the fact that the plasminogen pool was never exhausted under long-lasting urokinase therapy. The plasminogen levels during a 14-day, or even longer, urokinase therapy were reduced, but always measurable.

CONCLUSIONS

The results show that it was possible to dissolve 1 – 6-day-old venous thromboses in about 75% with a standardized streptokinase-heparin therapy. Moreover, it was possible to dissolve 1 – 6-week-old venous occlusions in about 40%. These data correspond with the results of other groups (Widmer *et al.*, 1977; Theiss *et al.*, 1975). The results of the urokinase therapy in 1 – 6-day-old deep vein thromboses

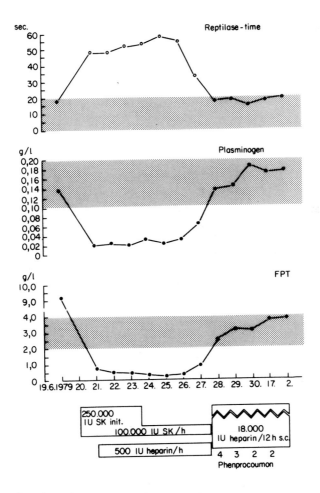

Fig. 2a. Reptilase time, plasminogen and fibrinogen (FPT) during the 7-day streptokinase therapy and the following anticoagulation therapy.

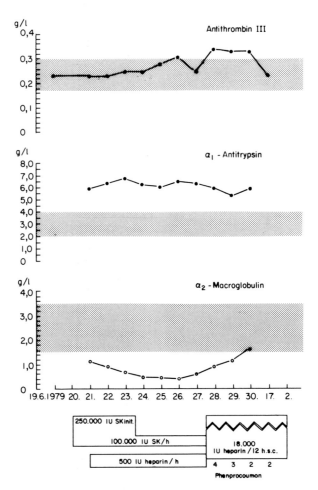

Fig. 2b. Antithrombin III, α_1 antitrypsin, α_2 macroglobulin during the 7-day streptokinase therapy and the following anticoagulation therapy.

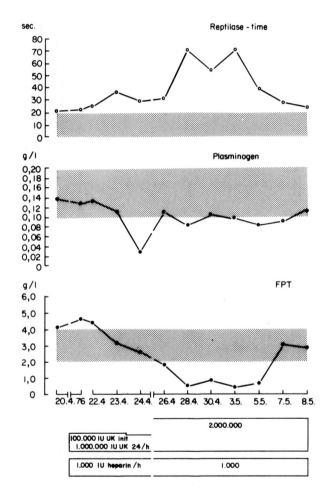

Fig. 3a. Reptilase time, plasminogen and fibrinogen (FPT) during 18 days of urokinase therapy with 1 000 000 IU UK/24 h and 2 000 000 IU UK/24 h (Pat. D.U.).

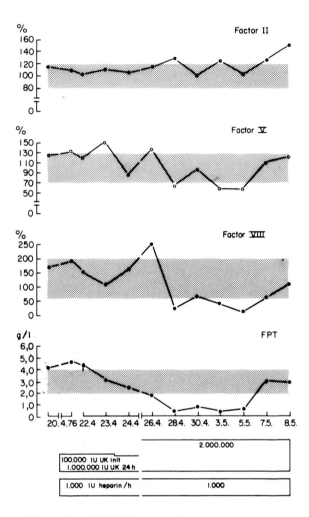

Fig. 3b. Factor II, factor V and VIII, fibrinogen (FPT) during 18 days of urokinase therapy with 1 000 000 IU UK/24 h and 2 000 000 IU UK/24 h (Pat. D.U.).

were not satisfying. A complete recanalization could only be achieved in one of seven patients. These results are evidently the sequel of the short duration of treatment in these patients because the results in older, 1 - 6-week-old thromboses were much better with the same therapeutic scheme and a longer-lasting treatment. In all, seven of 35 patients with 1 - 6-week-old venous thromboses achieved a complete recanalization and 19 of these patients achieved partial recanalization. These results in older phlebothromboses correspond with the observations reported by Tilsner (1974) that the results of fibrinolytic therapy, with urokinase in a similar dosage regimen, could be considerably improved by a long-term fibrinolytic therapy of 7 - 14 days.

The two therapeutic schemes are difficult to compare but both the streptokinase regimen and the urokinase regimen proved effective. So far as it is possible to draw conclusions about the different therapeutic schemes and the patients treated, we can say that fibrinolytic therapy with urokinase should be performed longer than with streptokinase. Moreover, the indication for fibrinolytic therapy in deep vein thrombosis should not be restricted to 6 days. Randomized studies on the treatment of deep vein thrombosis with different urokinase and strepto-kinase dosage regimens are necessary to achieve in future optimal dosage regimens with a good therapeutic effect.

REFERENCES

May, R. (1979). "Chirurgie der Bein- und Beckenvenen." Thieme, Stuttgart.
Theiss, W., Kriessmann, A. and Wirtzfeld, A. (1975). *Dtsch. med. Wschr.* **100**, 1887.
Tilsner, V. (1979). *Vasa* 3, 458.
Wenzel, E., Holzhüter, H., Muschietti, F., Angelkort, B., Ochs, H. G., Pusztai-Markes, S., Nowak, H. and Stürner, H. (1974). *Dtsch. med. Wschr.* **99**, 746.
Widmer, L. K., Madar, G., Widmer, M. Th., Schmitt, H. E. and Duckert, F. (1977). *In* "Akute tiefe Becken- und Beinvenenthrombosen" (H. Ehringer, ed.) Huber, Bern.

BIOCHEMICAL COMPARISON OF INTERMITTENT STREPTOKINASE AND INTERMITTENT STREPTOKINASE PLASMINOGEN THERAPY

V. V. Kakkar, G. H. Barlow, N. A. G. Jones and P. Webb

Thrombosis Research Unit, King's College Hospital Medical School, London, UK

INTRODUCTION

There is no doubt that thrombolytic therapy is highly effective in dissolving thrombo-emboli. However, this form of treatment has not been adopted for treating the great majority of patients suffering from thrombo-embolic disease for the following reasons: the drugs administered to produce a thrombolytic effect (such as urokinase and streptokinase) are expensive when compared with heparin; secondly, the therapy is considered to be potentially dangerous because of the serious haemorrhage which may occur, the possibility of reactions such as pyrexia, and lastly, strict laboratory control is necessary to regulate the dose of lytic agent.

To overcome these drawbacks, several new approaches are at present being investigated. We have already reported encouraging results when an intermittent streptokinase infusion has been combined with administration of purified, pre-treated homologous plasminogen (Kakkar *et al.*, 1975). Thirty patients who presented with extensive deep vein thrombosis were included in this study. Complete lysis of all thrombi was observed in approximately 60% of the patients, partial but extensive lysis in 23% and the thrombi remained unchanged in 17%.

Serono Symposium No. 37, "Vascular Occlusion: Epidemiological, Pathophysiological and Therapeutic Aspects", edited by M. Tesi and J. Dormandy, 1981. Academic Press, London and New York.

We have now introduced further modifications in our regimen of intermittent streptokinase infusion. We would like to present the biochemical changes occurring on a twice a day regimen of streptokinase.

MATERIALS AND METHODS

Materials

Plasminogen was kindly supplied by Laboratoire Choay (Paris) and streptokinase (Kabikinase) by KabiVitrum Ltd (London). The chromogenic substrate, S2251, was purchased from Kabi Diagnostica (Stockholm). The Soybean trypsin inhibitor was purchased from Sigma Chemical Co. (London). The Quantichrom ATIII kits were kindly supplied by Abbott Diagnostics (Langen).

Patients

Nine patients with established deep vein thrombosis have been studied. They were given streptokinase with or without plasminogen according to a randomized allocation, five on streptokinase alone and four on combination therapy. If the patients were to have plasminogen, 90 mg of plasminogen in 60 ml normal saline were given intravenously over 30 min before streptokinase infusions. On the first day, a loading dose of 600 000 units of streptokinase in 60 ml normal saline was given intravenously over 30 min. On subsequent days, a dose of 300 000 units was given twice daily.

Plasma Samples

Blood samples were taken (a) prior to daily treatments, (b) immediately after the daily infusion of plasminogen and (c) immediately after the infusion of streptokinase. The samples were obtained by an indwelling central venous catheter and were collected in sodium citrate at a final concentration of 0.38%. The blood was divided into equal portions, to one of which aprotinin (Bayer) was added (500 units/ml). Platelet poor plasma was prepared by centrifugation at 2000×8 for 20 min at $+4\,^{\circ}$C. Plasma samples without aprotinin were used for all determinations except fibrinogen and FDP.

Antiplasmin was determined by the method described by Teger-Nilsson *et al.* (1977) using the chromogenic substrate, S2251. The assay was automated and performed on the Abbott Biochromatic Analyser 100 (Abbott-Langen) (ABA-100).

Antithrombin III was determined on the ABA-100 using the Quantichrom III diagnostic kit. This kit uses the chromogenic substrate, S2160, for its analysis.

Fibrinogen was determined essentially by the thrombin method of Blomback and Blomback (1956).

Fibrinogen and fibrin degradation products (FDP): Serum obtained during the determination of fibrinogen was used to determine FDP levels. The method was the tanned red cell inhibition immunoassay (TRCH II, Wellcome Reagents, London).

Fibrinolytic activity levels were measured in the plasma on heated and unheated fibrin plates, prepared according to Astrup and Mullertz (1952). It was also measured during the chromogenic substrate S2251 (Friberger and Knos, 1978).

Levels of the plasmin (ogen) streptokinase activator complex were determined using an automated analysis of the ABA-100 with the chromogenic substrate S2251. Plasma samples were incubated with Soybean trypsin inhibitor (SBTI), final concentration 0.5 mg/ml prior to analysis. As shown by Reddy and Marcus (1974), the addition of SBTI completely inhibits the enzymatic activity of plasmin but has no inhibitory effect on the activator complex.

Thrombin clotting time was measured by standard techniques (Hardisty and Ingram, 1956).

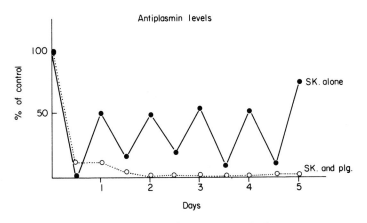

Fig. 1. Antiplasmin values as a percentage of original control values.

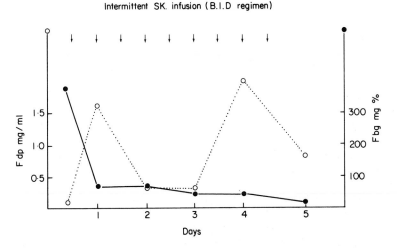

Fig. 2. Fibrinogen ●-● and FDP ○-○ levels during twice-a-day intermittent therapy with streptokinase only.

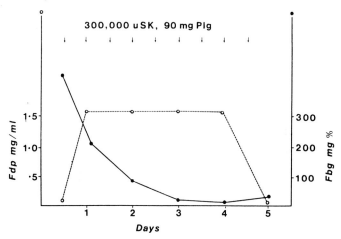

Fig. 3. Fibrinogen ●–● and FDP ○–○ levels during twice-a-day intermittent streptokinase and plasminogen therapy. Arrows indicate time of SK dose which is 30 min after administration of plasminogen.

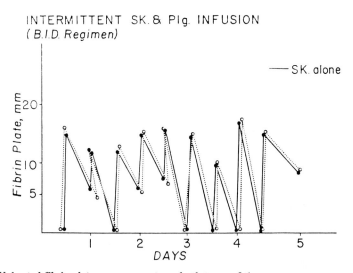

Fig. 4. Unheated fibrin plate measurements on both types of therapy.

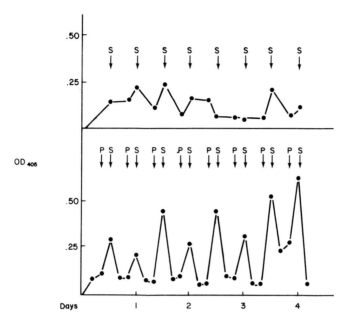

Fig. 5. Plasminogen activator levels in patients during therapy. Upper curve is that with streptokinase alone, bottom curve combination therapy. Arrows and letters mark position of receiving drug.

RESULTS

The average antiplasmin levels for both regimens are shown in Fig. 1. The value with streptokinase alone undulates between about 20 and 50% of normal, reaching the highest levels just prior to the initiation of a new dose, the value on the combination therapy drops to zero and remains there throughout the treatment regimen. The antithrombin III levels remain constant throughout the entire time of treatment independent of the dosing regimen.

The average results for the fibrinogen and FDP levels are shown in Fig. 2 for the streptokinase therapy and in Fig. 3 for the combination therapy. Both therapies bring about a marked decrease in the fibrinogen levels with the rate of disappearance somewhat faster with the streptokinase alone. The FDPs show a plateau effect with the combination therapy reaching a high level and remaining high throughout the dosing regimen. The streptokinase treatment shows a bimodal type response with a second elevation occurring on about day 3.

Fibrinolytic activity on unheated fibrin plates for both regimens is shown in Fig. 4. There is little difference seen in this parameter between the two different regimens. On heated fibrin plates which would eliminate most of the plasminogen activator activity, there was only a small response indicating little free plasmin present in either case.

In Fig. 5, the average levels of plasminogen activator for the two treatments is shown. The infusion of plasminogen prior to the streptokinase brings about a marked increase in the level of activator, which occurs following each infusion of the streptokinase. There appears to be a stepwise increase in the amount of activator present as the therapy progresses. The thrombin clotting time increased immediately following the loading dose and remained elevated throughout the treatment period fluctuating between 1.5 and 3 times normal.

DISCUSSION

These results are part of the growing evidence supporting the concept that intermittent streptokinase therapy, especially in combination with lys-plasminogen, has advantages over the classical approach.

The first potential improvement is in the antiplasmin levels. Our data with streptokinase twice a day are very similar to those reported by Verstraete *et al.* (1978) for their single dose therapy. However, the twice-a-day regimen in combination with lys-plasminogen appears to remove the antiplasmin activity completely for the duration of therapy.

The presence of large amounts of activator complex also has potential advantages. First, the higher levels should prevent formation of a hyperplasminaemic state and therefore lower the bleeding hazards. Secondly, the evidence of Amery (1969), suggesting that the complex absorbs to blood clots would mean that lysis within the thrombus could occur with low levels of plasmin and with the correct ratio of activator to plasmin, results in a substantial reduction in fibrinogenlysis. Thirdly, is the possibility for reduced antigenicity. The earlier observations that streptokinase is fragmented in the complex (Reddy and Markus, 1974) and that these fragments are less antigenic (Barlow *et al.*, 1976) could mean reduced antibody formation if the streptokinase is completely involved in complex formation. The other *in vitro* observation that the complex itself is less antigenic (Barlow *et al.*, 1975) would also support the potential for less antigenicity even though one clinical trial on the purified complex did not support this observation (Verstraete *et al.*, 1977).

The results discussed above can also help explain the strong fibrinolytic state in the patients as demonstrated by the high FDPs and marked reduction in fibrinogen with very low levels of measurable plasmin. The absence of anti-plasmin along with much of the available plasminogen in activator complex should let the small amounts of plasmin available be free for lytic action.

Finally, while these data would support the use of intermittent streptokinase plasminogen regimen from a biochemical standpoint, the effectiveness of the therapy will need to await additional therapeutic evaluation. The data would also indicate that there is a need for further biochemical exploration of the dosing ratio of streptokinase to plasminogen, in order to obtain the most effective balance between activator and proteolytic activities. Such further clinical studies are now in progress.

REFERENCES

Amery, A. (1969). Activation of the human fibrinolytic system by streptokinase. Therapeutic application in thromboembolic occlusions of the limb arteries and in myocardial infarction. Acco, Leuven, Belgium.

Astrup, P. and Mullertz, S. (1952). *Arch. Biochem. Biophys.* **46**, 346.
Barlow, G. H., Devine, E. and Finley, R. (1975). *Res. Comm. Chem. Path. Pharm.* **10**, 465.
Barlow, G. H., Finley, R. and Castellino, F. J. (1976). *Thromb. Res.* **8**, 237.
Blomback, B. and Blomback, M. (1956). *Arkiv für Chemi.* **16**,415.
Friberger, P. and Knos, M. (1978). *In* "Chromogenic Substrates", (M. F. Scully and V. V. Kakkar eds). Churchill Livingstone, Edinburgh.
Hardisty, R. M. and Ingram, G.I.C. (1956). "Bleeding Disorders" Blackwell Scientific Publications, Oxford.
Kakkar, V. V., Sagar, S. and Lewis, M. (1975). *Lancet* **2**, 674.
Reddy, K.N.N. and Markus, G. (1974). *J. Biol. Chem.* **249**, 4851.
Scully, M. F., Lane, D. A., Sagar, S., Thomas, D. P. and Kakkar, V. V. (1977). *Thrombos. Haemostas.* **37**, 162.
Teger-Nilsson, A–C., Friberger, P. and Gyzander, E. (1977). *Scand. J. Clin. Lab. Invest.* **37**, 403.
Verstraete, M., Vermylen, J., Amery, A. and Vermylen, C. (1966). *Br. Med. J.* **1**, 454.
Verstraete, M., Vermylen, J., Holleman, W. and Barlow, G. H. (1977). *Thromb. Res.* **11**, 227.
Verstraete, M., Vermylen, J. and Schetz, J. (1978). *Actuel. Probl. Angiol.* **37**, 95.
Ziemski, J. M., Marchlewski, S., Meissner, A. J., Rudowski, W., Kolakowski, L., Lopaciuk, S. and Latallo, Z. S. (1978). *Actuel. Probl. Angiol.* **37**, 187.

THE ANTITHROMBOTIC ACTION OF HEPARAN SULPHATE

D. P. Thomas, E. A. Johnson and T. W. Barrowcliffe

National Institute for Biological Standards and Control, London, UK

INTRODUCTION

Heparin is a long-established and highly-effective antithrombotic drug, particularly for the prophylaxis and treatment of venous thrombo-embolic disease (Thomas, 1978). However, heparin suffers from certain disadvantages, chiefly the relatively high incidence of haemorrhagic complications associated with its use. This undesirable side-effect occurs mainly when the drug is given by intravenous injection, where the rate of significant haemorrhagic complications can be as high as 10–15% (Mant *et al.*, 1977). Anticoagulants in general, and heparin in particular, are an important cause of iatrogenic deaths. Indeed, it has been claimed that heparin is responsible for a majority of drug deaths in patients who are reasonably healthy (Porter and Jick, 1977). Even subcutaneous administration of low dose heparin is associated with a significantly higher incidence of post-operative haematoma, in patients receiving the drug as prophylaxis against deep vein thrombosis (DVT) (Multicentre Trial, 1975). Heparin is undoubtedly effective, but reservations concerning its safety have prevented heparin from achieving its full therapeutic potential. This is particularly the case with prophylactic administration, where there is understandable reluctance on the part of many physicians to use a drug which may produce undesirable haemorrhagic side-effects in patients who are otherwise well.

These drawbacks associated with ordinary heparin have been largely responsible for the recent interest in heparin fractions and analogues. With increased understanding of the mode of action of heparin, and particularly its role in potentiating the action of the main inhibitor of clotting (antithrombin III), there has also been

Serono Symposium No. 37, "Vascular Occlusion: Epidemiological, Pathophysiological and Therapeutic Aspects", edited by M. Tesi and J. Dormandy, 1981. Academic Press, London and New York.

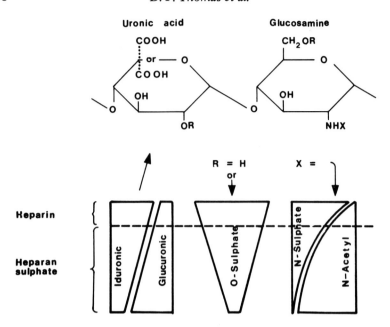

Fig. 1. A schematic illustration of the structural relationship between heparin and heparan sulphates.

the recognition that it is possible to prepare heparin fractions which selectively potentiate anti-Xa (Barrowcliffe *et al.*, 1978).

We have compared another glycosaminoglycan with heparin, both *in vivo* and *in vitro*. Heparan sulphate (HS) is a near relative of heparin; like heparin, it has glucosamine as the amino sugar as opposed to galactosamine in chondroitins (Fig. 1). HS is widely distributed in the body, and is known to be present on cell surfaces (Kraemer, 1977). Heparan has a lower sulphate content than heparin, and like heparin, heparan sulphate also exhibits considerable heterogeneity.

In this study, we have examined the effect of HS *in vitro* in anti-Xa clotting assays, and correlated this with the ability of HS to prevent experimental venous thrombosis.

MATERIALS AND METHODS

Heparan Sulphate

Heparan sulphate was prepared from a heparan-rich fraction of porcine mucosal glycosaminoglycan kindly provided by Laboratori Derivati Organici, Milan, Italy. Solvent fractionation of the barium salts was followed by ion-exchange chromatography and then fractional precipitation of the calcium salt. The hexosamine was 98% glucosamine, $[\alpha]_D = +59°C$, and the ratio of SO_3^- to CO_2^- was 1.75 (heparins > 2). The mean molecular weight by gel permeation chromatography was about 7500.

Heparin

Sodium and calcium salts of mucous heparin were used (Leo Laboratories, London, England; Laboratoire Choay, Paris, France).

Assays

Clotting assays using the anti-Factor Xa (anti-Xa) and activated partial thromboplastin time (APTT) methods were carried out as described previously (Andersson *et al.*, 1976). Pooled platelet-free human plasma was used as substrate, from blood collected on acid citrate dextrose. The plasma was spun at high speed (48 000 *g* for 30 min) and stored at −30°C for no longer than 3 months.

Anti-Xa clotting assays were carried out using the technique of Denson and Bonnar (1973). The levels of anti-Xa activity induced by HS were read against a standard curve prepared using the rabbit's control plasma and ordinary heparin. Anti-Xa amidolytic assays were carried out using the synthetic substrate S-2222 (Kabi, Stockholm, Sweden). Bovine Factor Xa (Diagnostic Reagents Ltd., Thame, Oxon., England) was allowed to react for 1 min with heparinized plasma, the substrate (1 mmol) was then added and the reaction was terminated with acetic acid after a further 4 min. Absorbances were read at 405 nmol.

In vivo assays for detecting thrombosis were carried out using the bioassay model for stasis thrombosis of Wessler *et al.* (1959). Human serum (1.32 ml/kg) was injected into marginal ear veins of rabbits, and previously isolated jugular veins were ligated 10 s after infusion of the serum. The venous segments were opened after 10 min stasis and examined for the presence or absence of thrombi. Thrombi were scored on the scale of 0 to 4+, the latter representing complete clotting of all the blood contained within the segment. Before serum was

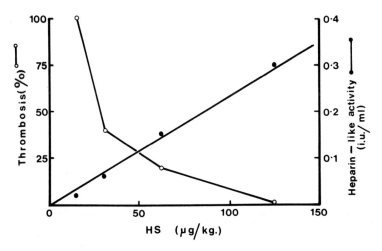

Fig. 2. Inhibition of thrombosis *in vivo* by heparan sulphate (HS). Each point represents the mean values for 6 rabbits. Heparin-like activity was measured by an anti-Xa clotting assay. Thrombus formation was determined on a scale where 100% represents complete clotting of the blood in the isolated venous segment.

injected, heparan sulphate was administered via a marginal ear vein, and a blood sample taken. HS was injected at four dose levels, over a range 15 to 125 µg/kg, with six rabbits being studied at each dose level.

Table I. Specific activity (µ/mg) of heparan sulphate citrated platelet-poor plasma. Results given are means and ranges.

Assay	HS
APTT	20.0
Anti-Xa:	
Clotting	77.0 (72–84)
Amidolytic	16.8 (12.6–20)
(S–2222)	

RESULTS

Heparan sulphate (HS) was found *in vitro* to have low potency by APTT assay, and very little activity in an anti-Xa amidolytic assay. However, by anti-Xa clotting assay, HS had a specific activity about half that of heparin (Table I).

HS was injected into rabbits (15-125 µg/kg) and tested for its ability to impair formation of stasis thrombi in a standard model. Concentrations of HS as low as 30-60 µg/kg impaired the formation of stasis thrombi. Increasing doses of HS produced a linear response, in terms of increasing anti-Xa clotting activity (Fig. 2). In this model 15 µg/kg did not prevent thrombosis, whereas 125 µg/kg prevented thrombosis completely. Also in this model, a level of heparin-like activity of around 0.2 IU/ml by anti-Xa assay was associated with a 50% reduction in the formation of thrombi. Low levels of heparin-like activity by anti-Xa assay were associated with little or no change in the plasma as measured by APTT, and the presence or absence of thrombi correlated much better with the anti-Xa level.

DISCUSSION

Heparan sulphate is usually considered to be a weak anticoagulant, and previous workers have suggested that HS is some 70 times less active than heparin as a conventional anti-coagulant (Teien *et al.*, 1976; Cofrancesco *et al.*, 1979). However, Hatton and colleagues showed that HS markedly accelerated the inactivation of thrombin by antithrombin III (Hatton *et al.*, 1979). When measured by esterase activity, HS was almost as effective as heparin in potentiating the inactivation of thrombin by antithrombin III. We have previously demonstrated that HS has significant anti-Xa clotting activity *in vitro* (Thomas *et al.*, 1979); we have now shown that HS prevents stasis thrombosis in experimental animals. At about 50 µg/kg, only one in four rabbits developed thrombosis, and this means that the ability of HS to prevent venous thrombosis in this model is comparable with that of heparin itself (Gitel *et al.*, 1977). Furthermore, these results confirm that the prevention of stasis thrombosis experimentally can be directly related to the enhancement of a natural inhibitor of clotting, and not primarily to an effect on overall clotting.

Our results are not necessarily at variance with those of Teien *et al.* (1976). The sulphur content and sulphur-carboxylate ratio show that the HS we used had approximately 1.75 sulphate groups per disaccharide unit (heparin has 2-2.5). The HS used by Teien *et al.* evidently had a significantly lower degree of sulphation, and the assays they used to evaluate its activity did not include anti-Xa clotting assays. We have also examined a standard HS sample from beef lung tissue, kindly provided by Professor Cifonelli of the University of Chicago, which has less than 0.5 sulphate per disaccharide unit. This material has proved to have very much lower activities than our HS, by both APTT and anti-Xa clotting assays. Preparations of HS appear to be even more heterogeneous than those of heparin.

The mechanism by which HS exerts its anti-Xa effect is not yet known. Preliminary studies suggest that HS binds to purified At III, but to a much lesser extent than heparin. The discrepancy between clotting and synthetic substrate assays suggests a mechanism of action different from that of heparin, and it may well be that an inhibitor of Xa other than At III is involved.

The current interest in heparin fractions is largely based on the assumption (still unproven) that a heparin fraction with high specific activity would carry a lesser risk of undesirable side-effects. For example, a heparin fraction prepared by gel filtration or selective absorption on to an At III column may have a specific anti-Xa activity of, say, 750 IU/mg. Clearly, it becomes theoretically possible to administer smaller doses of such a drug. Instead of giving 50 mg of heparin, a comparable effect on anti-Xa activity could be achieved with only 10 mg. Another approach is to use other glycosaminoglycans which, although they have a lower specific activity than heparin when measured by conventional clotting assays, nevertheless have a relatively marked effect by anti-Xa assay. For example, mucosal heparin has an anti-Xa/APTT ratio of 1.0-1.2, which means that the drug has more or less equal potency when measured by either assay. A drug which has a specific activity of 75 IU/mg by anti-Xa, but only 25 IU/mg by APTT, would have a ratio of 3.0. While this drug would be a poor "Heparin" when measured against standard heparin in an APTT assay, nevertheless it may be a useful drug when used for the prophylaxis of DVT. Our results indicate that not only has HS a highly favourable anti-Xa/APTT ratio *in vitro*, but that it is also effective as an antithrombotic drug experimentally. Therefore, HS appears to have the therapeutic potential of heparin, but without a comparable effect on overall clotting. It may therefore give the protection that is achieved with heparin, but with fewer haemorrhagic complications. It is concluded that HS with a high anti-Xa/APTT ratio is worthy of clinical trial as an antithrombotic drug, particularly for the prophylaxis of venous thrombosis.

REFERENCES

Andersson, L. -O., Barrowcliffe, T. W., Holmer, E., Johnson, E. A. and Sims, G. E. C. (1976). *Thrombosis Research* **9**, 575.

Barrowcliffe, T. W., Johnson, E. A. and Thomas, D. P. (1978). *British Medical Bulletin* **34**, 143.

Cofrancesco, E., Radaelli, F., Pogliani, E., Amici, N., Torri, G. G. and Casu, B. (1979). *Thrombosis Research* **14**, 179.

Denson, K. W. E. and Bonnar, J. (1973). *Thrombosis et Diathesis Haemorrhagica* **30**, 417.

Gitel, S. N., Stephenson, R. C. and Wessler, S. (1977). *Proceedings of the National Academy of Sciences, USA* **74**, 3028.

Hatton, M. W. C., Berry, L. R. and Regoeczi, E. (1978). *Thrombosis Research* **13**, 655.

International Multicentre Trial (1975). *Lancet* **2**, 45.

Kraemer, P. M. (1977). *Biochemical and Biophysical Research Communications* **78**, 1334.

Mant, M. J., Thong, K. L., Birtwhistle, R. V., O'Brien, B. D., Hammond, G. W. and Grace, M. G. (1977). *Lancet* **1**, 1133.

Porter, J. and Jick, H. (1977). *Journal of the American Medical Association* **237**, 879.

Teien, A. N., Abildgaard, Y. Höök, M. (1976). *Thrombosis Research* **8**, 859.

Thomas, D. P. (1978). *Seminars in Hematology* **15**, 1.

Thomas, D. P., Merton, R. E., Barrowcliffe, T. W., Mulloy, B. and Johnson, E. A. (1979). *Thrombosis Research* **14**, 501.

Wessler, S., Reimer, S. M. and Sheps, M. C. (1959). *Journal of Applied Physiology* **14**, 943.

LONG-TERM PROGNOSIS OF ATHEROSCLEROSIS OBLITERANS IN VARIOUS REGIONS USING CONSERVATIVE OR SURGICAL TREATMENT

H. Heine, L. Heinemann, C. Norden and H. Schmidt

Central Institute for Cardiovascular Research of the Academy of Science GDR, Berlin-Buch, German Democratic Republic

We investigated 1193 patients with peripheral arterial disease, 331 patients with cerebrovascular insufficiency and 220 patients with post-myocardial infarction for several years. The mortality rate per observation year for PAD was 5.8%, for IHD–9.6% and for CVD–3.6%. The majority of patients died due to cardiovascular disease and of these, 45% died due to myocardial infarction. From the 145 which died in the myocardial infarction group, 92% died due to cardiovascular disease (103 persons or 70% because of a recurrent AMI).

Risk factors and additional cardiovascular disease are closely related and influence the prognosis, i.e. compare survival rates of patients suffering from CVD and PAD in Fig. 1.

There were 390 patients with PAD who received long-term anticoagulant therapy and 803 patients had control treatment. There are no significant differences between the two groups with regard to age, clinical stage, number and size of obliterations and additional cardiovascular disease at the beginning. The average control interval was 7 years. The prognosis of patients using anticoagulants was better; the yearly mortality rate for patients with anticoagulants was 4% and in the control group 11% i.e. at the end of the follow-up period 32% *vs* 62% (Fig. 2).

The incidence of myocardial infarction and stroke was higher in the control

Serono Symposium No. 37, "Vascular Occlusion: Epidemiological, Pathophysiological and Therapeutic Aspects", edited by M. Tesi and J. Dormandy, 1981. Academic Press, London and New York.

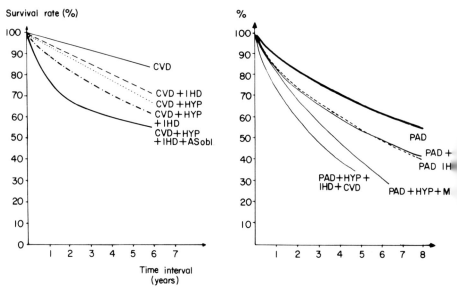

Survival rate of patients with extracranial CVD/PAD and additional cardiovascular diseases

Fig. 1. Survival rate of patients with extracranial CVD and PAD compared with additional diseases.

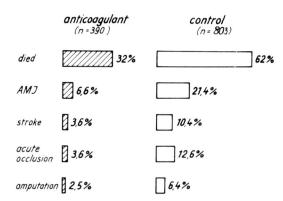

Fig. 2. Survival and acute cardiovascular complications in anticoagulant therapy and control group.

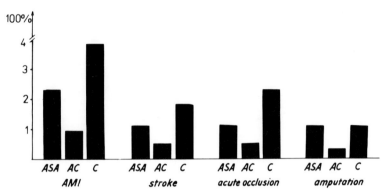

Fig. 3. Annual complication rates (%) in patients using anticoagulants (AC), acetylsalicylic acid (ASA) and with basic cardiovascular treatment (C).

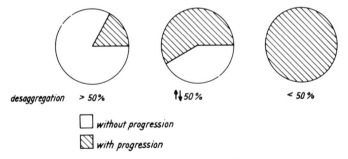

Fig. 4. Desaggregation rate and progression of atherosclerosis.

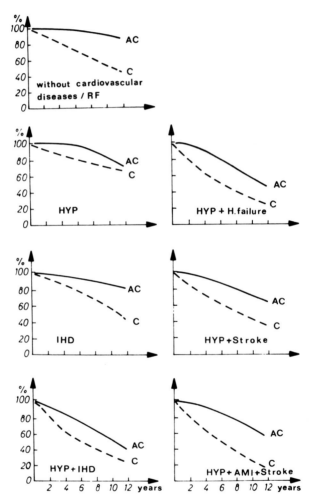

Fig. 5. Survival in anticoagulant (AC) and control group (C) and dependence on additional cardiovascular diseases and risk factors (RF).

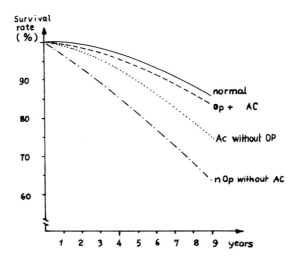

Fig. 6. Survival rates of patients suffering from CVD depends on anticoagulants (AC) and surgery (OP).

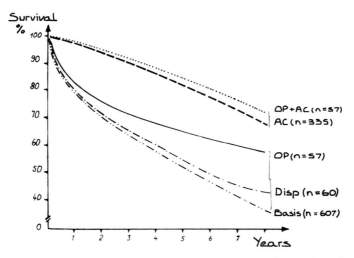

Fig. 7. Survival rates of different conservative and surgical groups. AK= anticoagulants, OP + AK = vascular surgery followed by anticoagulants, OP = surgery alone, Disp = dispensaire treatment, Basis = basic cardiovascular treatment.

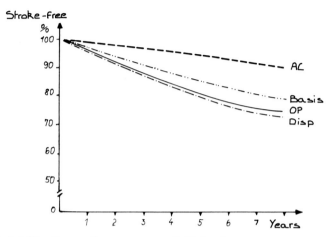

Fig. 8. Probability of preventing acute myocardial infarction.

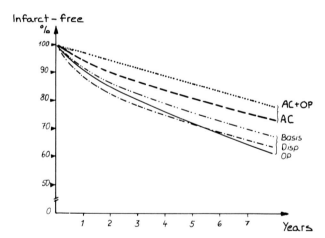

Fig. 9. Probability of preventing stroke.

group. From our preliminary results of a comparative study with acetylsalicylic acid (ASA) we conclude that: it is more effective to use anticoagulants or ASA when compared to standard cardiovascular treatment (Fig. 3). The greater the desaggregation rate of thrombocytes, the more retarded is the progression of atherosclerosis (Fig. 4). When we analyse the survival rate compared with risk factors and additional disease, we get the same results: i.e. a better prognosis in AC-therapy than in the control group (Fig. 5).

What differences in long-term prognosis exist between surgical treatment and conservative therapy (basic cardiovascular treatment without anticoagulant therapy)? Figure 6 shows the influence of anticoagulant therapy on survival in cerebrovascular disease as an example. The most effective therapy in cases of extracranial CVD is vascular surgery followed by anticoagulant treatment.

Similarly, in patients suffering from PAD, the best effect was found in those with vascular bypass operation and anticoagulant therapy or anticoagulant treatment alone (Fig. 7). Significantly worse results were found in the other groups. The yearly survival rate shows that only 4.8% of cases using anticoagulants died, compared with 8.3% in the pure surgical group, 11% in the dispensary group and 11.6% in the group with basic cardiovascular treatment. The survival rate of patients with anticoagulant treatment was especially good after surgical therapy (3.2% yearly mortality). Figures 8 and 9 demonstrate that in cases of surgical treatment followed by anticoagulants, the probability of myocardial infarction decreases in comparison with the other three groups.

In summary, we emphasize that surgical treatment and anticoagulants both have positive effects on survival, development of acute cardiovascular complications and subjective symptoms. In all possible cases, we recommend vascular surgery. But surgery alone does not prevent the progression of atherosclerosis. Combination with long-term treatment with Ac or ASA results in the best long-term prognosis.

DEFIBRINATION AND ITS POSSIBLE APPLICATION IN PREVENTION AND TREATMENT OF VASCULAR OBSTRUCTIONS

Z. S. Latallo

Institute of Nuclear Research, Warsaw, Poland

Clinical observations on the effect of snake bites, particularly by Malayan pit viper *Agkistrodon rhodostoma* (Reid and Thean, 1963) and *Bothrops atrox* (Ghitis and Bonelli, 1963) revealed that one of the major features consisted of a long-lasting state of defibrination. This phenomenon appeared to be due to the presence of specific enzymes in the venoms of these snakes, which were able to convert fibrinogen into fibrin and hence were named thrombin-like enzymes. The enzymes were isolated, purified and endowed with generic names, ancrod and batroxobin respectively. Although similar, they are not identical. Both are glyco-proteins of a molecular weight estimated as 30 000 daltons for ancrod (Esnouf and Tunnah, 1967) and 36 000 daltons for batroxobin (Stocker, 1978). Ancrod and batroxobin are both immunogenic but, as shown by Barlow *et al.* (1973), immunologically distinct proteins.

Extensive studies on animals, especially on the toxicity, teratogenecity, etc. followed by trials on human volunteers, allowed the introduction of the enzymes into clinical use. At present, the following preparations are produced: ancrod — Arvin (Berk Pharmaceuticals), Venacil (Abbott, USA); batroxobin — Defibrase (Pentapharm). Potency of these preparations is expressed in different units — batroxobin units (BU) for Defibrase and Twyford units for ancrod. Both enzymes are highly stable in solution at a rather wide range of pH, even at higher than ambient temperatures.

Serono Symposium No. 37, "Vascular Occlusion: Epidemiological, Pathophysiological and Therapeutic Aspects", edited by M. Tesi and J. Dormandy, 1981. Academic Press, London and New York.

In vitro effect on fibrinogen consists of splitting off only fibrinopeptide A resulting in formation of des A-fibrin clot. In human plasma, no other clotting factors except fibrinogen and factor XIII are affected. The latter seems to be activated to some extent by batroxobin (from *B. atrox moojeni*) but not by the enzyme (from *B. atrox marajoensis*). Ancrod is generally considered as inactive toward factor XIII, but Gaffney and Brasher (1974) provided some evidence indicating that it also might activate this factor. This discrepancy, as well as some others, is perhaps due to the fact that in contrast to the *Bathrops atrox* group of snakes much less is known about possible differences in subspecies of *Agkistrodon rhodostoma.*

This is where the similarity of these thrombin-like enzymes to thrombin ends. In contrast to the latter, neither ancrod nor batroxobin is inhibited by antithrombin III (AT III) or by AT III complex with heparin or by hirudin. What is perhaps most important from the point of view of clinical application is that these snake venom enzymes do not induce platelet aggregation release reaction and do not cause clot retraction in platelet-rich plasma (Brown *et al.*, 1972; Niewiarowski *et al.*, 1975). Inhibition of these enzymes in blood is rather slow and is ascribed mainly to α_2-macroglobulin (Egberg, 1974). It could be achieved rapidly by adding specific antisera. Both are inhibited by dyflos — di-isopropyl fluorophosphate (Collins and Jones, 1972), which characterizes them as serine proteases. They are not inhibited by soy bean trypsin inhibitor nor by aprotinin. The enzymes are capable of hydrolysing some synthetic substrates with distinctly different specificity. Among chromogenic substrates, the most sensitive for ancrod is Tos-Gly-Pro-Arg-pNA (Chromozym TH, Penta-pharm) whereas for batroxobin H-D-Phe-Pip-Arg-pNA (S-2238, Kabi) (unpublished data).

Intravenous or subcutaneous administration of the thrombin-like enzymes in man results in a gradual decrease in plasma fibrinogen accompanied by the appearance of circulating soluble fibrin monomer complexes (SFMC). These complexes, as judged by measuring their titre with either ethanol or protamine sulphate gelation tests, appear in blood in large quantities at the initial stage of defibrination and disappear within some hours when the fibrinogen level reaches very low values (Latallo and Lopaciuk, 1973). Studies with radioactively labelled fibrinogen in man indicate that most radioactivity is retained in the spleen, some in the liver but not in lungs (Straub and Harder, 1971). Studies in dogs (Egberg, 1973) have shown that the glomerular filtration rate was not markedly affected by batroxobin and most radioactivity was excreted with urine. Only small amounts of fibrinogen-related material were found in liver and spleen.

A sharp rise in SFMC is immediately followed by the appearance of large amounts of fibrinogen degradation products (FDP) in patients' blood (Straub and Harder, 1971; Latallo and Lopaciuk, 1973) and it coincides with a marked fall in plasminogen. Although *in vitro* experiments exclude a possibility of direct activation of plasminogen by ancrod or batroxobin and no increased fibrinolytic activity can be detected in patients plasma, a secondary fibrinolytic reaction is apparently responsible for the massive production of FDP. This is well documented by the results of studies on plasminogen half-life and plasmin-antiplasmin complexes during treatment with batroxobin (Collen and Vermylen, 1973; Collen *et al.*, 1975).

As already mentioned, the defibrinating enzymes do not affect platelets directly. However, at the initial stage of treatment, a transient and moderate fall in platelet count could be observed. The platelets reappear in circulation within a few hours and their survival time remains normal (Latallo and Lopaciuk, 1973). Haemostatic function of platelets seems to be fully retained, perhaps due to the fact that the platelet fibrinogen is not affected by the enzymes. At least no change in batroxobin treated patients was observed (Lopaciuk *et al.*, 1975). It should be noted that administration of platelet inhibitors during defibrination greatly enhances bleeding tendency (Olson and Johnson, 1972).

Besides clotting and haemostatic function, fibrinogen plays an important role in haemorheology. Reduction of its concentration in blood results in decrease of blood and plasma viscosity and thus facilitates the blood flow. A rather sharp change in viscosity already becomes apparent at fibrinogen level below 100 mg% (Pitney and Regoeczi, 1970; Ehrly, 1973; Völker, 1975). This phenomenon is actually considered to play a major role in the treatment of cases with impaired peripheral circulation especially those due to the blockage of small arteries and capillaries.

The rate at which defibrination occurs depends on the amount of enzyme given and its route of administration. A state of deep hypofibrinogenaemia occurs within 6–10 h after i.v. injection of 1–2 units of either of the enzymes per kg body weight. It could be easily maintained for several days or even some weeks provided the dose is repeated at 12–24 h intervals. Adjustment of the dose of enzyme based on monitoring the fibrinogen content in patients' plasma allows one to obtain a desired degree of hypofibrinogenaemia.

From the above discussion it becomes apparent that the defibrinating enzymes could be applied in a variety of pathological states. Three major aims for their use however, could be identified:

(a) to prevent thrombus formation and/or propagation;
(b) to improve blood flow especially in capillaries and to thus increase tissue oxygenation;
(c) to enhance natural or iatrogenically (SK, UK) induced fibrinolytic or thrombolytic processes.

Hence, various groups of clinicians became interested and a considerable number of experimental studies on animal models as well as exploratory trials in man began. The number of patients already subjected to treatment with either ancrod or batroxobin could be presently estimated well above one thousand. An excellent and very comprehensive review on all aspects concerning the thrombin-like enzymes and their action was recently published by Stocker (1978).

The list of possible indications which were or still are under investigation is rather long and comprises such states as:

(1) peripheral arterial occlusions;
(2) deep-vein thrombosis with or without pulmonary embolism;
(3) prevention of rethrombosis following surgery or fibrinolytic therapy;
(4) central retinal vein thrombosis.
(5) myocardial infarction;
(6) coronary arterial stenoses;

(7)   sickle cell anaemia;
(8)   priapism;
(9)   anticoagulation and thrombosis prevention in venous surgery;
(10) extracorporeal haemodialysis;
(11) artifical heart-lung life support;
(12) transplant rejection.

The list presented above is not complete. One can imagine other possible indications. Most attention has been focussed on the first three groups of patients, peripheral vascular obstruction, DVT and prevention of DVT. The treatment of the first group was primarily aimed at improving blood flow and tissue oxygenation and, therefore, the treatment schedules were such as to obtain a rather moderate state of hypofibrinogenaemia (usually in the range of 60–100 mg of plasma fibrinogen). The results were rather favourable but not in all studies. Tilsner (1975) compared heparin and ancrod in their efficacy at relieving rest pain in patients with arterial occlusions stage 3 to 4 (according to Fontaine). The treatment was successful in 29 out of 41 ancrod patients and only two out of 25 of heparin cases. Double-blind clinical trials with batroxobin and placebo in 20 patients suffering from intermittent claudication (Martin et al., 1975) however, did not show significant difference. The cases submitted for it were at an earlier Fontaine stage and doses of batroxobin rather low. A study of Meissner et al. (1977) clearly indicates that a highly significant improvement of the muscle rest blood flow is achieved with batroxobin treatment in patients at the third to fourth stage of the Fontaine scale. Their unpublished results indicate not only fast but a surprisingly long-lasting relief of the rest pain in these cases.

Treatment of DVT needs induction of more pronounced hypofibrinogenaemia (0–60 mg% of plasma fibrinogen) since its aim, at least in part, is halting the thrombus growth. The impression one gets from reviewing the available data is that the treatment is less effective than thrombolytic therapy, but less dangerous in respect of bleeding and other complications (Tibbutt et al., 1974). The therapy with ancrod also had fewer side-effects than with heparin (Kakkar et al., 1969; Davies et al., 1972). It might become a procedure of choice in patients with contraindications to thrombolytic therapy. A combined treatment with batroxobin and SK (Latallo and Lopaciuk, 1973; Latallo et al., 1975) should be potentially most effective but involves a high risk of bleeding and needs further studies.

An important field of application concerns the use of ancrod or batroxobin as a follow-up to thrombolytic therapy (Lopaciuk et al., 1975). Although Tibbutt et al., (1977) did not find any advantages in this procedure over conventional oral anticoagulant therapy in a controlled trial on 26 patients, this regimen should be taken into consideration for patients with a high risk of rethrombosis and in those with incomplete thrombolysis.

Prevention of DVT in high-risk patients, especially after surgery, has been recently dominated by subcutaneous treatment with heparin. There still remain some areas where neither heparin nor other drugs show a prophylactic effect, e.g. high incidence of DVT and pulmonary embolism after hip fracture. A recent randomized double-blind study of Lowe et al. (1978) on 105 patients comparing ancrod with placebo has shown a highly significant prophylactic effect of the enzyme with a P value of less than 0.001 for major and bilateral DVT. Five days' treatment with a daily dose of 280 units of ancrod subcutaneously starting on the day of operation was carried out. An extensive review of these and other studies on above listed indications with a list of references can be found in Stocker's (1978) article.

One of the major problems in the study of any new drug is obviously the safety of its applications. A retrospective study has been started on this subject by the Task Force on Clinical Use of Snake Venom Enzymes of the International Committee on Thrombosis and Haemostasis in 1976. The study was still in progress at the time of this symposium. There have been 587 questionnaires collected from ten participating centres. Preliminary analysis of the first 210 patients (Latallo, 1978) indicate that application of ancrod or batroxobin involves very small risk of bleeding complications provided it is not combined with thrombolytic therapy and the contraindications are taken into account.

The tentative list of contraindications consists of the following:

Congenital or acquired abnormalities of the clotting and haemostatic system, it also includes continuous treatment with oral anticoagulants and potent anti-aggregating agents.

Treatment with inhibitors of fibrinolysis or with dextran within last 24 h.

Presence of active lesions in the gastrointestinal, genito-urinary or respiratory tract.

Cerebral insufficiency or evidence of a lesion associated with a risk of intra-cranial haemorrhage.

Minor surgical procedures which could provide a source of occult bleeding (e.g. liver or renal biopsy, artery punctures etc.) within 7 days.

Major surgical procedures within last 7 days.

Implantation of artificial artery prosthesis within last 4 months or other arterial surgery within last 14 days.

Suspected dissecting aortic aneurysm.

Liver or renal insufficiency of a severe degree.

Bacterial endocarditis.

Endotoxaemia.

Pregnancy at any stage, post-partum period of not less than 5 days.

These contraindications concern treatment aimed at obtaining very low fibrinogen levels (0 – 60 mg%). Most of them do not have to be applied when the purpose of therapy is to increase blood flow. Analysis of the data collected up to now also shows that in spite of the fact that the potency of the two enzymes is expressed in different units, equivalent doses of either result in lowering fibrinogen in plasma to a similar level.

Resistance to treatment occurs usually after 4 – 6 weeks of administration but does not involve any overt clinical manifestations, except increase in fibrinogen content. According to Vinazzer (1975), the half-life of the antibody to ancrod is 97 days. Patients resistant to ancrod could be defibrinated by batroxobin and vice versa. Side-effects are rare, consisting mainly of local skin irritation, skin rash was observed in four, fever reaction in six, migraine in nine and general shock in two out of 587 cases analysed.

In conclusion, the thrombin-like enzymes ancrod and batroxobin, due to their specific ability for selective removal of fibrinogen from circulating blood, certainly have great potential. At present, these drugs appear to be relatively safe. Their beneficial action has been observed in a variety of pathological states but there is still lack of a solid proof of their efficacy. The only exemption is perhaps their prophylactic effect against DVT after fracture of femoral neck surgery (Lowe *et al.*, 1977). Still, the list of indications is open and the need for randomized controlled clinical trials is urgent.

REFERENCES

Barlow, G. H., Lewis, L. J., Finley, R., Martin, D. and Stocker, K. (1973). *Thrombos. Res.* **2**, 17–22.
Brown, C. H., Bell, W. R., Shreiner, D. P. and Jackson, D. P. (1972). *J. Lab. Clin. Med.* **79**, 758–769.
Collen, D., De Cock, F. and Verstraete, M. (1975). Symposium on Thrombin-like Enzymes. Abstract. July 15–17, Trier.
Collen, D. and Vermylen, J. (1973). *Thrombos. Res.* **2**, 239–250.
Collins, J. P. and Jones, J. G. (1972). *Europ. J. Biochem.* **26**, 510–517.
Davis, J. A., Merrick, M. V., Sharp, A. A. and Holt, J. M. (1972). *Lancet* **1**, 113.
Egberg, N. (1973). *Acta. phys. scand.* Suppl. 400.
Egberg, N. (1974). *Thrombos. Res.* **4**, 35–53.
Ehrly, M. (1973). *Herz Kreisl.* **5**, 135.
Esnouf, M. P. and Tunnah, G. W. (1967). *Br. J. Haemat.* **13**, 581–590.
Gaffney, P. I. and Brasher, M. (1974). *Nature (Lond.)* **251**, 53–54.
Ghitis, J. and Bonelli, V. (1963). *Ann. Intern. Med.* **59**, 737.
Kakkar, V. V., Flanc, C., Howe, C. T., O'Shea, M. and Flute, P. T. (1969). *Br. Med. J.* **1**, 806–810.
Latallo, Z. S. (1978). *Thrombos. Haemost.* **39**, 768–774.
Latallo, Z. S., Lopaciuk, S. and Meissner, J. (1975). *In* "Defibrinierung mit thrombinähnlichen Schlangengiftenzymen" (M. Martin and W. Schoop, Eds), 181, Huber, Bern-Stuttgart-Wien.
Latallo, Z. S., Lopaciuk, S. (1973). *Thrombos. Diathes. Haemorrh.* Suppl. 56, 253–255.
Lopaciuk, S., Meissner, J., Ziemski, J. M. and Latallo, Z. S. (1975). *In* "Defibrinierung mit thrombinähnlichen Schlangengiftenzymen" (M. Martin and W. Schoop, Eds) 191–199. Huber, Bern-Stuttgart-Wien.
Lowe, G.D.O., Campbell, A. F., Meek, D. R., Forbes, C. D., Prentice, C.R.M. and Cummings, S. W. (1978). *Lancet* **2**, 698–700.
Meissner, J. A., Karpowicz, M. and Konopka, L. (1977). *XII Congr. Warsaw. Europ. Surg. Res.* **9**, Abstract. Suppl. 1, 111.
Niewiarowski, S., Stewart, G. J., Nath, N., Sha, A. T. and Liebermann, G. E. (1975). *Am. J. Physiol.* **229**, 737–741.
Olson, P. and Johnson, H. (1972). *Thrombos. Res.* **1**, 135–146.
Pitney, W. R. and Regoeczi, B. (1970). *Br. J. Haemat.* **19**, 67–81.
Reid, H. A. and Thean, P. C. (1963). *Lancet* **1**, 621.
Stocker, K. (1978). *In* "Handbook of Experimental Pharmacology", Vol. 46, Fibrinolytics and Antifibrinolytics (F. Markwardt, Ed.), 451–484.
Tibbutt, D. A., Williams, E. W., Walker, M. W., Chesferman, D. N., Holt, J. M. and Sharp, A. A. (1974). *Br. J. Haematology* **27** 407–414.

Tibbutt, D. A., Chesfermann, C. N., Williams, E. W., Faulkner, T. and Sharp, A. A. (1977). *Thromb. Haemost.* 37, 222–232.

Tilsner, V. *In* "Defibrinierung mit Thrombinähnlichen Schlangengiftenzymes". (M. Martin and W. Schoop, Eds) 225–230 Huber, Bern-Stuttgart-Wien.

Vinazzer, H. (1975). "Symposium on Thrombin-like Enzymes", Abstract. July 15–17, Trier.

THE ROLE OF DEFIBRINATING AGENTS IN THE TREATMENT OF VASCULAR DISORDERS

C. R. M. Prentice, G. D. O. Lowe, J. J. F. Belch and C. D. Forbes

University Department of Medicine, Royal Infirmary, Glasgow, Scotland

The main action of ancrod and defibrase is to reduce the plasma fibrinogen level. The clinical relevance of this was noted by Reid and Chan (1968), who observed that patients in Malaya bitten by *Agkistrodon rhodostoma* had non-clotting blood due to total depletion of fibrinogen, but suffered no major haemorrhagic complications. This least observation must be qualified since defibrinated patients do undergo an increased risk of haemorrhage, although this is not common. Ancrod and defibrase cause defibrination by splitting Arg-Gly bonds of the A α-chain of fibrinogen leading to release of fibrinopeptide A, but not fibrinopeptide B (Holleman and Coen, 1970). The des A-fibrin so formed is less robust in structure compared to thrombin-formed fibrin (Kwaan and Grumet, 1975) and is more susceptible to fibrinolysis (Turpie *et al.*, 1971; Kwaan and Barlow, 1971).

Although ancrod and defibrase are not direct plasminogen activators, the fibrin formed by them undergoes rapid proteolysis for form FDP. These have a structure identical to plasmin-formed FDP, suggesting that destruction of this fibrin is mediated by plasmin (Prentice *et al.*, 1974). Although the precise mechanism of secondary fibrinolysis is not well understood, the depletion of plasminogen (Turpie *et al.*, 1971) and increased turnover of plasminogen (Collen and Vermylen, 1973), together with fast antiplasmin depletion, confirm that plasminogen activation has taken place.

Serono Symposium No. 37, "Vascular Occlusion: Epidemiological, Pathophysiological and Therapeutic Aspects", edited by M. Tesi and J. Dormandy, 1981. Academic Press, London and New York.

EFFECT ON VISCOSITY

Fibrinogen is a major determinant of plasma viscosity (Wells *et al.*, 1964). The defibrinating enzymes cause depletion of plasma fibrinogen with consequent reduction in plasma and blood viscosity (Ehrly, 1972) and reduction in red cell tendencies to aggregate (Schmid-Schönbein *et al.*, 1978). Reduction in blood viscosity leads to increased blood flow, which may be important in tissues rendered ischaemic secondary to vascular stenosis or obliteration. Additionally, high fibrinogen and viscosity values may increase the risk in a patient having surgery of post-operative deep vein thrombosis (Dormandy and Edelman, 1973).

It can thus be seen that the defibrinating agents produce a variety of haemostatic changes, summarized in Table I, which may produce a substantial anti-thrombotic effect, affecting platelet behaviour as well as the coagulation and fibrinolytic enzyme systems.

Table I.   Anti-thrombotic actions of ancrod.

(1)	*Reduces fibrinogen level causing*:
	(a) Decrease in plasma and whole blood viscosity especially at low shear rates.
	(b) Decrease in the quantity of fibrin laid down in thrombus.
	(c) Decrease in circulating platelet aggregates.
	(d) Reduction in red cell aggregation.
(2)	*Increases F.D.P. levels causing*:
	(a) Impaired fibrin polymerization.
	(b) Reduced platelet aggregation.
(3)	*Facilitates fibrinolysis causing*:
	(a) Reduced level of alpha-2 antiplasmin.
	(b) Enhancement of cation of streptokinase or urokinase.

CLINICAL PHARMACOLOGY

The clinical pharmacology of defibrinating agents has been well reviewed by Stocker (1978). Ancrod and reptilase must be given parenterally, either by the intravenous or subcutaneous routes. The elimination of ancrod following i.v. administration into rabbits is a multi-exponential function, with an initial phase half-life of 3–5 hours, and a later slower phase half-life of 9–12 days, at which time some 6–10% of the enzyme remains (Regoeczi and Bell, 1969). Ancrod binds to α 2-macroglobulin which is responsible for major inactivation of the enzyme (Egberg, 1974). The dose of ancrod depends on the rate at which it is wished to cause defibrination. When administered by the i.v. route, a dose of 2–4 units/kg. body weight can be given over the first 12 h, followed by 1–2 units/kg. b.w. every 12 h thereafter. Doses subsequent to the initial one can be given by bolus injection, since there is not the danger of causing massive fibrin formation in the presence of a high fibrinogen substrate.

Subcutaneous injection of ancrod can be initiated by a dose varying from 2-4 units /kg b.w. over the first 24 h, followed by 1-2 units/kg b.w. daily (Lowe *et al.*, 1978b). This method causes fibrinogen to fall to a mean of about 50-80 mg fibrinogen per 100 ml of plasma. Clearly, at this level of fibrinogen, there is less danger of haemorrhage than during total defibrination.

Monitoring of ancrod or reptilase dosage is carried out by a simple clot observation test, as described by Reid *et al.* (1963), or by rapid estimation of clottable fibrinogen such as by the method of Clauss (1957). The danger of haemorrhage is only appreciable in the "no-clot" situation indicating substantial fibrinogen depletion, and even in this case dangerous haemorrhage is not often seen, although substantial bruising may occur.

CLINICAL ASPECTS

Defibrination therapy can be divided into treatment of arterial and venous disorders.

Arterial Disorders

Peripheral Arterial Disease
The reduction in plasma and blood viscosity caused by defibrination leads to increased blood pressure and flow in the legs of patients with peripheral arterial disease (Ehrly and Schroeder, 1977; Dormandy *et al.*, 1977; Lowe *et al.*, 1979). Two different categories of patients with peripheral arterial disease who have been studied are those with ischaemic rest pain (Fontaine's Stage III) and those with severe intermittent claudication.

Ischaemic rest pain. Two trials of ancrod in patients with ischaemic rest pain showed benefit and in the second study, patients with rest pain preferred ancrod to Ronicol in a cumulative sequential analysis study (Wolf *et al.*, 1975; Wolf, 1976). Numerous publications testify to a beneficial effect of therapeutic defibrination in hypoxic ischaemia. The clinical end-points have been avoidance of surgical amputation or, if amputation becomes necessary, limitation of tissue removal to a smaller area than would otherwise have been necessary (Ehrly, 1975). However, these trials have not been controlled and so it is difficult to discount the beneficial effects of a period of in-hospital treatment with bed rest.

We have recently carried out a double-blind controlled study of i.v. ancrod *vs* saline placebo in patients with rest pain, which is reported by Dr Lowe in this book (Lowe *et al.*, p.133). In brief, there was no significant difference in benefit between the ancrod and saline-treated patients as regards reduction of pain or avoidance of subsequent surgical measures. The most interesting finding was a 50% improvement of pain in the saline treated patients, as well as in the ancrod patients. This major placebo effect must not be underestimated in patients having therapy for peripheral arterial disease.

Intermittent claudication. Intermittent claudication is a notoriously difficult condition to study since the symptoms fluctuate widely over the weeks or even days. The early reports of defibrination therapy showed clinical benefit in patients with intermittent claudication, and Dormandy *et al.* (1977) also claimed that ancrod was effective in an uncontrolled study. However, a double-blind controlled study by Martin *et al.* (1976) with batroxobin showed no difference in patients with intermittent claudication with respect to both the walking distance or post-stenotic pressure.

Ischaemic Heart Disease

There have been no substantial trials on the use of ancrod for the treatment of myocardial infarction. Leube *et al.* (1972) allocated 60 patients with acute myocardial infarction into two groups receiving heparin or ancrod. There was no significant difference in the mortality rate of about 18% at 40 days. However, the small scale of this study is insufficient to test any treatment in acute myocardial infarction. A trial of subcutaneous ancrod *vs* placebo in patients with crescendo angina pectoris showed significantly greater benefit, as judged by reduction of glyceryl trinitrate, from ancrod (Leube and Sondern, 1975). In view of the recent study which showed that streptokinase had a beneficial effect on mortality at six weeks in the treatment of acute myocardial infarction (European Co-operative study, 1979), perhaps the role of ancrod in myocardial infarctions should be reassessed. One of the major effects of streptokinase in this study was to reduce fibrinogen levels to a mean of 50 mg/ml and it was perhaps this fibrinogen lowering effect which was responsible for the benefit. Ancrod or batroxobin may be able to achieve the same results at a lower cost.

Venous Disorders

Deep Vein Thrombosis

Established deep vein thrombosis. Three trials have shown that heparin and ancrod appear to be equally effective as an anticoagulant for the treatment of deep vein thrombosis but both heparin and ancrod are less effective than streptokinase in restoring venographic patency to the circulation (Kakkar *et al.*, 1969; Tibbutt *et al.*, 1974; and Davies *et al.*, 1972). The results of these three trials suggested than ancrod might be more easy to administer than heparin. The study of Tibbutt *et al.* (1974) provided the curious information that although streptokinase caused substantial lysis as assessed by venography, the clinical results of treatment by either streptokinase or ancrod were equal when assessed three months after treatment. This point needs further investigation. Additionally, Davies *et al.* (1972) found that there were complications in only three of sixteen patients treated with ancrod compared with seventeen of the streptokinase-treated patients.

Deep vein thrombosis prophylaxis. Many anticoagulants have been used for the prophylaxis of deep vein thrombosis post-operatively or in hospital conditions where the patient is immobile. Of these, the regimen of low dose subcutaneous heparin has been most widely studied and used, and one could well ask why another prophylactic agent should be tested. One condition where the current anticoagulants have failed is in fractured neck of femur patients who are notoriously prone to thromboembolic complications post-operatively. We think that a regimen of subcutaneous ancrod for prophylaxis following fractured neck of femur repair might be useful because the reduction in circulating fibrinogen will cause limitation of thrombus growth. There is additionally a logistic advantage in that a daily subcutaneous injection of ancrod given for 3-4 days post-operatively will provide significant lowering of the fibrinogen level to 100 mg% or less for 8-10 days post-operatively.

This should be compared with the 20 or 30 injections of subcutaneous heparin to be given to every patient on heparin prophylaxis. In a dose-ranging trial, Lowe *et al.* (1978b) compared 14 control patients with 28 patients treated with one of four low dose subcutaneous ancrod regimens. In all groups of patients given ancrod, there was a significant fall in fibrinogen and also a lowering of plasma and blood viscosity by 10-15%. We have now completed a clinical trial in fractured neck of femur patients to assess its value (Lowe *et al.*, 1978b). In this study, there was significantly less extensive deep vein thrombosis in the ancrod treated patients than the controls. We are currently studying a similar regimen of subcutaneous ancrod for the prevention of deep vein thrombosis after replacement hip surgery.

Other indications for defibrinating agents. There is a possibility that ancrod might be useful in renal diseases, such as some types of glomerulonephritis or transplanted kidneys undergoing rejection, where fibrin deposition is a problem. In a study of experimental glomerulonephritis in rabbits (induced by injections of bovine serum albumin) Naish and Peters (1974) found that rabbits pre-treated with ancrod had significantly better results than the control animals. This was assessed by mortality, improvement in the renal function and the amount of fibrin seen histologically within the glomeruli when the animals were sacrificed.

The use of ancrod or batroxobin in a variety of other conditions where fibrin formation may cause adverse effects is being studied. These conditions include central retinal vein thrombosis, priapism, stickle-cell anaemia, prevention of rethrombosis following surgery or fibrinolytic therapy and extra corporeal circulations.

Ancrod may be useful when used in combination with thrombolytic agents. Ancrod, by causing defibrination, might augment the action of plasminogen activators such as streptokinase or urokinase as the level of fibrinogen, a competitive substrate with fibrin for the action of plasmin, would be reduced within the circulation. We have carried out a small dose-ranging study in this field (Forbes *et al.*, 1976) and found that ancrod could be given in combination with streptokinase without haemorrhagic complications.

CONCLUSIONS

I have tried to outline the areas where ancrod and batroxobin may have potential as an antithrombic agent. The drugs are promising in some fields and, at the laboratory level, are interesting agents with a potent pharmacological action. At present, there are no definite indications for these drugs, although their extensive use for patients with arterial disease means that further controlled appraisal is required here. In the treatment of established deep vein thrombosis, these drugs appear to be as effective as heparin and safer. In the prophylaxis of deep vein thrombosis, the drugs merit further investigation, particularly in the field of orthopaedic surgery.

REFERENCES

Clauss, A. (1957). *Acta Haematologie.* **17**, 237.
Collen, D. and Vermylen, J. (1973). *Thrombosis Research.* **2**, 239.
Davies, J. A., Merrick, M. V., Sharp, A. A. and Holt, J. M. (1972). *Lancet* **1**, 113.
Dormandy, J. A. and Edelman, J. B. (1973). *British Journal of Surgery.* **60**, 187.
Dormandy, J. A., Goyle, K. B., and Reid, H. L. (1977). *Lancet* **2**, 625.
Egberg, N. (1974). *Thrombosis Research.* **4**, 35.
Ehrly, A. M. (1972). *Biorheology* **9**, 151.
Ehrly, A. M. (1975). *Folia Angiologica* **23**, 377.
Ehrly, A. M. and Schroeder, W. (1977). *Angiology* **28**, 101
European Co-operative Study Group for streptokinase treatment in acute myocardial infarction (1979). *New England Journal of Medicine.* **301**, 797.
Forbes, C. D., Barbenel, J. and Prentice, C. R. M. (1976). *Haemostasis* **5**, 348.
Holleman, W. H. and Coen, L. J. (1970). *Biochimica et Biophysica Acta* **200**, 587.
Kakkar, V. V., Flanc, C. Howe, C. T., O'Shea, M. J. and Flute, P. T. (1969). *British Medical Journal* **1**, 806.
Kwaan, H. C. and Barlow, G. H. (1971). *Thrombosis Diathesis Haemorrhagica Supplement* **47**, 361.
Kwaan, H. C. and Grumet, G. N. (1975). *In* "Thromboembolism" (A. N. Nicolaides, ed.) 251. Medical and Technical Publishing Company, Lancaster.
Leube, G., Kuhn, J. J. and Hartert, H. (1972). *Medizinische Welt* **23**, 601.
Leube, G. and Sondern, W. (1975). *Folia Angiololica* **23**, 411.
Lowe, G. D. O., Campbell, A. F., Meek, D. R., Forbes, C. D., Prentice, C. R. M. and Cummings, S. W. (1978a). *Lancet* **2**, 698.
Lowe, G. D. O., Morrice, J. J., Fulton, A., Forbes, C. D., Prentice, C. R. M. and Barbenel, (1978b) *Thrombosis and Haemostasis* **40**, 134.
Lowe, G. D. O., Forbes, C. D., Dunlop, D., Lawson, D. H., Pollock, J. G., Prentice, C. R. M. and Drummond, M. M. (1980) (in press). *Angiology.*
Lowe, G. D. O., Morrice, J. J., Forbes, C. D., Prentice, C. R. M., Fulton, A. J. and Barbenel, J. (1979). *Angiology.* **30**, 594.
Martin, M., Hirdes, E., and Auel, H. (1976). *Thrombosis Research.* **9**, 47.
Naish, P. F. and Peters, D. K. (1974). *Clinical Science and Molecular Medicine.* **46**, 16.
Prentice, C. R. M., Edgar, W. and McNicol, G. P. (1974). *British Journal of Haematology.* **27**, 77.
Regoeczi, E. and Bell, W. R. (1969). *British Journal of Haematology.* **16**, 573.
Reid, H. A., Chan, K. E. and Thean, P. C. (1963). *Lancet* **1**, 621.
Reid, H. A. and Chan, K. E. (1968). *Lancet* **1**, 485.
Schmid-Schönbein, H., Weiss, J., Volgar, E., Klose, H. J., and Malotta, H. (1978). *Zeitschrift fur Allgemeinmedizin (Stuttgart)* **54**, 1635.
Stocker, K. (1978). *In* "Fibrinolytics and anti-fibrinolytics" (F. Markwardt, ed.) 451. Springer-Verlag.
Tibbutt, D. A., Williams, E. W., Walker, M. W., Chesterman, C. N., Holt, J. M. and Sharp, A. A. (1974). *British Journal of Haematology* **27**, 407.
Turpie, A. G. G., Prentice, C. R. M., McNicol, G. P. and Douglas, A. S. (1971). *British Journal of Haematology* **20**, 217.
Wells, R. E., Gaweonski, T. H., Cox, P. J. and Perera, R. D. (1964). *American Journal of Physiology* **207**, 1035.
Wolf, G. K., Vinazzer, H. and Tilsner, V. (1975). *Folia Angiologica* **23**, 391.
Wolf, G. K. (1976). *European Journal of Clinical Pharmacology* **9**, 387.

PREVENTION OF COMPLICATIONS IN ATHEROSCLEROTIC
OCCLUSIONS OF LOWER EXTREMITIES

J. Linhart, J. Spáčil and A. Broulíková

Institute for Clinical and Experimental Medicine, Prague, Czechoslovakia

INTRODUCTION

Long-lasting ischemic disease of lower extremities may cause various complications. However, those complications resulting from advanced ischemia of the foot, such as ischemic rest pain and/or necrosis, are most dangerous and may bring about loss of the limb. Therefore, therapeutic measures capable of increasing blood flow to the ischemic foot were analysed.

METHODS

In all, one hundred consecutive patients aged 53 ± 12 years were examined. They suffered from chronic ischemia of lower extremities due to arterial obliterations. The diagnosis was made by angiography or physical non-invasive examination based on history, palpation, positional test and Doppler ultrasound measurements. Blood flow through the foot was measured by venous occlusion plethysmography using a mechanical water-filled instrument with water temperature of 32 °C. Skin capillary flow in the foot was measured using I-131 clearance. A treadmill was employed to assess constant walking speed of 2 km/h in the observations concerning the effect of muscular exercise on peripheral hemodynamics. There was partial overlapping of patients in the individual subgroups.

Serono Symposium No. 37, "Vascular Occlusion: Epidemiological, Pathophysiological and Therapeutic Aspects", edited by M. Tesi and J. Dormandy, 1981. Academic Press, London and New York.

RESULTS AND DISCUSSION

Intravenous infusions containing procaine, tolazoline and nicotinic acid were in all applied to 52 patients covered with blankets, so as to prevent dissipation of heat (Linhart, *et al.*, 1974). Calculated local vascular resistance in the foot decreased and there was a significant increase in total foot blood flow as well as in subcutaneous capillary flow by 42% and 36%, respectively ($P < 0.001$ in both instances) (Fig. 1). It is thus evident that the vasodilator infusions may be of value in the treatment of patients with advanced ischemia of the foot who are not suitable candidates for reconstructive surgery.

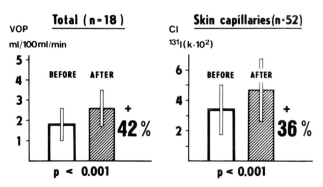

Fig. 1. The effect of infusion of vasodilator drugs on total blood flow (left) and skin capillary flow (right) in the foot in patients with peripheral arterial occlusions.

It has been established that isometric handgrip increases systemic blood pressure. In addition, our observations have shown that ankle blood pressure distal to arterial occlusion rises in proportion to the increase in systemic pressure (Spáčil and Linhart, 1978). An elevation of foot blood flow by 32% ($P < 0.001$) has been demonstrated in 11 patients during the pressure reaction. However, the possible therapeutic effect of the procedure has not yet been clarified.

In 16 patients with advanced foot ischemia, walking slowly at a speed of 2 km/h, we have observed an increase in capillary blood flow through the instep skin by 110% ($P < 0.001$) as compared to the recumbent posture (Spáčil *et al.*, 1976). This may in part be explained by concomitant pressure changes. In the standing subject, peripheral arterial and venous pressure increases as a result of the hydrostatic forces. With the slow walking speed, arterial blood pressure distal to the occlusion changes only slightly, whereas venous pressure drops due to the action of muscle pump. The high arteriovenous pressure difference contributes to better perfusion of the tissues. Thus, slow walking is a suitable type of exercise treatment for many patients with advanced foot ischemia or even circumscript tissue necrosis.

In addition to other procedures, the above therapeutic principles were employed in a long-term control program. All 100 patients were periodically invited for check-ups once in 4–6 months, even if their condition was stabilized or if they were asymptomatic. The investigation included clinical examination,

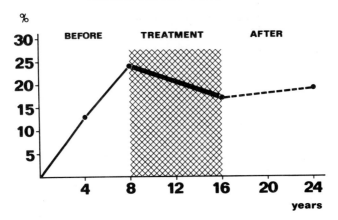

Fig. 2. The percentage of ischemic skin complications in 100 patients before treatment, during the long-term control program (treatment) and after its termination.

positional test of vascular function and control of biochemical parameters. Therapy was adjusted according to the findings. Moreover, the patients were encouraged to visit our department for immediate treatment in case of complications such as abrupt decrease in walking distance, inflammatory changes or accidental traumatic lesion.

During the spontaneous course of the disease in the pre-treatment period of 8 years, the percentage of ischemic skin complications increased with time (Fig. 2). When the program was started, the percentage curve changed abruptly so that during the 8 years of the program complications developed only in 19 patients and healed rapidly in all but one diabetic subject in whom bilateral amputation was necessary. Eight years after termination of the program, questionnaire information could only be obtained from 30 patients. It suggested that the local findings in the extremities remained satisfactory while 50% of the respondents had evidence of ischemic heart disease.

CONCLUSIONS

Total and capillary foot blood flow can be increased by infusions of vasodilator substances. Walking at a speed of 2 km/h also increases capillary blood flow in the ischemic foot skin. Both procedures are of definite clinical value whereas the therapeutic position of the handgrip-induced hypertension with concomitant increase in foot flow remains unclear.

A long-term control program employing the above measures was instituted in 100 patients for 8 years. As a result, 81% patients remained free of skin ischemia, and 18 of 19 subjects with ischemic skin complications healed rapidly. It is concluded that with rational approach a great number of patients can be maintained in a satisfactory condition for long periods of time.

REFERENCES

Linhart, J., Frič, M. and Spáčil, J. (1974). *Angiologia III*, 65–68.
Spáčil, J., Hlavová, A., Linhart, J. and Přerovský, I. (1976). *VASA* 5, 323–328.
Spáčil, J. and Linhart, J. (1978). *VASA* 7, 131–137.

THE EFFECT OF ANTI-AGGREGATING DRUGS ON PATENCY OF SUBSTITUTES IN ARTERIAL SYSTEM

J. Pirk, V. Ružbarský, J. König, M. Krajíček, P. Pavel and P. Firt

Institute for Clinical and Experimental Medicine Surgical Department, Prague, Czechoslovakia

INTRODUCTION

In recent years, research in vascular surgery has increasingly concentrated on the possibility of reconstructing small arteries with low-flow rates. Almost 100% of synthetic grafts with a diameter less than 5 mm and a correspondingly low blood flow rate become occluded in the early post-operative stage. Therefore, the best material for these reconstructions are still vein autografts. However, even veins are subject to changes, often called subendothelial proliferation, which lead to a progressive narrowing of the arterial lumen and late occlusions in some of these reconstructions.

The results of our earlier experiments (Pirk, *et al.*, 1978) support the hypothesis that the underlying mechanism of subendothelial proliferation is platelet aggregation on the inner, surgically damaged, surface of the vein graft. Thrombosis is a cause of early occlusion of synthetic grafts. If our hypothesis about subendothelial proliferation holds true, its development could be inhibited by reducing the tendency of blood platelets to aggregate with anti-aggregating drugs.

Serono Symposium No. 37, "Vascular Occlusion: Epidemiological, Pathophysiological and Therapeutic Aspects", edited by M. Tesi and J. Dormandy, 1981. Academic Press, London and New York.

MATERIAL AND METHODS

A bilateral aorto-iliac bypass was constructed in 17 mongrel dogs of either sex and weighing 30 kg. An autologous jugular vein was used on one side and a Czechoslovak knit polyester prosthesis, 4 mm in diameter, on the opposite side. Their lengths ranged between 10 and 12 cm with all anastamoses constructed end-to-side. To approximate the blood flow to that of an aortocoronary bypass, we diminished the lumen of external pelvic arteries by ligation 2 cm distal to the peripheral anastomosis. Blood flow and pressure were recorded in all bypass reconstructions. The dogs were divided into three groups depending on medication

Group 1: 6 dogs – controls without medication.
Group 2: 5 dogs – medication, 250 mg acetylsalicylic acid (ASA) 3 times daily, was started 3 days pre-operatively and continued throughout the experiment.
Group 3: 6 dogs – received the following mixture: 250 mg ASA, 75 mg dipyridamole, 5 drops DH ergotoxine (1 mg/ml) and 20 mg papaverine twice a day. This medication was started 3 days pre-operatively and continued throughout the experiment.

Table I. The initial values of flow (ml/min) and blood pressure (mmHg).

Group	1	2	3
Veins	58.3	52.5	57.5
Prosthesis	63.7	50.0	52.5
Pressure	129.1	130.0	124.1

Table II. The results of control arteriography.

Group	1	2	3
Vein patent	4	4	5
Vein occluded	2	1	1
Prothesis patent	0	1	5
Prothesis occluded	6	4	1

RESULTS

The initial values of blood pressure and flow are given in Table I. The values for vein and synthetic grafts showed no significant differences within each group or between separate groups. Control arteriography was performed a week after the operations; its results appear in Table II. Despite the low number of dogs, the different patency of synthetic grafts in groups 1 and 3 is significant. The dogs were killed after 12 weeks and samples taken for histology.

In the control group, all synthetic grafts became occluded by fibrous tissue, whose formation seems to have been caused by thrombus organization. The lumen of the vein grafts was distinctly diminished due to mural thrombus organization and subendothelial proliferation. Group 2, given ASA, exhibited only one patent synthetic graft in which the healing process was associated with abundant cellular growth and a low fibrous pseudo-intima without endothelial cover. The findings in the occluded synthetic grafts of group 2 and controls were alike. The vein grafts showed a low, and in places focal, endothelial proliferation. Mural thrombosis, if present, was lower than in controls and had a focal pattern, i.e. it did not occur along the whole course of the graft. Group 3, given the anti-aggregating mixture, was characterized by a low or absent subendothelial proliferation without thrombosis in vein grafts.

DISCUSSION

Our experiments confirmed the well-known fact that vein autografts continue to be the best material for arterial reconstructions in low-flow areas. They also suggest that the results of bypass reconstructions in low-flow areas could be improved by drugs inhibiting mural thrombosis, and reducing or preventing platelet adhesion and aggregation.

The antiaggregating effect of ASA has been known for years. Great amounts are needed for inducing its antiaggregating effect. Folts reports to have given dogs 35 mg/kg b.w. (Folts *et al.*, 1976), which corresponds to 2 - 3 g in man. Our results in group 2, where the dogs received only 25 mg/kg of ASA, agreed with their reported observations. There was only one patent prosthesis. Moschos demonstrated that ASA and dipyridamole possess antiaggregating effects when given separately, but when combined, the same effect could be induced by much lower doses (Moschos *et al.*, 1972). In view of this potential, we decided to add papaverine and DH-ergotoxine, whose antiaggregating effect has thus far been documented only *in vitro* (Švehla, 1968). We also chose these drugs for their beneficial effect on the cardiovascular system.

Despite the low number of dogs, the different patency of synthetic grafts in groups 1 and 3 is significant. The situation is somewhat different in vein reconstructions, in which the antiaggregating compounds have no effect on their early post-operative patency. This is because flow values of about 40 ml/min are considered a critical limit. On the other hand, the activity of antiaggregating medication would manifest itself only at flow rates below this limit. Our flow rates ranged between 50 to 60 ml/min. Histological examination showed that ASA is capable of reducing mural vein thrombosis and subendothelial proliferation. This is probably due to a much less thrombogenic inner surface of the vein compared with synthetic grafts. Therefore, at lower flux rates, that antiaggregating effect of ASA alone is sufficient.

REFERENCES

Folts, J. D., Crowell, E. B. and Rowe, G. G. (1976) *Circulation* **54**, 365.

Moschos, Ch. B., Lahiri, K., Peter, A., Jesrani, M. U. and Regan T. J. (1972). *Am. Heart. J.* **84**, p. 525.

Pirk, J., Radevič, B., Ružbarský, V., Firt, P., and Hejhal, L. (1978). *Czechoslovak Medicine* **1**, 44.

Švehla, C. (1968). *Časopis lékařů českých* **107**, 93.

SECTION V
SURGICAL THERAPY

AORTIC JUXTARENAL OCCLUSIONS

G. Agrifoglio, G. B. Agus, P. Castelli and U. Tambussi

Institute of Vascular Surgery of the University of Milan, Italy

In recent years, a renewed interest has been placed on juxtarenal aortic occlusions as an indication of atherosclerotic disease (Courbier *et al.*, 1974; Faenza *et al.*, 1971; Frantz *et al.*, 1974; Frøysaker *et al.*, 1973; Hobson *et al.*, 1975; Kieffer; Liddicoat *et al.*, 1975; Malan and Ruberti, 1970; Nunn and Kamal, 1972; Starrett and Stoney, 1974).

In the past, their frequency has certainly been undervalued: this could explain the lack of larger reports on this matter. The terminology itself is changing originally defined as infrarenal aortic or high abdominal aortic obstruction, today different kinds of aortic obstruction are unified under the term "juxtarenal".

We divided the juxtarenal obstruction into five main types (Fig. 1).

Type A. The most frequent; the occlusion is placed across the aorta as a bar, just below the renal arteries.

Type B. A narrow segment of subrenal aorta is still patent thanks to lumbar collaterals.

Type C. The occlusion is infrarenal and can narrow one or both of the renal arteries.

Type D. The occlusion is suprarenal with total obstruction of a renal artery and a possible stenosis of the other.

Type E. The occlusion is subrenal with typical terminal aortic revascularization by the inferior mesenteric artery.

The starting point of thrombosis is in the distal aorta, which is seriously compromised, but its proximal extension is generally slow. However, even if patients in these conditions are asymptomatic for a relatively long time (Bergan and Trippel, 1963), the disease evolution is progressive and dramatic with a high

Serono Symposium No. 37, "Vascular Occlusion: Epidemiological, Pathophysiological and Therapeutic Aspects", edited by M. Tesi and J. Dormandy, 1981. Academic Press, London and New York.

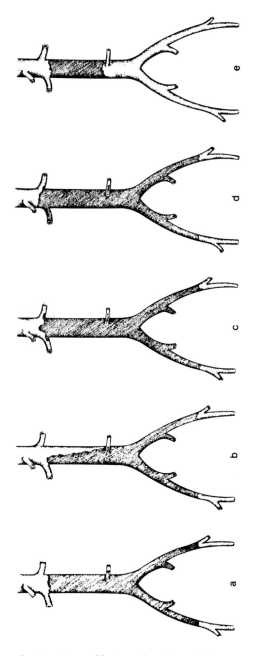

Fig. 1. Illustration of various types of juxtarenal aortic occlusions.

percentage of direct extensions of thrombosis to the visceral arteries (Bergan and Trippel, 1963; Hobson *et al.*, 1975).

SURGICAL TECHNIQUES

Three aspects of surgical technique have been pointed out recently: the method employed for renal protection from ischemia or embolization, the technique of thromboendarterectomy (TEA) on the juxtarenal aorta and the kind of aortotomy through which it is performed, the possible alternative of an *in situ* intervention and *remote bypass procedures*.

With regard to the protection of the kidneys, vascular clamps or tourniquets are placed on the renal arteries before the TEA of the supra- and infrarenal segment of aorta, in order to avoid an embolization of atheromatous or thrombotic material (Bergan and Trippel, 1963; Thurlbeck and Castlemen 1957). In addition, other common methods employed are suprarenal clamping limited to 25–30 min, osmotic diuresis by mannitol, hypothermia, pre-operative arterial pressure preservation and heparinization.

The method of performing the TEA, its extension and above all, the cleavage plane to employ, is a more complex matter. One problem is whether to perform a longitudinal or transverse aortotomy just below the renal arteries. The points of agreement between authors who practise one or other technique is reflected in our experience. It is governed by the clinical picture of obstruction verified angiographically and the intra-operative evaluation of the condition of the aortic wall and of the renal arteries by digital palpation. Furthermore, a pressure gradient of at least 25 mmHg (Constantini *et al.*, 1977) indicates the necessity of a direct intervention on the renal arteries.

In the occlusion of type A, where thrombosis is predominant, we perform a total transverse resection of the aorta about 2 cm below the renal arteries and beginning of an obliterated segment of aorta, in order to permit a better mobilization of the juxtarenal tract and an accurate suture of the distal aorta. The disobliteration generally can be performed by squeezing the obstructing thrombus. With intermittent flushing, any residual debris is removed from the aorta. Finally an end-to-end aortofemoral bypass is performed (Fig. 2).

In the occlusion of the other less frequent types generally the atherosclerotic lesions of the aortic wall are more important than in type A and may involve also the orifices of the visceral arteries. Therefore, we prefer to perform a longitudinal aortotomy from the level of the renal arteries; its lower extension is limited by any decision to perform disobliteration of the inferior mesenteric artery. The suprarenal aorta is clamped first. The TEA thus performed permits the removal of the lesions by the dissection of the right cleavage plane, avoiding the creation of intimal flaps in the renal arteries. Following completion of the suture of the proximal aortotomy, the clamp is moved under the renal arteries to perform the end-to-side anastomosis of the aortofemoral bypass (Fig. 3).

Remote bypass procedures have been used more recently as a possible alternative to the *in situ* intervention (Frantz *et al.*, 1974; Nunn and Kamal, 1972). It involves a bypass between the ascending or descending thoracic aorta and the iliac or femoral arteries. The aim is to avoid proximal anastomosis near a

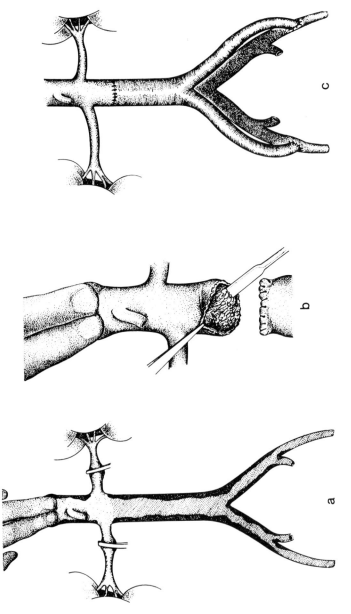

Fig. 2. Total transverse aortotomy utilized in dealing with Type A occlusions. Note renal clamping and subsequent end-to-end aortofemoral bypass.

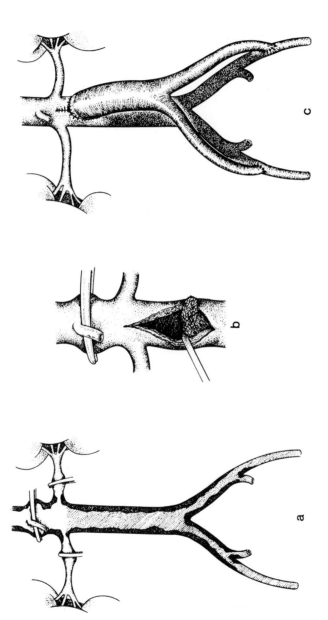

Fig. 3. Longitudinal aortotomy used for less common types of obstruction. End-to-side aortofemoral anastomosis performed.

seriously atherosclerotic infrarenal aorta. In our opinion, this type of bypass, besides ignoring the critical component of the aortic occlusion at such a level, i.e. the involvement of the visceral vessels, constitutes excessive surgical aggression. It is better, in selected cases, to employ an axillofemoral bypass such as we performed in one patient exposed to a high cardiologic risk and in a second patient in the presence of retroperitoneal fibrosis.

PATIENTS

During the period January 1971 to April 1979, 828 patients underwent operation for aorto-iliac occlusive disease. Of these, 63 (7.6%) were found to have total occlusion of the juxtarenal aorta. There were 52 men (82.5%) and 11 women (17.5%) with an age range of 41–72 years and a mean age of 56 years.

All patients presented with symptoms of vascular insufficiency of the lower

Table I. Fontaine's stage.

Stage	No.	%
II	41	69.4%
III	12	20.3%
IV	6	10.3%

Table II. Patency of the peripheral arteries.

Iliac	14.2%
Common femoral	22.4%
Superficial femoral	82.5%
Popliteal	72.4%
Tibial	66.6%

Table III. Institute of Vascular Surgery of the University of Milan. Operations for juxtarenal aortic occlusions. January, 1971–April, 1979.

Thrombectomy of the juxtarenal aorta and end-to-end aortofemoral bypass	26	41.2%
TEA of the juxtarenal aorta and end-to-end aortofemoral bypass	12	19.1%
Transaortic TEA and end-to-side aortofemoral bypass	23	36.5%
Axillofemoral bypass	2	3.2%

Table IV. Operations.

TEA of the renal arteries	2	3.1%
Aortorenal bypass	1	1.5%
TEA of the inferior mesenteric artery	6	9.5%
TEA of the common femoral artery	3	4.7%
TEA of the profunda femoral artery	7	11.1%
TEA of the superficial femoral artery	4	6.3%
TEA of the superficial and profunda femoral arteries	5	7.9%
Femoropopliteal Dacron bypass	1	1.5%
Lumbar sympathectomy	19	30.1%

extremities as reported in Table I graded by Fontaine's stages. In the second stage, thigh claudication was observed in 45% of patients; in 42%, thigh claudication was associated with calf claudication, while in only 13% was there calf claudication. Rest pain and trophic changes were less frequent than in the other sites of narrowing. Sexual impotence was present in 40% of male patients.

Hypertension related to demonstrable renal artery stenosis (2 patients) and total renal artery obstruction (1 patient) was present in 4.6% of patients. Renal lesions without hypertension were observed in two patients (3.1%). In three patients (4.7%) a clinical picture of abdominal angina was present: one of these underwent an intestinal resection. The condition of the peripheral circulation was good in most cases: its patency was documented angiographically in a lot of patients (Table II).

Table III shows the surgical techniques employed. In 26 patients, juxtarenal aortic thrombectomy and end-to-end aortofemoral bypass was performed. In 12 patients, the subrenal aorta was resected and end-to-end aortofemoral bypass performed, after juxtarenal aortic TEA. In 23 patients, juxtarenal aortic TEA and end-to-side aortofemoral bypass was carried out. In the remaining 2 patients, axillofemoral bypass had been performed, one because of cardiologic risk, the other because of retroperitoneal fibrosis. Table IV shows the operations.

RESULTS AND CONCLUSIONS

The immediate results were very good. Patients obtained a considerable improvement as regards symptoms of peripheral ischemia, especially in relation to the improved condition of the distal arterial tree. In 82.3% of the patients that were discharged, the peripheral pulses (pedal and/or posterior tibial) reappeared.

Table V. Follow-up of 32 patients (average period 1-8 years).

Survival	30	males 25 females 5	93.8%
Dead	2		6.2%
Asymptomatic	25		83.8%
Claudication	3		10.0%
Rest pain	2		6.7%
Tibial pulses			
- present	21		70.0%
- absent	9		30.0%
Improved erection	10		40.0%

There were no operative deaths. One patient died of acute renal failure after the operation. Another patient, who underwent an axillofemoral bypass because of poor general condition, died one month later. The last patient died of unknown causes 5 years later.

Thirty patients were followed up for a period that ranged from 1 to 8 years; 25 patients (83.3%) were asymptomatic; three patients (10%) developed claudication again because of bypass branch obliteration; two patients (6.7%) developed rest pain because of new lesions distal to the bypass. Tibial pulses were still present in 21 patients (70%). Furthermore sexual impotence disappeared in 10 patients after the operation (Table V).

REFERENCES

Bergan, J. J. and Trippel, O. H. (1963). *Archives of Surgery* 87, 60.
Costantini, S., Gabrielli, L., Castelli, P. and Papacharalambus, D. (1977). *L'Ospedale Maggiore* 2, 142.
Courbier, R., Jausseran, J. M. and Reggi, M. (1974). *Journal de Chirurgie* 3, 283.
Faenza, A., Coscia, M., Innocenti, P. and Pierangeli, A. (1971). 73rd Congresso Società Italiana Chirurgia, Napoli. 492-500.
Frantz, S. L., Kaplitt, M. J., Beil, A. R. and Stein, H. L. (1974). *Surgery* 75, 471.
Frøysaker, T., Skagseth, E., Dundas, P. and Hall, K. V. (1973). *Journal of Cardiovascular Surgery* 14, 317.
Hobson, R. W., Rich, N. M., Fedde, C. W. and Maj, F. (1975). *American Surgeon* 41, 271.
Kieffer, E. *In* "Encyclopedie Médico-Chirurgicale," 3, 24, 12, 43150. Chirurgie Vasculaire, Paris.
Liddicoat, J. E., Szabolcs, M. B., Dang, M. H. and De Backey, M. E. (1975). *Surgery* 77, 467.
Malan, E. and Ruberti, U. (1970). *Minerva Chirurgica* 25, 229.
Nunn, D. B. and Kamal, M. A. (1972). *Surgery* 72, 749.
Starret, R. W. and Stoney, R. J. (1974). *Surgery* 76, 890.
Thurlbeck, W. M. and Castlemen, B. (1957). *New England Journal of Medicine* 10, 442.

CLINICAL AND PROGNOSTIC EVALUATION AND THERAPEUTIC ATTITUDE IN ARTERIOSCLEROTIC LESIONS OF THE RENAL ARTERIES (179 PATIENTS)

S. Miani, P. Mingazzini, P. Mingazzini and R. Scorza

Department of Surgery, School of Medicine, University of Milan, Italy

The great development of aortographic examination, now almost routine in patients affected by atherosclerotic disease of the lower extremities, allowed the demonstration of the high frequency of atherosclerotic lesions. These typically occur in the proximal renal artery adjacent to the aorta but, more rarely, can spread distally or even involve the primary branches of the renal artery in both normotensive and hypertensive patients. This finding raises various questions.

1. Does a consistent and direct relationship exist between the presence and the severity of renal stenosis and the diastolic blood pressure levels?

2. When is renal surgical revascularization indicated in hypertensive patients?

3. In patients with renal stenosis but with no evidence of renovascular hypertension, is it justified to perform prophylactic surgery to avoid subsequent renal ischemia?

The purpose of this paper is to summarize the conclusions drawn from the study of a wide series of aortorenal aortographies, to discuss our surgical attitude, and to report long-term results in 108 of 179 patients affected by renal stenosis.

CLINICAL MATERIAL

All the 1636 aortograms performed at "Padiglione Zonda" between 1972 and 1977 for diagnosis of aortoiliac occlusive disease or renovascular hyper-

Serono Symposium No. 37, "Vascular Occlusion: Epidemiological, Pathophysiological and Therapeutic Aspects", edited by M. Tesi and J. Dormandy, 1981. Academic Press, London and New York.

Table I.   Total number of aortograms, 1636 (1972 / 1977).

| Renal artery lesions | : | 230 | | |

Occlusive arterial diseases (lower extremities)		Renovascular hypertension
179		51

Normotensive	Hypertensive
131	48

Table II.

		Hypertensive	
Arteriopathic patients with renal artery lesions	179	48	26.8%
Comparative arteriopathic sample without renal artery lesions	179	16	8.9%

Table III.   Patients (total number) 108.

Aortography time	X^a	Control time		
Normotensive	25	Normotensive	48	44.4%
Hypertensive	33	Normotensive (with drug therapy)	16	14.8%
Hypertensive	29	Hypertensive	24	22.2%
Normotensive	18	Hypertensive	8	7.4%
		Died in interval	12	11.1%

[a]X = average time interval between aortography and control (months).

tension were reviewed. X-rays of 179 patients demonstrated characteristic features of atherosclerosis of one or both renal arteries. Out of 179 patients, 131 were normotensive, whereas the diastolic blood pressure of 48 patients was above 100 mmHg (Table I). This incidence of hypertension is considerably higher than that of a control population of patients affected by atherosclerotic disease (Table II). Only six of the 179 patients, all belonging to hypertensive group, underwent an operation (in four cases corrective vascular surgery was undertaken: in two it was necessary to carry out a nephrectomy). In order to follow up the clinical course of the 179 patients, they were all called back. When direct patient follow-up was impossible reliable data were obtained from personal physicians; in this way the data of 108 patients were gathered (Table III).

Follow-up for the entire series averaged 26 months, ranging from 1 to 6 years. Table III shows that only eight patients (7.4%) developed a mild hypertension during the follow-up period. Of 40 initially hypertensive patients, 16 had a diastolic blood pressure (with drug therapy) in the normal range, whereas 24 patients (22%), even though receiving antihypertensive drug therapy, were found moderately hypertensive. Forty-eight patients (44%), initially normotensive, did not undergo any change in their pressure values at the control time (average control interval 25 months). Finally, 12 patients (11.1%) died; the cause of death in four patients being related to vascular disease.

DISCUSSION

The results of the study, on radiologically demonstrable renal artery stenosis in patients investigated by aortography, confirm that many subjects affected by narrowing of renal artery lumen often do not present with renovascular hypertension. A possible explanation of this behavior may be found in the fact that an atherosclerotic lesion developing chronically and extending to intrarenal arteries may cause a slow and gradual reduction of the amount of functioning renal parenchyma in parallel with the blood supply decrease, so that neither ischemia nor hypertension occurs (Eyler 1962). The question therefore arises whether it is right for these patients to undergo an operation and which kind of surgical management is more suitable with reference to the shape of the anatomical lesions.

In order to select the operative candidates, in addition to the investigative studies usually made in renovascular hypertension (excretory urogram, isotope renogram, selective angiography, bilateral ureteral catheterization), measurement of plasma renin activity (PRA) in the renal veins and in the inferior vena cava below the renal veins was also performed under basal conditions. In many cases, the PRA determination correctly detects a functionally significant stenosis of the renal artery. However, a normal renin ratio in the renal vein which is affected by stenosis is frequently found when the controlateral kidney is not capable of reducing the circulating volume of plasma.

In order to eliminate, or at least to reduce the false negative results, the infusion of trimetaphan has been recently used (Morganti *et al.*, 1975). The peripheral vasodilatation caused by this drug induces a redistribution of the circulating plasma volume, thus eliminating the volumetric component of the hypertensive disease. In this case, the values of P.R.A. tended to rise beyond the normal levels. In these conditions, the increased reninemia is the unique factor inducing hypertension. Other authors (Martorana *et al.*, 1979) suggest taking blood samples during acutely induced hypotension by sodium nitroprusside infusion.

On the other hand, it should be remembered that a reduction of renal blood supply necessarily involves a progressive decrease of the amount of functioning renal parenchyma. Therefore some authors (Constantini *et al.*, 1977) propose a thrombo-endoarterectomy of the proximal renal arteries when surgical revascularization of terminal aorta is required, even if there is no renovascular hypertension, when the pressure gradient between aorta and renal arteries evaluated intra-operatively is over 25 mmHg.

CONCLUSIONS

From the analysis of the clinical material and from the results of the follow-up of patients, it seems to us that patients affected by arteriosclerotic lesions of the renal arteries may be schematically classified into the following groups.

(1) Hypertensive patients with focal arteriosclerotic renal artery disease, without important lesions affecting the residual arterial tree.

(2) Patients who are affected by mild or no hypertension, with arteriosclerotic lesions of the renal arteries, which may or may not be associated with extra-renal arteriosclerotic disease.

(3) Patients affected by lesions of renal arteries, with associated major arteriosclerotic aortic disease (aneurysm, subrenal barrage), who need renal revascularization with abdominal aortic aneurismectomy or aortofemoral bypass.

We believe, and the results of this study seem to validate our conclusions, that only the first and the third group of the patients are to be considered candidates to surgical revascularization. On the contrary, we are convinced that for the second group of patients the best policy is a non-interventionist behavior. Many reasons support our attitude.

Wollenweber (1968) documented that no significant difference existed in the five-year survival rate of this kind of patient when treated surgically or medically.

In the 20% of the patients older than 50 years the arteriosclerotic renal artery stenosis are a consequence of long-standing essential hypertension and are of no importance in the development or maintenance of the patients' hypertensive state (Ernst *et al.*, 1973).

Finally, when the main renal trunk or the extrarenal arteries are the site of severe stenosis, important stenosis is found also in a great percentage of intra-renal arteries.

REFERENCES

Costantini, S., Gabrielli, L., Castelli, P. and Papacharalambus, D. (1977). *L'Ospedale Maggiore* 2, 142–144.
Ernst, C. B., Stanley, J. C., Marshall, F. F. and Fry, W. J. (1973). *Surgery* 859–867.
Eyler, W. R., Clark, M. D., Garman, J. E., Rian, R. L. and Meninger, D. E. (1962). *Radiology* 78, 879.
Martorano, G., Giberti, C., Carmignani, G., Belgrano, E. and Giuliani, L. (1979). *Surgery in Italy* 184–189.
Morganti, A., Leonetti, G., Terzoli, L., Bernasconi, M. and Zanchetti, A. (1975). *Boll. Soc. It. Card.* **XX** (10), 1159–1167.
Wollenweber, J., Sheps, S. G. and Davis, G. D. (1968). *American Journal of Cardiology* 60–71.

FOLLOW-UP OF 50 PATIENTS WITH CELIAC AXIS
COMPRESSION TREATED SURGICALLY

E. Zanella and L. Chiampo

Clinica Chirurgica Generale 2°, University of Parma, Italy

Celiac artery compression is challenged by some authors (Szilagyi *et al.*, 1972; Mihas *et al.*, 1977) as a definite clinical entity. Relief of epigastric pain and associated symptoms can occur after surgical release of the constricted artery (Bobbio *et al.*, 1967; Stanley and Fry, 1971; Van de Berg *et al.*, 1973; Watson and Sadikali, 1977; Joubaud *et al.*, 1977); these results are consistent with our suggestion that this syndrome is caused by the reduction of celiac axis blood flow (Zanella, 1976).

Our opinion is supported by the follow-up of 50 selected patients with celiac axis compression syndrome, confirmed by aortographic studies, surgically treated and followed-up for a period of 6 months to 12 years.

With reference to age, we have subdivided the patients into three groups: (1) younger than 40 years; (2) middle-aged between 41–65 years; (3) older than 66 years. The youngest patient was 18 years-old, the oldest 75 years-old (Table I).

The symptoms characterizing the clincial picture were epigastric pain (80%), weight loss (70%) and motor intestinal disorders (38%). The only significant sign, abdominal bruit in the epigastric area, was present in 26% of the examined subjects, chiefly in the young patients. The bruit could be demonstrated by means of phonoarterio-graphic recording, also used to study restoration of normal celiac axis blood flow after surgical decompression.

Twenty of our patients, as is typical, also had symptoms of biliary disorders, with epigastric pain, biliary colic, nausea and vomiting. Transient icterus occurred in three patients. Two patients had several symptoms of pancreatic insufficiency, in particular steathorrea and upper abdominal pain with leftsided radiation. A

Serono Symposium No. 37, "Vascular Occlusion: Epidemiological, Pathophysiological and Therapeutic Aspects", edited by M. Tesi and J. Dormandy, 1981. Academic Press, London and New York.

Table I. Age distribution of the 50 operated patients.

Age		No.	%
Young :	$<$ 40 years	15	30
Middle age:	41–65 years	28	56
Old:	$>$ 65 years	7	14

similar clinical picture was described by Cornil *et al.* (1970) and Zanella and Chiampo (1979).

The patients with biliary or pancreatic symptoms had a compression not only of the celiac axis but also of the common hepatic and splenic arteries. The most common causes of celiac axis compression were the *median arcuate ligament* of diaphragm, the *celiac nervous plexus* and *periarterial fibrosis*, while unusual causes were lymph nodes and tumors. The diagnosis can be confirmed only by means of aortography and the lateral films characteristically demonstrate the feature of celiac compression.

Our experience allows us to assert that some angiographic pictures are correlated to a particular cause of compression hence it is possible to propose pre-operatively, a suspected diagnosis of the mechanism of compression. The manifold causes of celiac axis compression have determined different operative treatments. When we found constricting fibers only we dissected the arcuate ligament of the diaphragm from the anterior wall of the aorta to the origin of the celiac axis. When compression by neurofibrous tissues was present the constricted artery was relieved by excision of the hypertrophied celiac ganglion and nerve bundles. Periarterial fibrous tissue was removed by sharp dissection around not only the celiac artery but also the common hepatic, splenic and sometimes superior mesenteric arteries.

RESULTS

The follow-up of 50 surgically treated patients was performed by periodical checks over a period of 6 months to 12 years. The results (Table II) were judged as follows: *excellent*, when patients had become asymptomatic and the symptoms disappeared; *good*, when reduction of the most severe symptoms, in

Table II. Follow-up results.

	No.	%
Excellent	21	42
Good	23	46
Poor	6	12
Total	50	100

particular abdominal pain and weight loss, had occurred and *poor*, if the clinical picture was partially modified with persistent post-prandial pain but weight gained.

One patient became asymptomatic after celiac decompression, but complained of severe epigastric pain and weight loss two years later. Repeated arteriogram showed a relapsing compression of the celiac axis. At a second laparotomy, a dense coat of fibrous tissue was found around the celiac and hepatic arteries which was lysed with resolution of the clinical syndrome.

The young patients frequently and permanently became asymptomatic after decompression. In this group, an abnormally high origin of the celiac axis appeared to be a congenital factor for the arterial entrapment. Another cause of compression was the variation in the arrangement of the crura of the diaphragm with an abnormally low projection of their level of attachment. Decompression of the celiac axis and concurrently involved hepatic and splenic arteries produced relief of both gastric and biliary symptoms, especially motor disorders of the biliary tract.

CONCLUSIONS

The good results of surgical correction of celiac artery compression, followed over a period of 12 years in 50 patients, seem to confirm our opinion that the syndrome is ischemic more than neurogenic in origin. The nearly complete and prolonged relief of pain and weight loss seems to be due more to the restoration of celiac blood flow than to the interruption of the celiac plexus and its fibres. The division of sympathetic fibers and ganglia alone does not render prolonged relief of visceral pain. The best results have been found in young patients, when only extrinsic compression without a parietal lesion was present.

Finally, we have noticed that concurrent biliary or pancreatic disorders subsided after restoration of celiac and collateral blood flow. This emphasizes that ischemia may play an important role in the pathogenesis of dysfunction of the liver and of the pancreas.

REFERENCES

Bobbio, A., Zanella, E. and Chiampo, L. (1967). *Minerva Chirurgica* 22, 1024.

Cornil, A., Lewalle, L. and Dreze, Ch. (1970). *Acta Gastroenterologica* 33, 51.

Joubaud, F., Pillet, J. and Boyer, J. (1977). *Semaine des Hôpital de Paris* 53, 157.

Mihas, A. A., Laws, H. L. and Jander, H. P. (1977). *American Journal of Surgery* 133, 688.

Stanley, J. C. and Fry, W. J. (1971). *Archive of Surgery* 103, 252.

Szilagyi, D. E., Rian, R. L., Elliott, J. P. and Smith, R. E. (1972). *Surgery* 72, 849.

Van de Berg, L., Lombard, R., Guffens, J. M. and Dreze, Ch. (1973). *Angèiologie* 25, 371.

Watson, W. C. and Sadikali, F. (1977). *Annals of International Surgery* 86, 278.

Zanella, E. (1976). *Scritti in onore del prof. E. Malan*. 317. Ed. Morell, Como.

Zanella, E. and Chiampo, L. (1979). *Minerva Medica* 70, 1175.

THE ROLE OF SUPERFICIAL TEMPORAL ARTERY—
MIDDLE CEREBRAL ARTERY ANASTOMOSES IN THE
PREVENTIVE VASCULAR SURGERY FOR TIA AND
FOR STROKE

R. Rodríguez y Baena, G. Brambilla, G. Sangiovanni, F. Rainoldi and D. Locatelli

Clinica Neurochifurgica, University of Pavia, Italy

The idea of creating an alternative to the direct surgical treatment of a pathological vessel by performing a bypass between two other vessels of a smaller
calibre but anatomically sound, came about in 1967, when M. G. Yasargil performed the first termino-lateral anastomosis between the superficial temporal
artery and the middle cerebral artery in a dog, under the operating microscope.

The post-operative angiography in 33 animals, 2 - 4 months after the operation, demonstrated bypass patency in 76% of the cases. During the same year,
Donaghy and Yasargil, encouraged by the results obtained in the field of experimental microsurgery, performed the first bypass in a human between the superficial temporal artery and a cortical branch of the middle cerebral artery.

This new operation quickly became more popular. After the nine initial cases
communicated in 1970 (Yasargil), the literature reports an average number of
2500 patients operated on all over the world.

SURGICAL PROCEDURE

The superficial temporal artery runs in the subcutaneous tissue between
skin and "galea capitis" supplying the frontal, temporal and parietal regions

Serono Symposium No. 37, "Vascular Occlusion: Epidemiological, Pathophysiological and
Therapeutic Aspects", edited by M. Tesi and J. Dormandy, 1981. Academic Press, London
and New York.

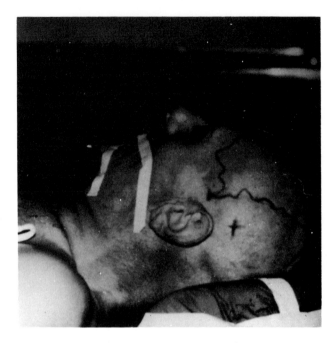

Fig. 1. The superficial temporal artery has been drawn on the scalp and (+) will be the electron point for the craniectomy in order to isolate the angular artery on the "cortex" (6 cm above the external auditory channel).

of the head. After angiographic evaluation of the superficial temporal artery calibre (1.2 mm minimum for a successful bypass) the vessel is identified by palpation and marked on the scalp (Fig. 1). A rectilinear incision is made and the sharp dissection of the frontal or parietal branch of the superficial temporal artery is begun. Some perivascular connective tissue is spared in order to manipulate the vessel without damaging the "vasa vasorum".

After the temporal muscle incision, a T-shape craniectomy incision is made about 6 cm above the external auditory channel; the dura is opened and the operating microscope brought to bear on the surgical field. Now the sharp microdissection of the cortical vessel from the arachnoid membrane begins. This artery must have a minimum external diameter of 0.8 mm in order to have a reasonable guarantee of a long-term bypass patency.

Two temporary microclips interrupt the blood flow in the vessel and an elliptical window is made in the artery wall about 1.5–2 mm in length (Fig. 2). Both vessels are now ready for the termino-lateral anastomosis which is performed by 10–12 interrupted sutures of 10.0 monofilament nylon. If the surgical procedure has been correct, after the microclips are removed, gentle compression for 2–3 min is usually sufficient to stop any bleeding from the suture line. The dura is left partially opened as is the temporal muscle and before suturing the surgical wound, a drain is sometimes placed under the "galea capitis" for the first 24 h (Fig. 3).

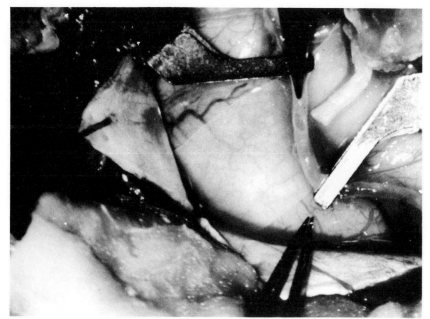

Fig. 2. The isolated cortical artery between two microclips: the elliptical window is visible and nearby is the superficial temporal artery tip prepared for the anastomosis.

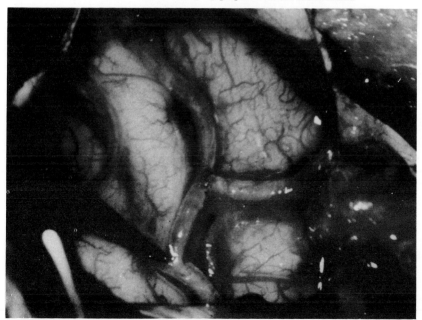

Fig. 3. The bypass is completed: after the microclips' removal there is no bleeding from the suture line and the vessels are patent and increased in calibre.

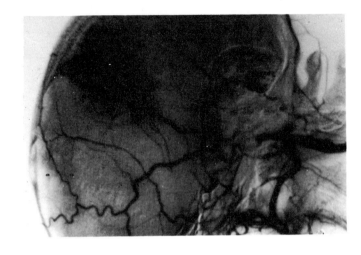

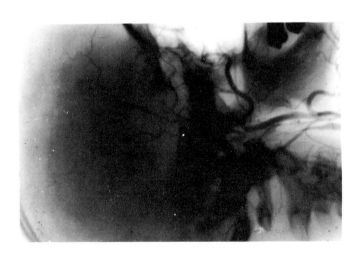

Fig. 4 a (left) and b (right). Pre- and post-operative angiography.

POST-OPERATIVE CONTROL

Every patient undergoes a repeat angiography 40–60 days post-operatively. In Fig. 4a, a complete occlusion of the internal carotid artery is visible just above the bifurcation; this is the angiographic pattern before the operation. Figure 4b shows post-operative (60 days) carotid angiography in the same patient with a satisfactory filling of the middle cerebral artery complex through the bypass (Figs 4a, b).

RESULTS

Up to the month of June 1979, 24 extra-intracranial bypass operations have been performed in the Neurosurgical Clinic of Pavia University: six patients with severe neurological deficits (established stroke) did not improve at all, while a total of 18 patients showed a real improvement: 15 had an excellent result, six a good result.From a radiological point of view, we found the best results in complete occlusion of the internal carotid artery; that is quite easily explained by the pressure gradient existing between the two vessels.

Today the clinical improvement after the cerebral revascularization is justified by the fact that in the ischemic area there is a great number of neurons still alive but functionally interrupted. It seems that an additional blood flow through the anastomosis brings back these neurons to their normal electrical activity.

Moreover, if we consider the total lack of mortality and of significant morbidity (two cases of skin necrosis with spontaneous resolution) it is reasonable to consider the extra-intracranial arterial bypass a real help in the treatment and in the prophylaxis of TIAs and strokes.

REFERENCES

Austin, G., Laffin, D. and Hayward, W. (1975). *Microneurosurgery* **47**, 67.
Rodríguez y Baena, R., Brambilla, G. L., Papandrea, G. P. and Paoletti, P. (1979). *Current Advances in Basic and Clinical Microcirculatory Research* **225**, 228.
Yasargil, M. G. (1969). *Microsurgery applied to Neuro-surgery.* **82**, 118.

PROFUNDOPLASTY: INDICATIONS, SURGICAL TECHNIQUES AND FOLLOW-UP*

P. Balas, E. Bastounis, N. Xeromeritis, J. Kambilafkas, C. Stamatopoulos
and P. Ioannidis

*First Department of Surgery, Athens University Medical School and "Hygia"
Medical Center, Greece*

The value of the profunda femoris artery as a major source of collateral blood supply to the distal part of the leg, thus securing adequate flow to prevent tissue loss and claudication, despite complete occlusion of the superficial femoral artery has now been well established (Cormier, 1969; Cohn *et al.*, 1971; Martin *et al.*, 1972; Bernhard *et al.*, 1976; Modgill *et al.*, 1977). In this paper we present our experience of profundoplasty, its indications and surgical techniques during the follow-up period from January, 1970 through June, 1979.

MATERIAL AND METHODS

Two hundred and one cases were submitted to profundoplasty between January, 1970 through September, 1979. In 83 cases, a simple profundoplasty was performed while in 118 cases, a profundoplasty in combination with a proximal arterioplasty was performed. All the patients had atherosclerotic arterial occlusive disease. The age of the patients was between 28 and 86 years with most of the patients in their sixth decade. The male/female ratio was 10:1.

The following five patterns of atherosclerotic involvement of the profunda femoris artery were established in our patients on the basis of arteriographic pictures and the operative findings (Table I).

Serono Symposium No. 37, "Vascular Occlusion: Epidemiological, Pathophysiological and Therapeutic Aspects", edited by M. Tesi and J. Dormandy, 1981. Academic Press, London and New York.

Table I. Patterns of atherosclerotic involvement of the profunda and other arterial segments.

Patterns	Arterial segments involved
1	Isolated stenosis of the origin of the profunda
2	Involvement of the main trunk of profunda + common femoral + proximal arteries.
3	Involvement of the main trunk profunda + stenosis or occlusion of common and superficial femoral and distal arteries.
4	Pattern 3 with occlusion of the superficial femoral or proximal arteries.
5	Extensive involvement of profunda + involvement of other arterial segments.

1. Isolated stenotic lesion at the origin of the deep femoral artery.

2. Atherosclerotic changes of the main trunk of the profunda and common femoral arteries in combination with proximal occlusive changes.

3. Atherosclerotic changes of the main trunk of the profunda with stenosis or occlusion of the common and superficial femoral arteries.

4. The same pattern as in 3 with complete occlusion of the superficial femoral artery with or without inflow aorto-iliac disease.

5. Extensive involvement of the profunda in association with involvement of other arterial segments.

The indications for performing profundoplasty, isolated or combined with other arterioplastic procedures, were as follows:

1   Incapacitating claudication.

2   Rest pain.

3   Ulcerations or impending gangrene of the foot.

The operative procedures depended on the arteriographic and operative findings. General anaesthesia was employed in most of the cases, especially in the combined procedures, but many cases of simple profundoplasty were performed under local anaesthesia.

Three categories of arterioplastic procedures were employed.

1. *Simple profundoplasty.* In these cases, a thromboendarterectomy of the common femoral artery and sometimes the external iliac, or the superficial femoral artery extending to the profunda femoris artery, was performed. In order to accomplish an extensive exposure of the profunda the superficial femoral artery was mobilized medially. The profunda was mobilized distally in order to find, by means of palpation, a soft segment, indicative of the absence of severe atherosclerotic changes, to place the distal clamp. Thromboendarterectomy was carried out distally until a relatively normal segment was reached. The endarterectomized segment of the common, superficial and profunda femoris arteries were usually covered by a dacron, venous or arterial patch. The arterial patch was taken from the occluded segment of the superficial femoral artery after stripping off the

Table II. Simple profundoplasty.

Technique	No. cases
Endarterectomy without patch	11
Endarterectomy + Dacron simple patch	18
Endarterectomy + Dacron pantaloon patch	2
Endarterectomy + Gore-Tex patch	3
Endarterectomy + simple vein patch	29
Endarterectomy + pantaloon vein patch	8
Endarterectomy + simple arterial patch	12
Total	83

Table III. Combined arterioplastic procedures with profundoplasty.

Procedure	No. cases
Aorto–Femoral	
Lateral	8
Bilateral	52
Femoro–Femoral	24
Axillo–Femoral	18
Femoro–Popliteal	16
Total	118

outer part of the arterial wall from the atheromatous core. The surgical techniques of the simple profundoplasty are shown in Table II. The pantaloon patch arterioplasty was used in cases of endarterectomy of the common, superficial and profunda femoris arteries.

2. *Proximal arterioplastic procedures in combination with profundoplasty.* These included uni-or bilateral aorto-femoral dacron bypass, femoro-femoral and axillo-femoral prosthetic bypass grafts.

3. *Distal arterioplastic procedures in combination with profundoplasty.* In these cases, a femoro-popliteal vein bypass was usually used. The profundoplasty in our series was limited only to the first part of the profunda. The combined procedures are shown in Table III.

RESULTS

The immediate follow-up results refer to the hospitalization period which extended up to 2–4 weeks after surgery. The long-term follow-up extended from 1–8 years after surgery. The immediate post-operative results were considered as: (a) Improvement, if the symptoms of claudication, rest pain and

Table IV.   Immediate post-operative results.

Clinical Symptoms and Findings	No. cases	Results		
		Improvement	Symptoms free	Failure
		No. (%)	No. (%)	No. (%)
Intermittent claudication	126	69 (54.76)	50 (39.68)	7 (5.56)
Rest pain	61	16 (26.22)	38 (62.29)	7 (11.47)
Gangrene	55	24 (43.64)	22 (40)	9 (16.36)

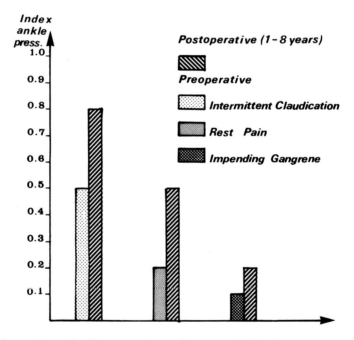

Fig. 1. Comparison and ankle pressure (pre- and post-operative) in three groups considered.

ulceration were ameliorated. (b) Symptom-free, if the symptoms disappeared and the trophic changes were healed with or without minor amputations. (c) Failure, if no improvement was accomplished or the symptomatology became worse resulting in necrosis and amputation of the foot. The immediate post-operative results are shown in Table IV. In some cases, the immediate results were extremely impressive, with the foot not only warm but weak pulses palpable as well.

Table V. Comparative study of the ankle pressure index in the follow-up period of 1–8 years.

Group of patients according to symptomatology	Mean value of Ankle Pressure Index	
	Pre-operative	Follow-up period
Claudication	0.50 ± 0.02	0.83 ± 0.04
Rest pain	0.22 ± 0.03	0.50 ± 0.03
Trophic changes	0.11 ± 0.02	0.32 ± 0.02

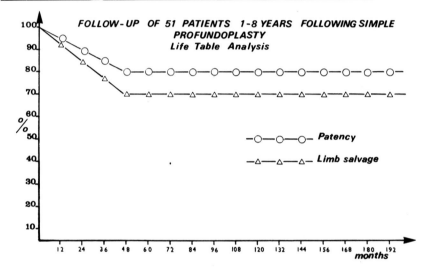

Fig. 2.

In some cases, mainly in simple profundoplasty and femoro-femoral bypass, during the immediate post-operative period, the area of angioplasty was checked by arteriography in order to determine the patency and appearance of the arteries and prostheses. Also, by measuring the ankle pressure pre- and post-operatively, we made an objective evaluation of the arterial circulation of the feet. The overall mortality was 2.0% during the early post-operative period. Three of the patients died due to myocardial infarction and one because of a dissecting aneurysm. In some cases, minor amputations of the toes were combined with a revascularization procedure or were performed subsequently.

The long follow-up, extending between 1 and 8 years, was accomplished only in 51 patients who had simple profundoplasty. This follow-up included a careful clinical examination, measurement of the index of ankle pressure and sometimes the performance of an arteriogram. The degree of increase of the ankle pressure is shown in Fig. 1 and Table V. By applying the method of the "life table analysis", it was found that the patency rate in the area of the arterioplasty was 78% while the leg salvage reached 70% at the end of the eighth year of follow-up (Fig. 2).

DISCUSSION

Simple profundoplasty has become popular in the last decade as a salvage arterioplastic procedure and for the improvement of claudication. The experience of other authors (Martin and Jamieson, 1974; Modgill *et al.*, 1977; Bernhard, 1979), and our own, justifies the expansion of the indications for profundoplasty in vascular practice not only as a single procedure but also as an important adjunct to inflow or outflow procedures.

The immediate results in our series compare favourably with those of Bernhard (1979). Limb salvage, after a follow-up of up to 8 years, was found to be 70%, while Bernhard (1979) reported a salvage rate of 67% on a follow-up for five years.

Profundoplasty alone is a simple but rewarding procedure to both patient and surgeon, but it has to be performed with an extremely fine surgical technique in order to accomplish a satisfactory outflow through the distal part of this important arterial circuit of the leg and also to provide a long-standing patency in the area of profundoplasty. The patency rate of 78% in our series on a follow-up of up to eight years is indicative of our painstaking technique in performing the procedure.

REFERENCES

Bernhard, V. M., Ray, L. T. and Militello, J. P. (1976). *S.G.O.* **142**, 840.
Bernhard, V. M. (1979). *Surg. Clin. N.Am.* **59**, 681.
Cohn, L. H., Trueblood, W. and Crowley, L. G. (1971). *Arch. Surg.* **103**, 475.
Cormier, J. M. (1969). Chirurgie de l'artére femoral profonde. In Techniques Chirurgicales Sec. 43070. Encyclopedie Medico-Chirurgicale, Paris.
Martin, P. and Jamieson, C. (1974). *Surg. Clin. N.Am.* **54**, 95.
Martin, P., Frawley, J. E., Barabas, A. P. and Rosengarten, D. S. (1972). *Surgery* **71**, 182.
Modgill, V. K., Humphrey, C. S., Shoesmith, J. H. and Kester, R. C. (1977). *Br. J. Surg.* **64**, 362.

THERAPY OF PERIPHERAL EMBOLISM

G. Tuscano, O. Maleti and R. Gibellini

*Cattedra di Anatomia Chirurgia e Corso di Operazioni Della Universita'
di Modena, Italy*

Arterial embolism represents one of the most frequent surgical emergency
situations in vascular surgery. The sudden interruption of the blood flow in
a limb due to arterial occlusion, besides prejudicing the limb's function and
vitality, can endanger the patient's life. In this report, we are exhibiting the
results and analysis of treatment in 126 cases of arterial embolism operated
on from 1970 to 1978.

Peripheral emboli were observed in 144 patients, their ages ranging from 30
to 86 years (the average age = 65), 98 were male and 46 female. In 15 cases,
both limbs were simultaneously involved. The most frequent aetiological factors
were cardiac disorders (70%). In 29 cases, the arm was involved (20.1%): in 115,
the leg (79.9%). The time interval between the initial occurrence of the symptoms and treatment is shown in Table I.

Arteriography was very rarely performed for the diagnosis and localization
of the involved area since clinical investigation often proved sufficient. In the
majority of cases we resorted to surgery, 21 cases were treated medically and
in four cases a primary amputation was necessary. The most frequent operation,
under local anaesthesia, was the Fogarty thromboembolectomy via a femoral
or brachial approach; supplementary incisions were very rarely carried out.
After surgery, only those patients afflicted by a recurrent embolus, those operated on at a late stage, or those who had had pathological arteries, were subjected to anticoagulants. The treatment used is indicated in Table II.

Pre-operative arteriography was carried out when the blood flow was insufficient, in popliteal arterial occlusions and in embolectomies operated on at a

Serono Symposium No. 37, "Vascular Occlusion: Epidemiological, Pathophysiological and
Therapeutic Aspects", edited by M. Tesi and J. Dormandy, 1981. Academic Press, London
and New York.

Table I. Time interval between the initial occurrence
of the symptoms and treatment in 144 patients.

Time	No. of patients
0 – 24 h	93
24 – 48 h	25
2 – 4 days	4
5 – 8 days	7
more than 8 days	8
Not defined	7

Table II. Treatment of 144 patients with peripheral embolism.

Medical treatment	21 (14.58%)		
	Anticoagulant	17	
	Fibrinolytic	4	
Surgical treatment			
	(1) Embolectomies	126	
	Associated operations		
	Patch on the arteriotomy		8
	TEA		4
	Fem-pool. bypass		2
	Venous thrombectomy		2
	Cervical rib resection		1
	Aneurysm resection and graft		2
	Fasciotomy		6
	Lumbar ganglionectomy		2
	(2) Primary amputations	4	

Table III. Results of 126 embolectomies in 119 patients.

Limb recovering	83	(69.8)
Deaths	19	(15.9)
Amputations	17	(14.3)

late stage. Results are shown in Table III. The results depend on the period
of time elapsing before treatment. The reappearance of one or two peripheral
beats was considered as good and the absence of distal beats but limb preservation as fair. The causes of mortality are given in Table IV.

Arterial emboli are frequent and continuously increasing. Surgical treatment
is aimed at restoring the blood flow to pre-occlusive levels. In fact, Fogarty's

Table IV. Causes of mortality after embolectomy
and secondary amputation.

Deaths after embolectomy	19
Deaths after secondary amputation	8
Causes	
Cardiac insufficiency	20
Pulmonary embolism	2
Respiratory insufficiency	2
Revascularization syndrome	1
Cerebral ictus	2

technique enables us to save the limb even in high risk patients. An early diagnosis, together with other factors (age of the patient, site of the embolism, degree of ischaemia) govern the quality of the results. In embolectomies performed at a late stage, after 48 h, the risk of amputation increases. In order to verify the complete patency of disobliteration, we usually resort to pre-operative arteriography. The evaluation of surgical results on embolism should be based on the disappearance of the ischaemic symptoms, on the improvement of local conditions and the reappearance of pulsations.

However, as the pre-embolic condition of the limbs is, for the most part, unknown, the mortality and above all the rate of amputation are still the best parameters for evaluation. On examining the overall results of the series, we find that the overall mortality was 15.9%. In 68.8% of cases, we recorded a limb salvage, however, we must mention the considerable number of people above 60 years of age who underwent operations and the period of time elapsing from initial symptoms and treatment, which in the majority of cases, was more than 24 h.

Even if Fogarty's technique enables distal removal of the arterial occlusion, the rate of amputation and mortality is still high; this depends mostly on the heart disorder that causes the embolic dissemination in such patients; the only measure to further improve results is a more timely diagnosis and treatment.

REFERENCES

Conti, A. and Tuscano, G. (1978). *Minerva Chirurgica* 1097–1101.
Darling, R. C., Austen, W. G. and Linton, R. (1967). *Surg. Gynec. Obstet.* **142**, 106.
Fiorani and Coll., (1972). *Atti 74° Congr. Soc. It. Chir. Roma*
Fogarty, J. T. and Daily, P., (1971). *Am. J. Surg.* **22**,
Haimovici, H. (1970). *Arch. Surg.* **100**, 639.
Kartchener, N. M. (1972). *Arch. Surg.* **104**, 5532.
Thompson, J. E. (1970). *Surg.* **67**, 212.

LONG-TERM RESULTS OF FEMORO-TIBIAL BYPASS

A. Cavallaro, V. Sciacca, A. Allessandrini, M. Garofalo and S. Stipa

IV Cattedra di Patologia Chirurgica dell' Universita di Roma, Italy

INTRODUCTION

Since its clinical introduction in 1960–61 (Palma, 1960; McCaughan, 1961), femoro-tibial reconstructive surgery has gained increasing acceptance. Patency of one or more tibial vessels in legs amputated for ischemia was the anatomopathologic and angiographic basis of this kind of vascular surgery. Through the years, increasing practice has allowed very distal vascular reconstructive procedures to be performed: femoral-to-pedal artery bypass (Shieber, 1969); femoral-to-lateral plantar artery bypass (Baird *et al.*, 1970) and femoral-to-first interosseous dorsal artery bypass (Van Gestel *et al.*, 1974).

PATIENTS AND PROCEDURES

Our experience is based on 63 patients, submitted to reconstructive surgery of tibial arteries from November, 1969 to June, 1979. The age of patients ranged from 28 to 85 years (mean 56 years); they were 52 male (mean age 54 years) and 11 female (mean age 60 years). On 63 patients and 64 limbs, 82 operations were performed, with 12 limbs operated on twice and three limbs operated on three times.

Main associated diseases were: Diabetes – 24 (38%); heart disease – 21 (33%); lung disease – 12 (19%) and kidney disease – 9 (14%).

Thirty-four patients (54%) presented associated diseases, clinically relevant, distributed as follows: (1) associated disease – 14 patients; (2) associated disease

Serono Symposium No. 37, "Vascular Occlusion: Epidemiological, Pathophysiological and Therapeutic Aspects", edited by M. Tesi and J. Dormandy, 1981. Academic Press, London and New York.

– 10 patients; (3) associated disease – 6 patients and (4) associated disease – 4 patients.

Only seven patients (11%) were operated on for claudication (severe enough to prevent a normal lifestyle); operative indication was rest pain in 18 cases (28%) and gangrene in 39 (61%) .

In ten patients, homolateral lumbar sympathectomy had been performed previously (1 to 12 months) at other institutions, with the following results: no change, 5; worsening, 4 and short-lasting improvement, 1.

In 13 patients, tibial reconstruction represented the extension of a more cranial arterial reconstructive procedure: in two instances, iliofemoral TEA was performed once with tibial bypass. Seven times, an aorto-femoral reconstruction performed by us 1 to 12 months previously, in spite of a good anatomical result, did not achieve functional improvement and was then completed with a femoro-tibial bypass. Four times, failure of an aorto-femoral reconstruction obliged us to perform thrombectomy of a Dacron prosthesis and to extend distally the reconstruction on account of a poor deep femoral artery.

The majority of patients had atherosclerosis; in five it was possible, on the basis of microscopy studies, to establish the diagnosis of non-diabetic arteritis. One patient presented with an iatrogenic lesion of the popliteal artery. For preoperative evaluation, angiography was performed in all patients. Arteriograms, even with late exposure films, were judged inadequate if tibial vessels were not visualized or if Doppler flowmetry had revealed some kind of flow in distal leg arteries. Pre-reconstruction intra-operative angiography was almost always performed to decide if and how to do the operation. Graft material was mainly autologous reversed vein (saphenous and/or cephalic); a PTFE prosthesis was used only when suitable veins were not available (9 cases = 11%).

In the 82 operative procedures, proximal anastomosis was implanted as follows:

Common femoral artery	55 (4 PTFE)
Superficial femoral artery	3
Dacron aorto-femoral prosthesis	4 (1 vein; 3 PTFE)
Dacron femoro-femoral prosthesis	1 (PTFE)
Deep femoral artery	7
Popliteal artery	4 (1 sequential bypass)
Autologous vein femoro-popliteal bypass	4 (Jump-bypass; PTFE)
Autologous vein femoro-tibial bypass	4 (Jump-bypass)

Distal anastomosis was as follows.

Tibioperoneal trunk	7 (8.5%)
Peroneal artery	5 (7%)
Posterior tibial artery	38 (46%)
Plantar artery	3 (3.6%)
Anterior tibial artery	27 (33%)
Pedal artery	2 (1.9%)

After bypass completion, control arteriography was rarely done. Doppler flowmetry was always performed. The same non-invasive technique was used for evaluation of bypass behaviour during follow-up; arteriorgraphy was considered necessary only when Doppler control showed a deterioration of the reconstruction. Follow-up carried out by us in all patients but four (who died in the post-operative period from complications of associated diseases) ranged from 6 months to 120 months (mean 53 months).

RESULTS

Most failures were immediate or early, with fair stability of the patent recon-structions after the first year (Table I). A marked difference between diabetic and non-diabetic patients is evident within the first three months. From then on, the behaviour of the two groups is similar, except for a higher mortality among diabetics (Table II). The behaviour of the bypasses, according to the site of distal anastomosis, is shown in Table III.

Table I. Numbers of reconstructions failing with time.

Interval (months)	Bypasses at the be-ginning of the interval	Bypasses failed during the interval	Patients at the begin-ning of the interval	Patients with failed bypass du-ring the in-terval	Patients dead during the interval
0 – 3	82	28	63	15	4
3 – 6	48	2	48	2	1
6 – 12	41	4	41	4	1
12 – 24	34	0	34	0	0
24 – 36	33	2	33	2	0
36 – 48	20	0	20	0	1
48 – 60	14	0	14	0	1
60 – 72	8	0	8	0	0
72 – 84	4	0	4	0	1
84 – 96	3	0	3	0	1
96 – 108	2	0	2	0	0
108 – 120	2	0	2	0	0

In 39 patients with gangrene, a limited amputation was performed 16 times (15 transmetatarsal amputations, 1 Chopart amputation). Ten times, early bypass failure required a major amputation; 12 times trophic lesions healed after a successful arterial reconstruction. In spite of a patent bypass, one patient under-went leg amputation, for sepsis.

The state of the 59 patients who survived the post-operative period was satis-factory; at the end of the follow-up:

Patients	59
Limbs	60
Patent bypasses	38/60 (63%)
Saved limbs	48/60 (80%)
Asymptomatic	25/48 (52%)
Claudication	22/48 (46%)
Rest pain	1/48 (2%)

Table II. Comparison of diabetic and non-diabetic failure rates.

Interval (months)	Diabetes			Non-diabetes		
	Patients at the beginning of the interval	Patients with failed bypass during the interval	Patients dead during the interval	Patients at the beginning of the interval	Patients with failed bypass during the interval	Patients dead during the interval
0 – 3	24	6	3	39	9	1
3 – 6	17	0	0	31	2	1
6 – 12	13	1	1	28	3	0
12 – 24	10	0	0	24	0	0
24 – 36	10	0	0	23	2	0
36 – 48	7	0	1	13	0	0
48 – 60	7	0	0	7	0	1
60 – 72	4	0	0	4	0	0
72 – 84	1	0	1	3	0	0
84 – 96	–	–	–	3	0	1
96 – 108	–	–	–	2	0	0
108 – 120	–	–	–	2	0	0

The behaviour of the bypasses, according to the site of distal anastomosis is shown in Table III.

Table III. Failure rate according to site of anastomosis.

Interval (months)	Peroneal artery	Tibio-peroneal trunk	Anterior tibial artery above interosseous membrane	Anterior tibial artery beyond interosseous membrane	Pedal art.	Posterior tibial artery Upper third	Middle third	Lower third	Plantar artery
0 – 3	5 (1)	7 (1)	9 (2)	18 (5)	1	4 (3)	8 (2)	27 (11)	3 (3)
3 – 6	4	6	7	10	1	3 (1)	5	12 (1)	–
6 – 12	4 (1)	5	7	8 (2)	–	2	4	11 (1)	–
12 – 24	2	4	6	6	–	2	4	10	–
24 – 36	2	3	6 (1)	6	–	2	4 (1)	10	–
36 – 48	2	2	3	3	–	1	3	6	–
48 – 60	2	1	2	2	–	1	2	4	–
60 – 72	1	1	1	1	–	1	1	2	–
72 – 84	1	–	–	1	–	1	–	1	–
84 – 96	1	–	–	1	–	1	–	–	–
96 – 108	1	–	–	–	–	1	–	–	–
108 – 120	1	–	–	–	–	1	–	–	–

Bypass failure occurred in 22 patients (35 reconstructions). Early failure was attributable in most cases to an incorrect operative indication, rarely to a breakdown in surgical technique. Late failure was due to trauma in one case (long trip on a hard seat) and to prolonged hypotension in another case. Although it was iatrogenic in two cases (pseudoaneurysm following control angiography; sclerotherapy of a bypass diagnosed as a pulsating varix), in most cases late failure was due to the progression of the basic disease or to the deterioration of the graft material.

REFERENCES

Baird, R. J., Tutassaura, H. and Miyagishima, R. T. (1970). *Ann. Surg.* **172**, 1059.
McCaughan, J.J.Jr. (1961). *Angiology* **12**, 91.
Palma, E. C. (1960). *Min. Cardioang.* **8**, 36.
Shieber, W. (1969). *Mo. Med.* **66**, 191.
Van Gestel, R., Bomcke, C., Casaer, Y. and De Canniere, P. (1974). *Lyon Chir.* **70**, 348.

INTRA-OPERATIVE LIMB DEPURATION FOR PREVENTION
OF REVASCULARIZATION SYNDROME

C. Spartera, E. Pastore[1], D. Alfani[2], G. Cucchiara[2], N. Aissa,
V. Faraglia and G. R. Pistolese

[1] *Chair of Anaesthesiology, School of Medicine, L'Aquila. Department of
Vascular Surgery, [2] Department of Surgical Pathology, Second Surgical
Clinic, School of Medicine, University of Rome, Italy*

A high mortality rate has been demonstrated in revascularization surgery for
acute limb ischemia. This mortality rate ranges between 18 and 22% even if the
operation, performed by the Fogarty method, is carried out under local anesthesia and does not cause serious trauma to poor-risk patients (Castelli, 1977).
According to the literature, the most frequent cause of death is the "revascularization syndrome" (RS), resulting from toxic and metabolic changes after restoration of blood flow in the ischemic limb (Fiorani *et al.*, 1972). The parameters
governing the development of RS are: the embolus site; the severity and the duration of the ischemia (Pistolese *et al.*, 1977; Agrifoglio *et al.*, 1978); an evaluation
of all these factors will indicate the highest risk class.

Nearly always limb amputation has been chosen as the elective surgical procedure to avoid a severe, (often fatal) or a mild RS, which could be highly dangerous in a poor-risk patient. On the basis of experimental research (Eiken *et al.*,
1964; Stipa *et al.*, 1967; Danese *et al.*, 1973), several investigators advise new
intra-operative procedures, together with the usual medical treatment, to save as
many ischemic limbs as possible, without increasing the mortality rate (Larcan
et al., 1973; Vercellio *et al.*, 1977; Tufano *et al.*, 1978).

Serono Symposium No. 37, "Vascular Occlusion: Epidemiological, Pathophysiological and
Therapeutic Aspects", edited by M. Tesi and J. Dormandy, 1981. Academic Press, London
and New York.

MATERIAL AND METHOD

The authors describe a new method of limb depuration, employing the Redy Haemodialysis System with a RP610 polyacrylonitrile membrane, to prevent RS. The characteristics of this membrane are its high blood-dialysate exchange velocity and its permeability to micro and medium molecules. Thus, myoglobin, which has a molecular weight of 17 000, has a clearance of 18 ml/m.

Table I. Patient treated with intra-operative limb depuration.

Patient	Age (year)	Ischemic Limb	Duration & Degree of Ischemia	Revascular Results
A	42	lower bilat.	10h–severe	good bilat.
B	65	lower bilat.	2d–severe	good Rt partial Lf
C	54	lower Rt ven. thromb.	3d–severe	good
D	68	lower Rt	12h–severe	fair
E	76	lower Rt	7d–severe	good

A microfilter, placed in the input line of the blood circuit, traps clots and microaggregates, both of which play an important role in the pathogenesis of acute respiratory distress syndrome (ARDS). An oxygen flow of 10 l/m bubbles into the dialysate-infusate, in order to increase the PO_2 of the limb venous blood. A bicarbonate solution must also be infused through the output line of the circuit to increase the buffer action of the dialysis system. The dialysate-infusate, without potassium, is warmed to 35–36 °C. The depuration time ranges between 45 and 60 min, depending on the patient's general condition, the severity and extent of the ischemia and the blood flow in the circuit (100–300 ml/m).

Five patients with acute severe ischemia involving either one or both lower limbs have been treated after embolectomy by the Fogarty method with cannulation of the femoral vessels (Table I). The operation is performed under local anesthesia and neuroleptoanalgesia. Continuous control of the acid–base balance and serum electrolyte values are carried out before, during and after surgical treatment.

RESULTS

In all but one case, revascularization treatment was successful. In the case with bilateral ischemia (Case B) a complete revascularization was obtained only on the right side, while residual ischemia remained on the left side (Table I).

Intra-operative Assessments

Limb venous PO_2 during depuration (Fig. 1). The oxygen flow into the dialysate-infusate (cases B.C.D.E.) causes an increase in the blood PO_2 in the output

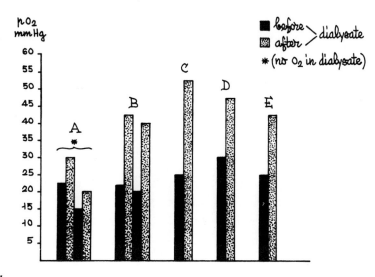

Fig. 1.

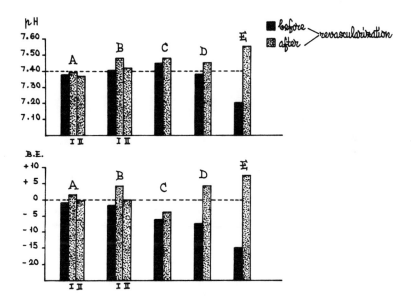

Fig. 2.

circuit line therefore effecting a partial oxygenation of the limb. In case A, no oxygen was added to the infusate.

Acid-base balance during depuration (Fig. 2). The systemic arterial blood pH and base-excess values, checked before and after revascularization, show a normal range in cases A and B; in cases C, D and E the initial metabolic acidosis was partially controlled (case C) or modified in metabolic alkalosis (cases D and E).

Systemic and limb serum potassium changes during depuration (Fig. 3). At the start of the depuration local potassium is always higher than systemic levels;

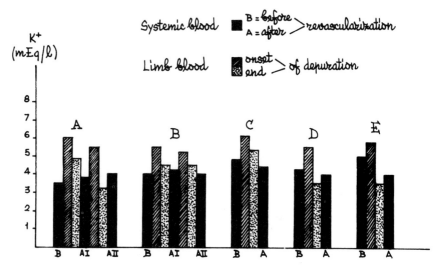

Fig. 3.

following depuration local values decrease and after revascularization no increases have been noted in the systemic serum potassium concentration.

Post-operative Assessment (Table II)

Serum potassium. No abnormal changes were noted following revascularization.

Acid-base balance. Mild post-operative alkalosis was induced by intravenous $NaHCO_3$ infusion in cases B.C.D.E. In case A, the acid-base balance was within normal values.

Renal function. Cases B.C.D. had a good recovery of renal function. Case A

Table II. Post-operative results after limb depuration.

Patient	Hyper-kalemia	Acid-base Balance	Renal Function	ARDS
A	no	normal range	acute failure (2 dialysis)	no
B	no	induced metabolic alkalosis	fair	no
C	no	"	fair	no
D	no	"	fair	no
E	no	"	hemo-myoglo-binuria no failure	no

suffered a renal failure which completely recovered on only two hemodialysis treatments. Case E showed hemo- and myoglobinuria without acute tubular necrosis.

ARDS. No patients showed evidence of acute respiratory distress syndrome.

COMMENTS

This method certainly achieves good control of serum potassium and metabolic balance thus reducing the most frequent cause of sudden cardiac arrest following revascularization of the ischemic limb (Cormier and Legrain, 1962). Furthermore, the employment of the microfilter prevents ARDS occurrence by trapping clots and microaggregates, thus preventing their entry into the pulmonary circulation.

The use of a polyacrylonitrile membrane constitutes a valuable means of depuration of metabolic toxic substances. Unfortunately, this method only partially solves the problem of renal failure due to tubular precipitation of myo- and hemoglobin (Haimovici, 1970), but with administration of bicarbonate infusions and diuretic drugs which induce high alkaline urine output, the risk of this frequent and often fatal complication is reduced.

Further favorable effects come about from the mechanical action of the circuit pump, which increases the limb blood flow and the capacity of the vascular bed and may clear the most distal clots and aggregates. Favorable results of revascularization can be expected if there are both high flow rates and low pressure in the extracorporeal circuit and if the clinical examination of the limb shows partial disappearance of the signs of ischemia during the depuration. The method we have used has shown satisfactory results even though it cannot be said to totally eliminate the eventual appearance of the syndrome. However, a severe syndrome will be reduced and a mild syndrome, which might be fatal in poor-risk patients, disappears.

REFERENCES

Agrifoglio, G., Vercelio, G. and Gabrielli, L. (1978). *Surgery in Italy.* **8**, 4.
Castelli, P. (1977). Atti 3rd Congr. Naz. Gruppo Ital. Chirurgia Vascolare, L'Aquila.
Cormier, J. M. and Legrain, M. (1962). *J. Chir.* **3**, 84, 473. Mars.
Danese, C. *et al.* (1973). *Arch. Surg.* **107**,
Eiken *et al.* (1964). *Arch. Surg.* **88**, 48.
Fiorani, P., Pistolese, G. R., Faraglia, V., Benedetti Valentini (1972). *Arch. Atti. Soc. Ital, Chir.* 74th Congr.
Haimovici, H. (1970). *Arch. Surg.* **100**, 639.
Larcan, A. *et al.* (1973). *J. Cardiovas. Surg.* **14**, 609.
Pistolese, G. R. *et al.* (1977). Atti 3rd Congr. Naz. Gruppo Ital. Chirurgia Vascolare, L'Aquila.
Stipa, S. *et al.* (1967). *J. Cardiovas. Surg.* **8**, 529.
Tufano, R. *et al.* (1978). *Minerva Anestesiologica* **44**, 59–63.
Vercellio, G. *et al.* (1977). Dati preliminari. Atti 3rd Congr. Naz. Gruppo Ital. Chirurgia Vascolare, L'Aquila.

PLASMA RENIN, ALDOSTERONE AND SARALASIN IN THE DETECTION AND MANAGEMENT OF ISTHMIC COARCTATION OF THE AORTA

P. Cugini,[1] T. Meucci,[1] A. Mancini,[1] D. Scavo,[1] A. Castrucci,[2] L. Boschi[2] and E. Massa[3]

[1]Patologia Medica, University of Rome; [2]Service of Cardiovascular Radiology, S. Camillo's Hospital of Rome; [3]Division of Cardiovascular Surgery, S. Filippo's Hospital of Rome, Italy

INTRODUCTION

Experimental studies revealed the participation of the renal pressor mechanism in the development of hypertension in dogs with artificial constriction of the thoracic aorta (Yagi et al., 1973; Sealy et al., 1973; Ferguson et al., 1977). The present investigation was performed to elucidate the possible use of renin-aldosterone profiles, and saralasin, an inhibitor of angiotensin II, in the management of the isthmic coarctation of the aorta (ICA) occurring spontaneously in human beings.

MATERIAL AND METHODS

Studies were carried out in eleven untreated hypertensive patients with ICA, eight males and three females, aged from 7 to 59 years. Diagnosis of ICA has been made on the basis of clinical and roentgenographic findings and confirmed by

Serono Symposium No. 37, "Vascular Occlusion: Epidemiological, Pathophysiological and Therapeutic Aspects", edited by M. Tesi and J. Dormandy, 1981. Academic Press, London and New York.

aortography. Each patient gave his informed consent. Investigations were performed according to the following protocol.

Pre-operative Studies

Each patient had a normal sodium and potassium diet for at least five days. Blood samples for simultaneous determinations of plasma renin activity (PRA) from aorta, peripheral and renal veins and of circulating plasma aldosterone (PA), were drawn when daily urinary sodium excretion appeared to be proportional to the Na intake. The technique for sampling of PRA by femoral catheterization, is described elsewhere (Scavo *et al.*, 1977).

Intra-operative Studies

All patients were treated by surgical repair of the aortic defect. The degree of coarctation was established by measuring intra-operatively the calibre of the lumen of the site of constriction. During the operation, the heart rate and arterial pressure has been monitored by means of a catheter placed in the radial artery and connected to a Stathan P23Dc transducer. Furthermore, a serial sampling of peripheral blood was made in order to correlate the haemodynamic parameters with the intra-operative changes in PRA.

Post-operative Studies

Patients were discharged without therapy. They had a physical examination every month in the outpatient section. Post-operative determinations of PRA and PA were performed in the erect position and on a normal sodium intake. The radioimmunological methods of Haber *et al.* (1969) and McKenzie and Clements (1974) were used to measure PRA and PA respectively. Student's *t* test was employed in the statistical analysis.

RESULTS

Pre-operative Findings

Biodata summarized in Fig. 1 show that five individuals in the present series of ICA patients exhibit high levels of peripheral PRA which are consistently associated with elevated concentrations of circulating PA. The rise of PRA is also evident in blood of renal veins, indicating that renin is hypersecreted in these patients. However, the data plotted in Fig. 2 clearly show that the renin hypersecretion is not linked to the mechanism of renal ischaemia, since no significant reduction in renal perfusion was found in ICA patients with hyperreninism.

The observation emerging from statistical analysis of data listed in Fig. 3 is that the activation of renin release seems to be independent of the severity of the obstruction to the aortic blood flow, no difference having been detected

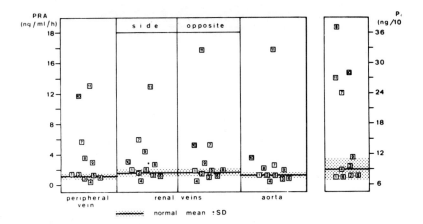

Fig. 1. Biodata in hypertensive patients with ICA.

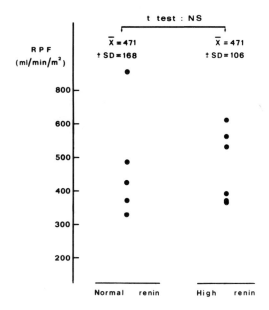

Fig. 2. Renal plasma flow (RPF) in normoreninaemic and hyperreninaemic patients with ICA.

between the normoreninaemic and hyperreninaemic group of ICA patients. Haemodynamic parameters depicted in Fig. 4 show convincingly the systematic involvement of the arterial regulating mechanism in ICA patients with associate hyperreninaemia.

Finally, the different responses to A–II blockade by saralasin displayed in

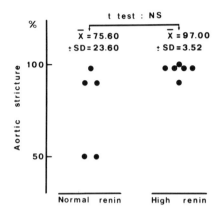

Fig. 3. Percent reduction of aortic lumen at the site of constriction in normoreninaemic and hyperreninaemic patients with ICA.

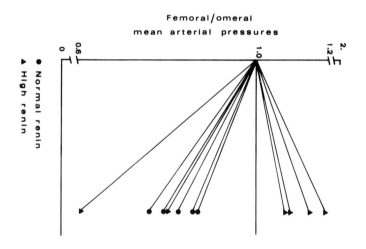

Fig. 4. Ratio between femoral and humeral arterial pressure in normoreninaemic and hyperreninaemic patients with ICA.

Fig. 5, strongly support the suggestion that the hyperangiotensinaemia plays an essential role in conditioning the rise of blood pressure in ICA patients with high renin.

Intra-operation Findings

Data given in Fig. 6, illustrate the relationship between the intra-operative kinetics of PRA and arterial pressure in two high renin ICA patients. The inspection of the biohumoral-haemodynamic curves reveals two typical behaviours. After aortic clamping, the patient with partial constriction shows a consistent

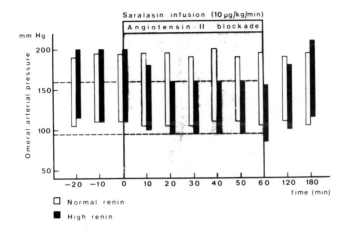

Fig. 5. Different effects of angiotensin–II blockade by competitive inhibitor, saralasin, in the presence of normoreninaemic and hyperreninaemic ICA.

rise of both PRA and PA, while the totally occluded patient appears to be insensitive to the sharp surgical closure of the aortic lumen. After removing the clamp, both patients exhibit a marked fall of high blood pressure. However, the patient who had the reactive increase of PRA shows a gradual return of renin-aldosterone levels to the baseline values. On the contrary, the other maintains the biohumoral variables on a straight line.

Post-operative Findings

The interrelationship shown in Fig. 7 is convincing evidence for the use of PRA–PA determinations, in clinical management of ICA, as biochemical markers of pathology promoting a renin-dependent hypertension.

One patient in the present series was not cured by the surgical correction of the coarctation. Contrary to other hyperreninaemic ICA patients, who became normoreninaemic after operation, the uncured individual failed to decrease circulating levels of PRA and PA. The negative result was due to the existence of unsuspected chronic nephroparenchymal disease. Laboratory data on renal function, including urography, radioisotope renograms, nephroscintigraphy and selective renal arteriography, were on the contrary, within the normal limits in hyperreninaemic patients who were ameliorated by surgical correction.

DISCUSSION

Results of the present investigation and previous studies (Morris *et al.* 1964; Brown *et al.*, 1965; Amsterdam *et al.*, 1969; Werning *et al.*, 1969; Van Way *et al.*, 1967; Sanchez *et al.*, 1977) clearly indicate that ICA patients are not a homogeneous category in regard to the dynamics of the renin-angio-tensin-aldosterone system (SRAA). However, the estimation of renin release supports

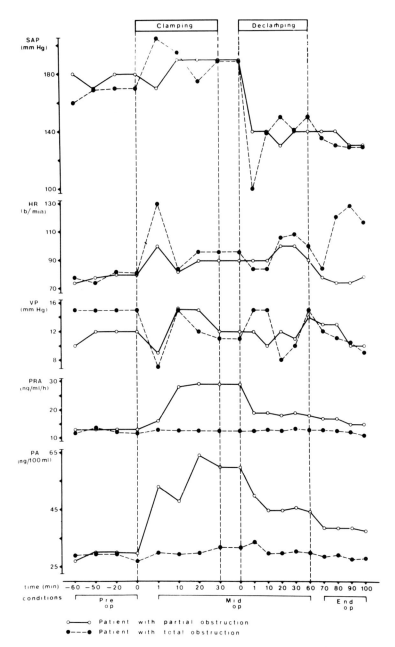

Fig. 6. Haemodynamic and biochemical changes related to the phases of surgical intervention in two distinct types of severity aortic constriction.

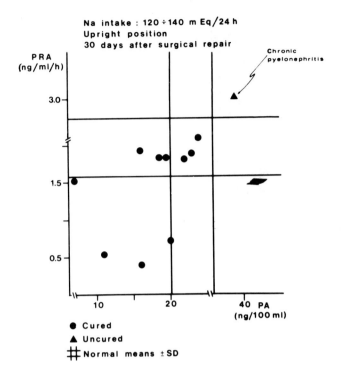

Fig. 7. Post-operative renin-aldosterone patterns related to the benefit of surgical repair of ICA.

the possibility that the renin secretion might be increased in patients affected by ICA. The occurrence of hyperreninism with secondary hyperaldosteronism in ICA seems to be dependent upon two distinct events.

The normalization of hyperreninaemia after surgical repair of the aortic defect in patients free of renal vasoparenchymal defects demonstrates a coarctation-dependent hyperactivation of renin release. The responsibility of a central mechanism for raising the renin secretion is emphasized by at least two fundamental observations. First, the fact that the renin hypersecretion in the presence of a congenitally narrowed thoracic aorta is not dependent on renal hypoperfusion. Secondly, the intra-operative finding recorded in the partially occluded patient, that PRA promptly increased and subsequently decreased at the time of vascular clamping and declamping respectively. This phenomenon was not, on the contrary, detected in the other patient in whom no further distension of aortic walls presumably occurred after clamping since the descending aorta was totally occluded at birth.

The other event underlying the increase of PRA and PA in ICA patients seems to be the possible coexistence of pathological disorders *per se* effecting the renin release In these circumstances, PRA and PA may be regarded as a biochemical tool for screening hyperreninaemic conditions associated with ICA (Table I) which interfere with the outcome of the surgical intervention.

In conclusion, the present investigation focussed on the biological significance of RIA determinations of PRA and PA in the diagnostic and prognostic phases of the ICA management. High renin-aldosterone profiles in young hypertensives

Table I.   Causes of activation of RAAS in isthmic
coarctation of the aorta.

Associated with hypertension

   renal artery stenosis (uni- or bilateral)
   nephroparenchymal diseases
   antihypertensive drugs affecting renin release
   aortic abdominal coarctation (prerenal)
   oral contraceptives.

Associated with normotension

   heart failure
   hepatic disorders.

---

lead us to suspect the presence of the coarctation of the descending thoracic
aorta, especially if the fundamental clinical sign of a pressure gradient between
the upper and lower extremities is not demonstrable. The biochemical surveillance of circulating PRA and PA in patients with diagnosed coarctation of the
aorta is important in order to select the cases and predict the surgical curability
in the presence of associated pathology.

REFERENCES

Amsterdam, E. A., Albers, W. H. and Christlieh, A. R. (1969). *Am. J. Cardiol.*
   23, 396.
Brown, J. J., Davies, D. L., Lever, A. F. and Robertson, J.I.S. (1965). *Br. Med.
   J.* **2**, 1215.
Ferguson, J. C., Barrie, W. W. and Schenk, W. G. (1977). *Ann. Surg.* **195**, 423.
Haber, E., Koerner, T., Page, L. B., Kliman, B. and Purnode, A. (1969). *J. Clin.
   Endocrinol. Metab.* **29**, 1349.
McKenzie, J. K. and Clements, J. A. (1974). *J. Clin. Endocrinol. Metab.* **38**, 622.
Morris, R. Jr., Robinson, P. R. and Scheele, G. A. (1964). *Can. Med. Ass. J.*
   90, 272.
Sanchez, G. C., Posadas, C., Millan, A., Kuri, J. and Serrano, P. D. (1977). *Arch.
   Inst. Cardiol. Mex.* **7**, 412.
Scavo, D., Cugini, P., Serdoz, R., Manconi, R., Meucci, T., Simonetti, G., Pas-
   sariello, R. and Rossi, P. (1977). *La Settimana degli Ospedali* **6**, 252.
Sealy W. C., Panijayanond, P., Alexander, J. and Scaber, A. V. (1973). *J. Thor.
   Cardiovasc. Surg.* **65**, 282.
Van Way, C. W., Michelakis, A. M., Anderson, W. I., Manlove, H. and Oates, J.
   A. (1976). *Ann. Surg.* **183**, 229.
Werning, C., Schonbert, M., Weidmann, P., Baumann, K., Gysling, E., Wirz, P.
   and Siegenthaler, W. (1969). *Circulation* **40**, 731.
Yagi, S., Kramsch, D. M., Madoff, I. M. and Hollander, W. (1968) *Am. J. Physiol.*
   215, 605.

THE RESULTS OF THORACIC SYMPATHECTOMY IN
RAYNAUD'S PHENOMENON

W. Montorsi,[1] C. Ghiringhelli[2] and F. Annoni

[1] *Universita' Degli Studi di Milano Istituto di Clinica Chirurgica III,*
[2] *Cattedra di Patologia Chirurgica III, Italy*

It is well known that by surgical intervention, it is possible to obtain sympathetic denervation of a limb affected by Raynaud's phenomenon (RP) with interruption of the vasomotor fibres at the level of the sympathetic chain. Over the last 20 years, initially in the surgical department directed by Professor Oselladore, then in those directed by Professor Montorsi and now also by Professor Ghiringhelli, we have operated on 203 patients suffering from RP. The evolution of surgical techniques over these years has been the direct result of an increased knowledge of the physiopathology of the sympathetic system and a critical examination of the results obtained.

From Fig. 1 it can be seen that over 20 years, we have carried out sympathectomies using three different techniques. At first, we used Smithwick's method (Fig. 1) which consists of a dissection of the anterior and posterior roots of the preganglionic fibres of the second and third ganglion and of the chain below the third thoracic ganglion. Later, we changed to gangliectomy using Adson's method (Fig. 2), i.e. the interruption of the communicating branches and of the intercostal nerves followed by the ablation of the thoracic chain from the second to the third ganglion by a paravertebral incision.

Since 1969, we have used Telford's techniques (Fig. 3). A supraclavicular cutaneous incision is made 2 cm above the upper edge of the clavicle from the sternocleidomastoid muscle to the trapezius. Taking the incision deeper, the clavicular branch of the sternocleidomastoid muscle is dissected, the external jugular vein tied and posterior body of the omohyoid muscle dissected revealing

Serono Symposium No. 37, "Vascular Occlusion: Epidemiological, Pathophysiological and Therapeutic Aspects", edited by M. Tesi and J. Dormandy, 1981. Academic Press, London and New York.

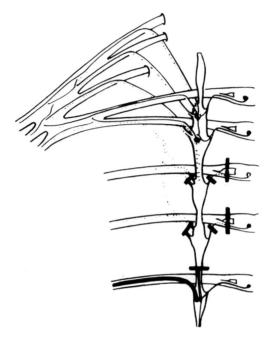

Fig. 1. Sympathetic denervation of the upper limb in Smithwick's sympathectomy.

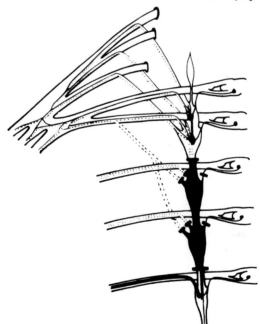

Fig. 2. Sympathetic denervation of the upper limb in Adson's gangliectomy.

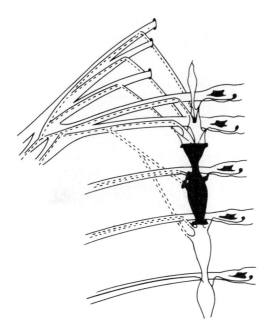

Fig. 3. Sympathetic denervation of the upper limb in Telford's gangliectomy.

the anterior scalene muscle. The phrenic nerve is mobilized and held aside in a medical position by means of a linen tie. It is now possible to dissect the anterior scalene muscle.

The subclavian artery is mobilized following ligature of the inferior thyroid artery so that the cervical pleura comes into view; this is lowered by dissection of the superior pleura fascia. This last manoeuvre finally exposes the cervico-thoracic ganglion which is situated lateral to the vertebral column, next to Chassaignac's tubercle. The operation consists of the ablation of the sympathetic chain from the distal portion of the cervicothoracic ganglion to the second thoracic ganglion inclusive. When possible the third ganglion is also excised.

If the three methods are compared (i.e. Smithwick's sympathectomy and Adson's and Telford's gangliectomies), it may be understood that the latter two techniques are very similar in their methods of denervation but that they differ in their approach to the operation site, which is paravertebral in the first case and supraclavicular in the second.

As far as clinical results are concerned, those obtained from sympathectomy are evaluated as shown in Table I. The results may be seen in Table II. It should be noted that the percentage of good and satisfactory results has improved progressively over the years as surgical techniques have changed. Another important point to note is that the improvement in surgical results corresponds to a progressive decrease in cases of primary RP. The reasons for this improvement lie in the following points.

As far as the comparison between Smithwick's and Adson's methods is con-

Table I. Criteria of definition of clinical results obtained from surgical denervation in Raynaud's phenomenon.

---

(1) Good result:

   Total or almost total disappearance of attacks of pain and/or cutaneous oedema; good hand temperature, dry skin, eventual healing of trophic lesions.

(2) Fair result:

   Decrease in attacks and pain, improvement in degree of oedema and skin appearance; slight improvement in hand temperature, stabilization of clinical symptoms at a less serious stage.

(3) Bad result:

   Persistance of attacks, pain and other clinical symptoms; failure to heal trophic lesions.

(4) Recurrence:

   Reappearance of pain on contact with cold; reappearance of vasomotor attacks; reappearance of sweating.

Table II. Clinical results obtained from sympathectomy in Raynaud's phenomenon.

Kind of procedure	Number of interventions	Result as Percentages		
		Good	Fair	Bad
Smithwick's sympathectomy				
Primary R. phenomenon	44	27	23	50
Secondary R. phenomenon	24	54	25	21
Adson's gangliectomy				
Primary R. phenomenon	29	24	40	36
Secondary R. phenomenon	29	40	40	20
Telford's gangliectomy				
Primary phenomenon	26	46	35	19
Secondary phenomenon	51	56	37	7
Total	203			

cerned, there is a major simplicity and efficacy of surgical technique.

In comparing the results between Adson's and Telford's gangliectomies, there is a more critical, and hence a more severe selection, of suitable cases for surgery. surgery.

Over the last year, in fact there has been an improvement in diagnostic methods and a deeper knowledge of the pathogenic mechanism of RP has been attained. Today this permits us to obtain good results in 53% of surgical cases, compared with poor results in only 10% of the cases.

The diagnostic tests that help in a satisfactory study of the patient, in a correct selection for surgery and in a higher percentage of favourable results following sympathectomy are first, those connected with a study of peripheral circulation and secondly those concerning the protective immunological balance of the patient. Whereas the first are generally well-known as technical procedures (thermography, plethysmography, rheography, Doppler's flowmeter test, viscosimetry,

Table III. Positive results of immunological tests in patients with Raynaud's phenomenon.

Immunological tests	Significance in Percentages
γ–Globulins $> 20\%$	45
RA Test	54
Waaler Rose	17
AMA	36
SMA	0
ANA	0

AMA: anti-mythocondrial antibodies; SMA: anti-smooth muscle antibodies; ANA: anti-nuclear antibodies.

Table IV. Correlation between positive results of immunological tests and clinical results of Telford's gangliectomy.

Immunological test in patients with Raynaud's phenomenon		Clinical result after sympathectomy	
		GOOD	BAD
All negative	2	2	=
Only RA test positive	2	1	1
All positive	3	=	3

determination of electrical cutaneous resistance and arteriography) it may be of use to give certain explanations on the nature and use of the immunological tests we carried out on a certain percentage of the patients who had already undergone surgery and had returned for a routine periodic check-up in the out-patients department. The same tests have been carried out on all patients who, over the last 6 months or so, have been under observation for possible surgery.

The screening tests are those shown in Table III with their relative signifi-cance. A positive result in these tests leads to the need for deeper study. Other tests, such as cryoglobulin and complement levels, immunocomplex research, may lead to a specific immunopathological diagnosis. The diseases that most frequently cause RP are the forms of secondary vasculitis, in particular SLE, scleroderma, cryoglobulinaemia and rheumatoid arthritis.

On analysing the correlation between the results of surgery and collagen disorders detected some time after surgery (Table IV), it became clear to us that all patients who were suffering from collagen disorders that were not clinically evident, had a bad clinical result, whereas all patients who were definitely not suffering from collagen disorders had good clinical results. Latent collagen disease is often not diagnosed unless it has reached a stage of advanced clinical symptoms. We believe it is for this reason that certain authors main-tain that the results of gangliectomy are more successful in secondary than in primary RP. In those patients in whom RP is accompanied by latent collagen disease, it can be said that the phenomenon can represent only a minor clinical manifestation and is a hidden warning of collagen disease.

As a result of all these considerations, which originated from the evaluation of out ample case records, we have now adopted certain criteria in the selection of patients for surgery, the validity of which will still have to be verified, but which would appear better than those we followed up to now.

(a)   We consider surgical operation possible only in patients who have suffered from RP for at least 3 years, regardless of its severity. Spontaneous remission of the symptoms is far from an exception, especially in young female patients.

(b)   RP must be very disturbing to the patient, in as much as it upsets his working activity and social relations.

(c)   The symptoms must prove resistant to medical therapy, carried out at sufficiently high doses over a long period of time, using vasoactive drugs or inhibitors of erythrocyte and platelet aggregation.

(d)   We always carry out immunological screening. If this proves negative we prescribe surgical treatment; if positive we never operate unless there are trophic lesions. In the latter case, sympathectomy always leads to an improve-ment in the lesions, even if the RP as such does not generally benefit from the operation. The patient must be informed in this case that although there is no alternative other than surgery, the results are limited.

It is possible that our severe methods of selection and our scrupulous adher-ence to these principles, are the reason for the continuous improvement in the results of our surgery. It will be interesting to evaluate the same results after a time lapse of several years.

BIBLIOGRAPHY

Abet, D., Bertoux, J. P., Vermyuck, J. P., Neven, P. and Pietri, J. (1979). *J. Chir.* **116**, 187.

Arnulf, G. (1976). *J. Cardiovasc. Surg.* **17**, 354.

Brands, L. C. (1975). *Plebologie* **30**, 205.

Ghiringhelli, C., Scarduelli, A. Albonico, C. and Doldi, S. B. (1964). *Chir. It.* **16**, Suppl. 2.

Devin, R., Brachereau, A. and Aubaniac, J. M. (1978). *Chirurgie* **104**, 225.

Gruss, J. D., Bartels, D. and Stojanovic, R. (1976). *J. Chir.* **112**, 307.

Kurchin, A. Zweig, A., Adar, R. and Mozes, A. (1977). *Wld J. Surg.* **1**, 667.

Montorsi, W. (1959). *Folia Angiologica* **6**, 198.

Montorsi, W. (1963). *Ann. Med.* **7**, 741.

Montorsi, W. (1966). Scritti in onore di Guido Oselladore 1965–1967.

Montorsi, W. (1974). *Min. Med.* **75**, 4087.

Montorsi, W., Ghiringhelli, C. and Curri, S. (1962). *In* "Grosser nel morbo di Burger, nel morbo di Raynaud e nella sclerodermia". Pleion, Milano

Montorsi, W., Ghiringhelli, C., Mascetti, M. and Gallo, G. (1960). *Min Cardio - Angiol.* **8**, 266.

Montorsi, W., Ghiringhelli, C., Mascetti, M. and Gallo (1960). *Min. Cardio - Angiol.* **2**, 538.

Perrin, M. Becker, F. and Brosset, E. (1978). *Societé de Chirurgie de Lyon*, **13**, 4.

Pratesi, F., Corsi, C., Deidda, C. and Nuti, A. (1976). *Praxis* **65** (44), 1375.

Rettori, R. and Ducros, R. (1979). *J. Mal. (Paris)* **4**, 23.

Romani, F., Talia, B., Pompei, G., Lo Russo, G. P. and Tuscano, G. (1979). *Min. Chir.* **34**, 5.

Salmon, J. and Gran, G. (1979). *Rev. Med. Liege* **14**, 10.